PHLEBOTOMY
ESSENTIALS

third edition

PHLEBOTOMY
ESSENTIALS

Third Edition

Ruth E. McCall BS, MT(ASCP)
Director of Phlebotomy and
Clinical Laboratory Assistant Programs
TVI Community College
Albuquerque, New Mexico

Cathee M. Tankersley BS, MT(ASCP), CLS (NCA)
Director of Phlebotomy Program
Phoenix College, Phoenix, Arizona
Clinical Educational Specialist
HemoCue, Inc., Mission Viejo, California
Laboratory Technical Supervisor
Valley Integrative Physicians
Phoenix, Arizona

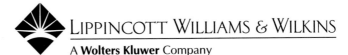

LIPPINCOTT WILLIAMS & WILKINS
A **Wolters Kluwer** Company
Philadelphia · Baltimore · New York · London
Buenos Aires · Hong Kong · Sydney · Tokyo

Executive Editor: John Goucher
Managing Editor: Emilie Linkins
Marketing Manager: Debby Hartman
Production Editor: Karen Ruppert
Designer: Risa Clow
Compositor: Graphic World
Printer: Quebecor

First Edition, 1993
Second Edition, 1998

Library of Congress Cataloging-in-Publication Data

McCall, Ruth E.
   Phlebotomy essentials / Ruth E. McCall, Cathee M. Tankersley.-- 3rd ed.
     p. cm.
   Includes bibliographical references and index.
   ISBN 0-7817-3452-5
   1. Phlebotomy. I. Tankersley, Cathee M. II. Title.

   RB45.15 .M33 2002
   616.07'561--dc21

                                                                    2002075992

To purchase additional copies of this book, call our customer service department at **(800) 638-3030** or fax orders to **(301) 824-7390**. International customers should call **(301) 714-2324**.

Visit Lippincott Williams & Wilkins on the Internet: http://www.lww.com. Lippincott Williams & Wilkins customer service representatives are available from 8:30 am to 6:00 pm, EST.

05 06 07
4 5 6 7 8 9 10

To my husband, John; my sons, Chris and Scott; my daughter-in-law, Tracy;
and my parents, Charles and Marie Ruppert; for their encouragement, patience, and support;
and to my grandchildren, Katie and Ryan, for regular doses of pure joy that kept me motivated.

RUTH E. McCALL

To my husband, Earl L. Tankersley, for his continuous encouragement,
and to a very special friend, Kees Van Elk, for his generosity and support.

CATHEE M. TANKERSLEY

CONTRIBUTORS

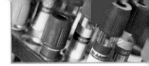

CONTRIBUTING AUTHOR
Brigitte Miedzybrocki BS, MT, ASCP
Lead Medical Technologist
Arizona Heart Hospital
Adjunct Faculty
Phoenix College
Phoenix, Arizona
(Chapters 11 and 14)

REVIEWERS

Doramarie Arocha, MS, MT(ASCP)
Medical Laboratory Sciences Instructor
The University of Texas Southwestern
    Medical Center
Dallas, Texas

Mary Banman, MT(ASCP), CLS(NCA)
Clinical Education
    Coordinator/Instructor
University of North Dakota
Grand Forks, North Dakota

Karen Brown, MS, MT(ASCP), CLS(NCA)
MLT Program Instructor
University of Utah School of Medicine
Salt Lake City, Utah

Kraig Chugg, MS, MT(ASCP)
Clinical Laboratory Sciences Instructor
Weber State University
Ogden, Utah

Donna J. Donaldson, MCLT, MT(ASCP)
Department of Diagnostic Services
Trident Technical College
Charleston, South Carolina

Elaine A. Dreisbaugh, MSN, BSN, RN, CPN
Nursing Instructor
Delaware County Community College
    (The Chester County Hospital)
Media, Pennsylvania

Robin Gail White, MLD(ASCP), MT(HEW)
JCL Hospital-North Mountain
Laboratory Operations Supervisor
Phoenix, Arizona

Gwen Lee
Phlebotomy Instructor
Baltimore City Community College
Baltimore, Maryland

Pamela B. Primrose, MT(ASCP)

Mary Jean Rutherford, MED, MT(ASCP) SC
Clinical Laboratory Sciences Instructor
Arkansas State University
State University, Arkansas

Julie Stiak, MED, BSMT
Director of the Healthcare Core
Phoenix College
Phoenix, Arizona

PREFACE

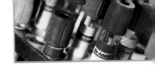

The goal of *Phlebotomy Essentials*, 3rd edition, as with previous editions, is to provide accurate, up-to-date, practical information and instruction in phlebotomy procedures and techniques, along with a comprehensive background in phlebotomy theory and principles. Although the text is comprehensive, the student-friendly writing style and format makes reading easy and locating information simple and quick. *Phlebotomy Essentials*, 3rd edition is appropriate for use as an instructional text for phlebotomist training programs in healthcare institutions and colleges, for cross training of nursing and allied health professionals, and as a reference for practicing phlebotomists and other healthcare workers looking to update their skills or study for national phlebotomy certification exams.

New to the 3rd edition are the following features:

- Full color illustrations throughout
- Key points and memory joggers to enhance student learning
- Case studies in applicable chapters to enhance student learning and encourage critical thinking
- Cutting edge technology, the latest safety regulations, and the latest safety equipment
- Expanded venipuncture chapter including venipuncture of the elderly and other special populations
- Expanded point-of-care testing and special procedures chapter directed at those who want to become multiskilled
- *Instructor Resource Guide* updated and presented on CD

The content of the book was designed in accordance with National Accrediting Agency for Clinical Laboratory Science (NAACLS) competencies. All procedures have been written to conform to Occupational Safety and Health Administration (OSHA) regulations, and, wherever applicable, standards developed by the National Committee for Clinical Laboratory Standards (NCCLS).

The authors wish to express their gratitude to the following: Bruce Knaphus for his photography, computer enhancement, and photo editing skills; Christopher McCall for his photography skills; Julie Stiak and Robin Inmon for manuscript review; Brigitte Miedzybrocki for serving as a contributing author; the manufacturers who allowed us to illustrate their products; the staff at Lippincott Williams & Wilkins, especially John Goucher, Heidi Weinkam, and Emilie Linkins; and most of all, our families for their continued support of our efforts.

RUTH E. McCALL
CATHEE M. TANKERSLEY

CONTENTS

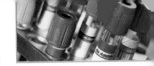

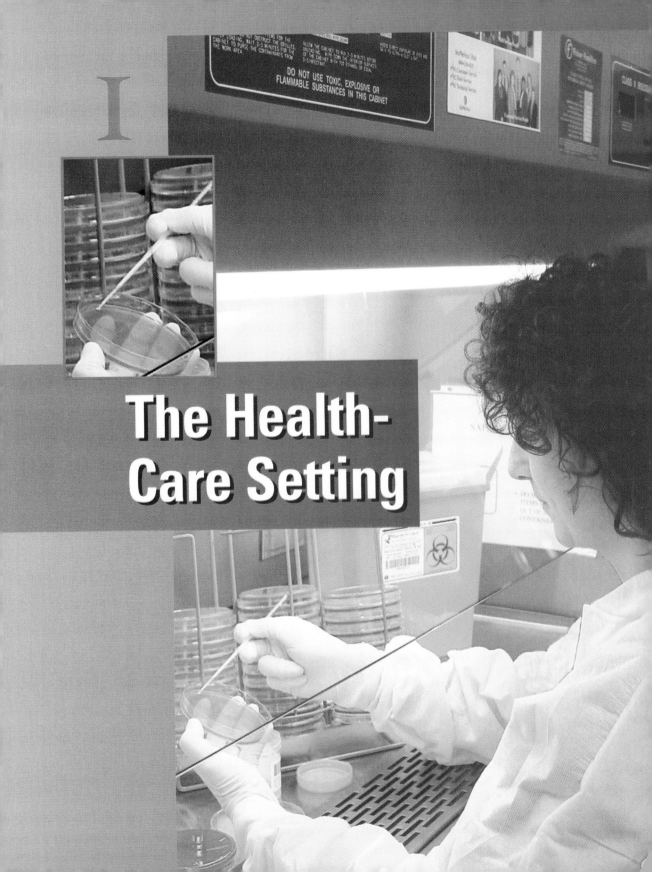

The Health-Care Setting

1

PHLEBOTOMY: PAST AND PRESENT AND THE HEALTH-CARE SETTING

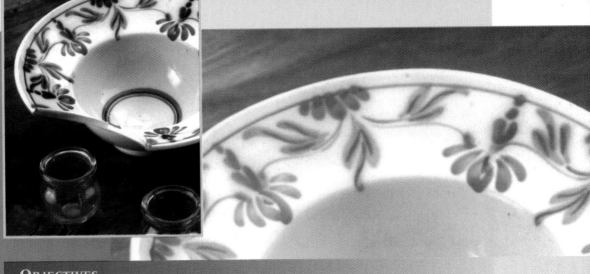

OBJECTIVES

Upon successful completion of this chapter, the reader will be able to:

1 Define the key terms and abbreviations listed at the beginning of this chapter.

2 Describe the evolution of phlebotomy and the role of the phlebotomist in today's healthcare setting.

3 Describe the traits that form the professional image and identify national organizations that support professional recognition of phlebotomists.

4 Describe the basic concepts of communication as they relate to healthcare and how appearance and nonverbal messages affect the communication process.

5 Describe proper telephone protocol in the laboratory.

6 Demonstrate an awareness of the different types of healthcare settings.

7 Compare types of third-party payers, coverage, and methods of payment to the patient, provider, and institutions.

8 Describe a traditional hospital organization and identify the healthcare providers in the inpatient facility.

9 List the clinical analysis areas of the laboratory and the types of laboratory procedures performed in the different areas.

10 Describe the different levels of personnel found in the clinical laboratory and how Clinical Laboratory Improvement Amendment regulations affect their job descriptions.

PHLEBOTOMY: AN HISTORICAL PERSPECTIVE

Since very early times, man has been fascinated by blood and has believed in some connection between the blood racing through his veins and his well-being. From this belief, certain medical principles and procedures dealing with blood evolved, some surviving to the present day.

An early medical theory developed by Hippocrates (460–377 BC) stated that disease was the result of excess substance, such as blood, phlegm, black bile, and yellow bile, within the body. It was thought that removal of the excess would restore balance. The process of removal and extraction became the treatment and could be done either by expelling disease materials through the use of drugs or by direct removal during surgery. One important surgical technique was **phlebotomy**—the process of blood-letting. Blood-letting involved cutting into a vein with a sharp instrument and releasing blood in an effort to rid the body of evil spirits, cleanse the body of impurities, or, as in Hippocrates' time, bring the body into proper balance. Literal translation of the word phlebotomy comes from the Greek words *phlebos,* meaning veins, and *tome,* meaning incision.

Some authorities believe phlebotomy dates back to the last period of the Stone Age, when crude tools were used to puncture vessels to allow excess blood to drain out of the body. A painting in a tomb showing the application of a leech to a patient evidences blood-letting in Egypt around 1400 BC. Early in the Middle Ages, barber-surgeons flourished. By 1210, the Guild of Barber-Surgeons was formed and divided the surgeons into Surgeons of the Long Robe and Surgeons of the Short Robe. Soon the Short Robe surgeons were forbidden by law to do any surgery except blood-letting, wound surgery, cupping, leeching, shaving, teeth extraction, and enema administration.

To distinguish his profession from that of the Long Robe surgeon, the barber-surgeon placed a striped pole from which a bleeding bowl (Fig. 1-1) was suspended outside his door. The pole represented the rod squeezed by the patient to promote bleeding and the white stripe on the pole corresponded to the bandages, which were also used as tourniquets. Soon, handsomely decorated ceramic bleeding bowls came into fashion and were passed down from one generation to the next. These bowls, which often doubled as shaving bowls, usually had a semicircular area cut out on one side to facilitate placing the bowl under the chin.

During the 17th and early 18th centuries, phlebotomy was considered a major therapeutic (treatment) process and anyone willing to claim medical training could perform phlebotomy. The lancet, a tool used for cutting the vein during a procedure called

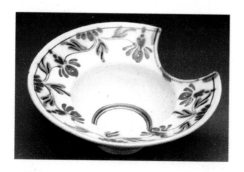

■ FIGURE 1-1 ■

Bleeding bowl. (Courtesy Robert Kravetz, MD, Chairman, Archives Committee, American College of Gastroenterology)

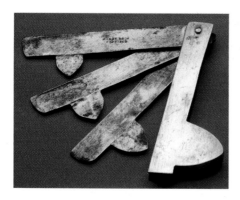

FIGURE 1-2

Typical fleams. (Courtesy Robert Kravetz, MD, Chairman, Archives Committee, American College of Gastroenterology)

venesection, was perhaps the most prevalent medical instrument of the times. The usual amount of blood withdrawn was approximately 10 mL, but excessive phlebotomy was common.

Key Point ➤ Excessive phlebotomy was thought to have contributed to George Washington's death in 1799, when he was diagnosed with a throat infection and the physician bled him four times in 2 days. It was because of Washington's request to be allowed to die without further medical intervention that the physician did not completely **exsanguinate** or remove all blood from him.

During this same period, phlebotomy was also accomplished by cupping and leeching. The art of cupping required a great deal of practice to maintain the high degree of dexterity necessary so as not to appear clumsy and frighten the patient away. Cupping involved the application of a heated suction apparatus, called the "cup," to the skin to draw the blood to the surface before severing the capillaries in that area by making a series of parallel incisions with a lancet or fleam. The typical fleam was a wide double-edged blade at right angles to the handle. Later versions (Fig. 1-2) had multiple blades that were folded into a brass case for easy carrying. The blades were wiped clean with only a rag and readily transmitted a host of bloodborne infections from patient to patient.

Fleams were used for general phlebotomy to open an artery or, more commonly, a vein to remove large amounts of blood. For more localized blood-letting, leeches were used. This procedure involved enticing the *Hirudo medicinalis*, a European medicinal leech, to the spot needing blood-letting with a drop of milk or blood on the patient's skin. After the leech was engorged with blood, which took about an hour, it was allowed to drop off by itself. By the mid-18th century, leeching was widely practiced in Europe, especially in France. Leeches were kept in special vessels that were filled with water and had perforated tops so that the leeches could breathe. Early leech jars were glass and, later, ceramic (Fig. 1-3). Within the last decade, leeches have made a comeback as defenders from the complications of microsurgical replantation (Fig. 1-4). The value of leech therapy lies in the components of the worm's saliva that contains a local vasodilator (substance that increases the diameter of blood vessels), a local anesthetic, and hirudin, an anticoagulant (substance that prevents clotting).

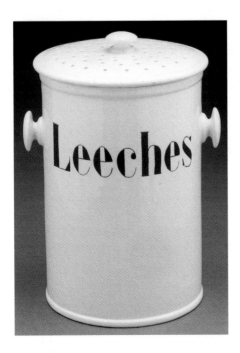

■ FIGURE 1-3 ■

Leech jar. (Courtesy Robert Kravetz, MD, Chairman, Archives Committee, American College of Gastroenterology)

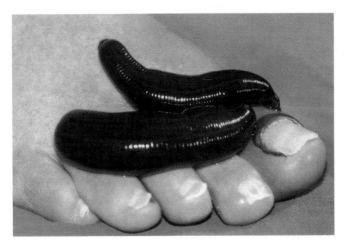

■ FIGURE 1-4 ■

Toe with leech. (Courtesy Robert Kravetz, MD, Chairman, Archives Committee, American College of Gastroenterology)

PHLEBOTOMY TODAY

The practice of phlebotomy continues to this day; however, principles and methods have improved dramatically. Today, phlebotomy is performed:

- To obtain blood for diagnostic purposes and monitoring of prescribed treatment
- To remove blood for transfusions at a donor center
- For therapeutic purposes, such as for a patient with **polycythemia,** a disease involving overproduction of red blood cells, or **hemochromatosis,** a rare disease characterized by excess iron deposits throughout the body

Phlebotomy is primarily accomplished by one of two procedures:

- Venipuncture, which involves collecting blood by penetrating a vein with a needle and syringe or other collection apparatus
- Dermal puncture, which involves collecting blood after puncturing the skin with a lancet or similar skin puncture device

The Role of the Phlebotomist in a Changing Healthcare Environment

The term phlebotomist is applied to a person who has been trained in various techniques to perform phlebotomy procedures. It is the responsibility of a phlebotomist to collect blood for laboratory analysis, which is necessary for the diagnosis and care of a patient. A well-prepared phlebotomist must have good manual dexterity, special communication skills, good organizational skills, and a thorough knowledge of laboratory test requirements and departmental policies. The most common duties and responsibilities of a phlebotomist are listed in Box 1-1.

Box 1-1

DUTIES AND RESPONSIBILITIES OF A PHLEBOTOMIST

- Prepare patients for collection procedures associated with laboratory samples.
- Collect routine skin puncture and venous specimens for testing as required.
- Prepare specimens for transport to ensure stability of sample.
- Maintain patient confidentiality.
- Transport specimens to the laboratory.
- Comply with all procedures instituted in the procedure manual.
- Promote good public relations with patients and hospital personnel.
- Assist in collecting and documenting monthly workload and recording data.
- Maintain safe working conditions.
- Perform laboratory computer operations.
- Participate in continuing education programs.
- Collect and perform point-of-care testing (POCT).
- Perform quality control checks on POCT instruments.
- Perform skin tests.
- Process specimens and perform basic laboratory tests.
- Collect urine drug screens.
- Perform electrocardiography.
- Perform front office duties, current procedural terminology coding, and so on.

Today, healthcare organizations are downsizing, reorganizing, and shifting the responsibilities for all healthcare providers in an effort to better serve the patient. The development of teams and the sharing of tasks have become necessary as healthcare organizations attempt to find the balance between cost-effective treatment and quality care. Advances in laboratory technology are making point-of-care testing (POCT) more common, centralized laboratory services are giving way to decentralized activities, and other health professionals are being cross-trained to perform venipunctures.

During this time of transition, the profession of phlebotomy maintains a standardized educational curriculum with a recognized body of knowledge. Structured programs exist in hospitals, vocational schools, and colleges that incorporate classroom instruction and clinical practice to prepare the student for national certification.

Official Recognition

Certification

Certification is evidence that an individual has mastered fundamental competencies in a particular technical area. Certification is a process that indicates the completion of defined academic and training requirements and the attainment of a satisfactory score on an examination. This is verified by the awarding of a title, signified by initials that a phlebotomist is allowed to display after his or her name. National agencies that certify phlebotomists along with the title and corresponding initials awarded are listed in Table 1-1.

Licensure and Registration

A license is a document or permit granted by the state indicating that permission has been granted for a person to perform a certain service after having met the education and experience requirements and successfully completing an examination. A health professional who has successfully passed a national certification examination or a state licensure examination will be put on a list called a registry. This listing is maintained as long as the health professional pays the registration fee annually (e.g., to the American Society of Clinical Pathology [ASCP] Board of Registry).

Table 1-1

Phlebotomist Certification Agencies and Title, and Initials Awarded		
Certification Agency	**Certification Title**	**Certification Initials**
American Society for Clinical Pathology (ASCP)	Phlebotomy Technician	PBT (ASCP)
American Society for Phlebotomy Technicians (ASPT)	Certified Phlebotomy Technician	CPT (ASPT)
National Credentialing Agency (NCA) for Medical Laboratory Personnel	Clinical Laboratory Phlebotomist	CLPlb (NCA)
National Phlebotomy Association (NPA)	Certified Phlebotomy Technician	CPT (NPA)
American Medical Technologists (AMT)	Registered Phlebotomy Technician	RPT (AMT)

Continuing Education

It is important for phlebotomists to participate in continuing education to keep their knowledge base and skills up-to-date. Many organizations sponsor workshops, seminars, and self-study programs that award continuing education units (CEUs) to those who participate. Some certifying and licensing agencies require CEUs or other proof of continuing education for renewal of credentials granted. Employers may offer in-service education or provide funds for employees to attend offsite programs offered by organizations such as The American Society for Clinical Laboratory Sciences (ASCLS) and The American Society for Phlebotomy Technicians (ASPT).

Public Relations and Client Interaction

As a member of the clinical laboratory team, the phlebotomist plays an important role in public relations for the laboratory. Positive public relations involves promoting good will and a harmonious relationship with staff, visitors, and especially patients. The phlebotomist is often the only real contact the patient has with the laboratory. In many cases, patients equate this encounter with the caliber of care they receive while in the hospital. A confident phlebotomist with a professional manner and a neat appearance helps to put the patient at ease and helps establish a positive relationship.

Recognizing Diversity

Despite similarities, fundamental differences among people arise from nationality, ethnicity, and culture, as well as from family background, life experiences, and individual challenges. These differences affect the health beliefs and behaviors of both patients and providers.

Culturally aware healthcare providers enhance the potential for more rewarding interpersonal experiences. This can lead to increased job satisfaction for them and increased patient satisfaction with the healthcare services they provide.

Critical factors in the provision of healthcare services that meet the needs of diverse populations include understanding the:

- Beliefs and values that shape a person's approach to health and illness
- Health-related needs of patients and their families according to the environments in which they live
- Knowledge of customs and traditions related to health and healing
- Attitudes toward seeking help from healthcare providers

By recognizing diversity the phlebotomist promotes good will and harmonious relationships that directly improve health outcomes, the quality of services, and public relations.

Professionalism

Professionalism is defined as the conduct and qualities that characterize a professional person. As part of a service-oriented industry, people performing phlebotomy must practice professionalism.

The overall impression conveyed by a person creates an image. The professional image is the way in which an occupation or a member of that profession is perceived. This image is formed from several characteristics or traits. The first characteristic deals with the superficial aspects of a person, for example, the way a person dresses or his or her manner of speaking. In fact, general appearance and grooming reflect directly on whether the phlebotomist is perceived as a professional. Conservative clothing, proper personal hygiene, and physical well-being contribute to a professional appearance. Institutional policies for attire are influenced by a federal standard that requires employers to provide protective clothing for laboratory workers, including phlebotomists.

Professionalism also involves personal behaviors or characteristics, including the following.

INTEGRITY

Professional standards of integrity or honesty require a person to do what is right regardless of the circumstances. For example, a phlebotomist often functions independently and may be tempted to take procedure shortcuts when pressed for time. A phlebotomist with integrity understands that following rules for collection is essential to the quality of test results—and respects those rules.

COMPASSION

A phlebotomist may show compassion and still remain professional. Compassion simply means being sensitive to a patient's or customer's needs and being willing to offer reassurance in a caring and interested way.

MOTIVATION

Phlebotomists with motivation find the workplace a challenge no matter what their tasks entail. Motivation is a direct reflection of a person's attitude about life. If phlebotomists have a positive attitude and a willingness to perform at their peak every day, the healthcare environment will consistently offer adventure and growth, especially during this exciting time of changing roles and responsibilities.

DEPENDABILITY

Dependability and work ethic go hand-in-hand. An individual who is dependable and who takes personal responsibility for his or her actions is extremely refreshing in today's environment and is a very desirable candidate for job opportunities in the healthcare setting or anywhere.

DIPLOMACY/ETHICAL BEHAVIOR

A phlebotomist should demonstrate diplomacy and ethical behavior at all times. Diplomacy means the phlebotomist uses effective communication skills and tact while dealing with the patient, even in stressful situations. Ethical behavior entails conforming to a standard of right and wrong conduct to avoid harming the patient in any way. Based on a system of principles called ethics, the professional can identify conduct that is morally desirable. A code of ethics, although not enforceable by law, leads to uniformity and defined expectation by the members of that profession. Professional organizations, such as ASCLS, have developed codes of ethics for healthcare professionals. The primary objective in any healthcare professional's code of ethics must always be the patient's welfare. As stated in the Hippocratic oath, "primum non nocere," or "first do not harm."

Patient Rights

The phlebotomist, as any other member of the healthcare team, must recognize the rights and privileges a patient has while in a hospital or other healthcare facility. These rights have been clearly defined in a document originally published in 1975 by the American Hospital Association called **A Patient's Bill of Rights.** This document, although not legally binding, is an accepted statement of principle that guides healthcare workers in their dealings with patients. It states that all healthcare professionals, including phlebotomists, have a primary responsibility for quality patient care, while also maintaining the patient's personal rights and dignity. Some of the rights especially pertinent to the phlebotomist are summarized in Box 1-2.

Box 1-2

A PATIENT'S BILL OF RIGHTS

- The right of the patient to always be treated with respect.
- The right to refuse to have blood drawn.
- The right to have the results of laboratory work remain confidential.
- The right to obtain from the physician the purpose of the testing and the results.
- The right to expect all communications and records pertaining to one's care should be treated as confidential.

Confidentiality

Patient confidentiality is seen by many as the ethical cornerstone of professional behavior in the healthcare field. It serves to protect both the patient and the practitioner. As a professional, the healthcare provider should recognize that all patient information is absolutely private and confidential. Information, such as a patient's test results, treatment, or condition, is not to be discussed any place where the information might be overheard. In addition, patient information should not be released to unauthorized people. Any questions relating to patient information, such as inquiries from a reporter in the case of a celebrity, should be referred to the proper person in administration. Unauthorized release of information concerning a patient is considered invasion of privacy. Information should only be given out with the written consent of the patient or when a healthcare provider is legally obligated to release the information.

Key Point ➤ Maintaining confidentiality is such an important issue in testing for HIV that the patient must sign a consent form before the test can be collected.

Communication Skills

Phlebotomy is both a technical and a people-oriented profession. Many different types of people or customers interact with phlebotomists. Often, the customer's perception of the healthcare facility is derived from the employees they deal with on a one-to-one basis, such as a phlebotomist. Customers expect quality service. If a phlebotomist lacks a good bedside manner (the ability to communicate empathically with the patient), he or she increases the chances of becoming part of a legal action should any difficulty arise while obtaining the specimen. Favorable impressions result when professionals respond properly to patient needs, and this occurs when there is good communication between the healthcare provider and the patient.

Communication Defined

Communication is a skill. Defined as the means by which information is exchanged or transmitted, communication is one of the most important processes that takes place in the healthcare system. This dynamic or constantly changing process involves three components: verbal skills, nonverbal skills, and the ability to listen.

Communication Components

VERBAL COMMUNICATION

Expression through the spoken word is the most obvious form of communication. Effective healthcare communication should be an interaction in which both participants are affected. It involves a sender (speaker), a receiver (listener), and, when complete, a process called feedback. It is through feedback that the listener or receiver is given the chance to correct miscommunication caused by personal bias or barriers.

Normal human behavior sets up many **barriers** to accurate verbal communication. These biases or personalized filters are major obstructions to hearing and understanding what has been said, as illustrated in the feedback loop in Figure 1-5. Examples of communication barriers are language limitations, culture diversity, emotions, age, and physical disabilities such as hearing loss. To encourage good verbal communication, the phlebotomist should use a vocabulary that is easily understood by his or her clients. To avoid creating suspicion and distrust in patients from other countries, the phlebotomist should be aware of cultural differences, and avoid clichés and nonverbal cues that could be misunderstood.

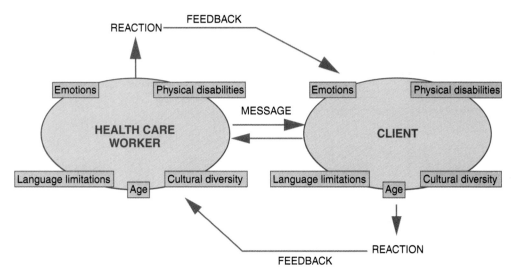

■ FIGURE 1-5 ■

Verbal communication feedback loop.

NONVERBAL COMMUNICATION

It has been stated that 80% of language is unspoken. Unlike verbal communication formed from words that are one-dimensional, nonverbal communication is multidimensional and involves the following elements.

Kinesics

The study of nonverbal communication is also called **kinesics** and includes characteristics of body motion and language such as facial expression, gestures, and eye contact. Figure 1-6 illustrates an exaggerated and simplified form of the six emotions that are most easily read by nonverbal facial cues. Body language, which most often is unintentional, plays a major role in communication because it is continuous and more reliable than verbal communication. In fact, if the verbal and nonverbal messages do not match, it is called a **kinesic slip.** When this happens, it has been shown that people tend to trust what they see rather than what they hear.

As health professionals, the phlebotomist can learn much about patients' feelings by observing nonverbal communication, which seldom lies. The patient's face often tells the health professional what the patient will not reveal verbally. For instance, when a patient is anxious, nonverbal signs may include tight eyebrows, an intense frown, narrowed eyes, or a downcast mouth (Fig. 1-6). Researchers have found that certain facial appearances, such as a smile, are universal expressions of emotion. Worldwide, we all recognize the meaning of a smile; however, strong cultural customs often dictate when it is used.

To communicate effectively with a person, it is important to establish good eye contact. A patient or client may be made to feel unimportant and more like an object rather than a human being if no eye contact is established.

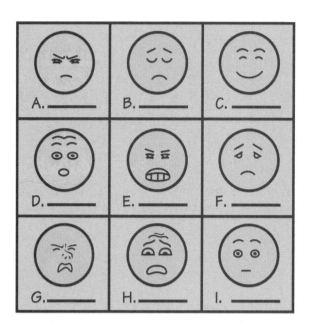

■ FIGURE 1-6 ■

Nonverbal facial cues. (Adapted from Northouse, P.G., & Northouse, L.L. (1992). Health Communication: Strategies for Healthcare Professionals (2nd ed.) (p. 127). Reprinted by permission of Appleton & Lange, Stamford, CT.)

Can you match the above sketches with the correct affects?
(1) happy, (2) sad, (3) surprise, (4) fear, (5) anger, (6) disgust.

Answers: A-5, B-2, C-1, D-3, E-5, F-2, G-6, H-4, I-3.

Proxemics

Proxemics is defined as the study of an individual's concept and use of space. This subtle but powerful part of nonverbal communication should be understood to relate better to the patient in a healthcare facility. Every individual has around him or her an invisible "bubble," defined as personal territory. The size of this bubble or territorial zone depends on the individual's needs at the time. Four categories of naturally occurring territorial zones and the radius of each are listed in Table 1-2. These "zones of comfort" are very obvious in human interaction. Entering personal or intimate zones is necessary in the healthcare setting and, if not carefully handled, the patient may feel threatened, insecure, or out of control.

Table 1-2

Territorial Zones and Corresponding Radii	
Territorial Zone	**Zone Radius**
Intimate	1 to 18 inches
Personal	1-½ to 4 feet
Social	4 to 12 feet
Public	More than 12 feet

Appearance

Most healthcare facilities have dress codes because it is understood that appearance makes a statement. The impression the phlebotomist makes as he or she approaches the patient sets the stage for future interaction. The right image portrays a trustworthy professional. Phlebotomists' physical appearance should communicate cleanliness and confidence. Lab coats, when worn, should completely cover the clothing underneath and should be clean and pressed. Shoes should be conservative and polished. Close attention should be paid to personal hygiene. Bathing and the use of deodorant should be a daily routine. Strong perfumes or colognes should be avoided. Hair and nails should be clean and look natural. Hair, if long, should be pulled back and fingernails should be short for safety's sake. Phlebotomists who deal with patients who are ill or irritable will find a confident and professional appearance helpful in doing their job.

Touch

Touching can take a variety of forms and convey many different meanings. For example, accidental touching could happen in a crowded elevator. Social touching could take place when a person grabs the arm of another while giving advice. Therapeutic touching is designed to aid in healing. This special type of nonverbal communication is a very important ingredient to the well-being of humans, and even more so in diseased humans.

Because medicine is a contact profession, touching privileges are granted to and expected for healthcare workers under certain circumstances. Whether a patient or healthcare provider is comfortable with touching is based on his or her cultural background. Because touch is a necessary part of the phlebotomy procedure, it is important to realize that, as a phlebotomist, patients are often much more aware of your touch than you are of theirs; there may even be a risk of the patient questioning the appropriateness of touching. Generally speaking, patients respond favorably when touch portrays a thoughtful expression of caring.

ACTIVE LISTENING

It is more difficult to communicate than to speak because effective communication requires that the listener participate. It is always a two-way process. The ordinary person can absorb verbal messages at about 500 to 600 words per minute, and the average speaking rate is only 125 to 150 words per minute. Therefore, the listener, to not be distracted, must use the extra time for active listening. Active listening means taking positive steps through feedback to ensure that the listener interprets what the speaker is saying exactly as the speaker intended. Listening forms the foundation for good interpersonal communication and is particularly valuable in building rapport with patients.

Effective Communication in Healthcare

It is not easy for the patient or the health professional to face disease and suffering every day. For many patients, being ill is a terrifying experience; having their blood drawn only contributes to their anxiety. Patients reach out for comfort and reassurance through conversation. Consequently, a phlebotomist must understand the unusual aspects of healthcare communication and its importance in comforting the patient.

Communication between the health professional and patient is more complicated than normal interaction. Not only is it often emotionally charged but it also involves, in many instances, other people who are very close to the patient and who may tend to be very critical of the way the patient is handled. Recognizing some of the elements in healthcare communication, such as empathy, control, trust, and confirmation, will aid the phlebotomist in successfully interacting with the patient.

ELEMENTS IN HEALTHCARE COMMUNICATION

Empathy

Defined as identifying with the feelings or thoughts of another person, empathy is an essential factor in interpersonal relations. It involves putting yourself in the place of another and attempting to feel like that person. Thoughtful and sensitive people generally have a high degree of empathy. Empathic health professionals help patients handle the stress of being in a healthcare institution. When a health professional recognizes the needs of the patient and allows the patient to express his or her emotions, this helps to validate the patient's feelings and gives the patient a very necessary sense of control.

Control

An important element relating to communication in the healthcare setting is control. Feeling in control is essential to an individual's sense of well-being. People like to think that they can influence the way things happen in their lives. A hospital is one of the few places where an individual gives up control over most of the personal tasks he or she normally performs. Many patients perceive themselves as unable to cope physically or mentally with events in a hospital because they feel fearful and powerless because of this loss of control. Consequently, the typical response of the patient is to act angry, which characterizes him or her as a "bad patient," or to act extremely codependent and agreeable, which characterizes him or her as a "good patient."

If a patient refuses to have blood drawn, the phlebotomist should allow him or her to express that statement of control and even agree with the patient. Patients who are allowed to exert that right will often change their minds and agree to the procedure, because then it is their decision. Sharing control with the patient may be difficult and often time-consuming, but awareness of the patient's need is important.

Confirmation

Too often busy healthcare givers resort to labeling patients when communicating with coworkers and even with patients themselves. They may say, for example, "oh, you're the one with no veins." Or "you're the bleeder, right?" Such communication is dehumanizing and is a subtle way of "disconfirming" patients. Each patient needs to be accepted as a unique individual with special needs. An example of initiating a confirming exchange with the patient in the first example could be, "Mrs. Jones, I seem to remember that we had a hard time finding a suitable vein last time we drew your blood." Or in the second case, "Mr. Smith, wasn't there a problem getting the site to stop bleeding after the draw last time?"

Trust

Another variable in the process of communication is trust. Trust, as defined in the healthcare setting, is the unquestioning belief by the patient that health professionals are performing their job responsibilities as well as they possible can. As is true with most professionals, healthcare providers tend to emphasize their technical expertise while sometimes completely ignoring the elements of interpersonal communication that are essential in a trusting relationship with the patient. Having blood drawn is just one of the situations in which the consumer must trust the health professional. Developing trust takes time and phlebotomists spend very little time with each patient. Consequently, during this limited interaction, the phlebotomist must do everything possible to win the patient's confidence by consistently appearing knowledgeable, honest, and sincere.

In summary, by recognizing the elements of empathy, control, trust, and confirmation, the phlebotomist can enhance communication with patients and assist in their recovery. Understanding these communication elements will help when used with other means of communication, such as the telephone.

TELEPHONE COMMUNICATION

The telephone is presently a fundamental part of communication. It is used 24 hours a day in the laboratory. To phlebotomists or laboratory clerks, it becomes just another source of stress, bringing additional work and uninvited demands on their time. The constant ringing and the interruption to the workflow often cause laboratory personnel to overlook the effect their style of telephone communication has on the caller. To maintain a professional image, every person given the responsibility of answering the phone should review proper protocol. He or she should be taught how to answer, put someone on hold, and transfer calls properly. To increase good communication, the telephone techniques shown in Table 1-3 should be followed.

THE HEALTHCARE SETTING

Virtually everyone in the United States becomes a healthcare consumer at some time in his or her life. For many, working through the bureaucracy involved in receiving healthcare can be confusing. Healthcare personnel who understand how healthcare is organized and financed, and their role in the system, can help consumers successfully negotiate the process with minimal frustration.

Healthcare Delivery

Two general categories of facilities, inpatient (nonambulatory) and outpatient (ambulatory), support all three levels (**primary, secondary,** and **tertiary**) of healthcare presently offered in the United States. See Box 1-3 for a listing of services and practitioners associated with the two categories.

Table 1-3

Proper Telephone Technique

1. **Answer promptly.** If the phone is allowed to ring too many times, the caller assumes the people working in the laboratory are inefficient or insensitive. When answering the phone, state your name and your department.
2. **Be helpful.** When a phone rings, it is because someone needs something. Because of the nature of the healthcare business, the caller may be emotional and need a calm, pleasant voice on the other end to respond to the request. To assist the caller and facilitate the conversation, ask how you can be of help. Keep your statements and answers simple and to the point to avoid confusion.
3. **Prioritize calls.** Callers should be informed if they are interrupting another call. Always ask if they can be put on hold in case it is an emergency that must be handled immediately. Coordinating several calls takes an organized person. Disconnecting a caller while transferring irritates the caller.
4. **Be prepared to record information.** Documentation is necessary when answering the phone at work to ensure that accurate information is transmitted to the necessary person. Have a pencil and paper close to the phone. Listen carefully, which means clarifying, restating, and summarizing the information received.
5. **Know the laboratory policies.** People who answer the telephone need to know the laboratory policies to avoid misinformation. Answers should be consistent. This helps to establish the laboratory's credibility, because a caller's perception of the lab involves more than accurate test results.
6. **Diffuse hostile situations.** Some callers are angry because of lost results or errors in billing. Agreeing with a hostile caller will immediately diffuse the caller. After the caller has been calmed down, an inquiry can be handled.
7. **Try to assist everyone.** It is possible to assist callers and show concern even if you are not actually answering their questions. Validate callers' requests by giving a response that tells them something can be done. Sincere interest in the caller will enhance communication and contribute to the good reputation of the laboratory.

Ambulatory Care and Homebound Services

Changes in healthcare practices that have significantly decreased the amount of time a patient spends in the hospital have led to innovative ways to serve healthcare, including the offering of a wide range of ambulatory services. These services meet the needs of patients who may still require healthcare provisions such as nursing care, lab tests, or other follow-up procedures after being discharged from the hospital. In addition, new health services are being developed for the fastest growing segment of the population, the elderly. Many homebound elderly require nursing care and physical therapy to be given and laboratory tests to be collected, where they reside, either in their homes or in long-term care facilities. A number of agencies employ nurses, respiratory therapists, phlebotomists and other healthcare workers to provide these services.

Public Health Service

One of the principal units under the Department of Health and Human Services is the Public Health Service (PHS). PHS agencies at the local or state level offer defense against infectious diseases that might spread among the populace. These agencies are constantly monitoring, screening, and educating the public (see Table 1-4 for examples of services provided by local health departments). Public health departments provide

---

Box 1-3

TWO CATEGORIES OF HEALTHCARE FACILITIES

Outpatient or **Ambulatory** Facilities
- Principal source of healthcare services for most people.
- Offer routine care in physician's office to specialized care in a freestanding ambulatory setting.
- Serve the **primary care** physician who assumes ongoing responsibility for maintaining patients' health.
- Serve the **secondary care** level physician (specialist) who performs routine surgery, emergency treatments, therapeutic radiology, and so on in same-day service centers.
- Examples are doctor and dentist offices, surgical centers, health clinics, and outpatient areas of the hospital.

Inpatient Facilities
- The key resource and center of the American healthcare system.
- Offer specialized instrumentation and technology to assist in unusual diagnosis and treatment.
- Serve the **tertiary care** (highly complex services and therapy) level practitioners.
- Usually require that patients stay overnight or longer.
- Examples are acute care hospitals, nursing homes, extended care facilities, hospice and rehabilitation centers.

---

their services for little or no charge to the entire population of a region, with no distinction between rich or poor, simple or sophisticated, interested or disinterested. Public health facilities offer ambulatory care services through clinics, much as with those in hospital outpatient areas, military bases, and Veterans Administration and Indian Health Service facilities.

As the country moves into managed care, integration between primary prevention and primary/ambulatory care is necessary. Because containment of healthcare costs is the driving force behind managed care, proactive public health programs can significantly contribute to reductions in overall healthcare costs.

Table 1-4

Examples of Services Provided by Local Health Departments	
Vital statistics collection	Tuberculosis screening
Health education	Immunization and vaccination
Cancer, hypertension, and diabetes screening	Operation of health centers
Public health nursing services	Venereal disease clinics

Healthcare Financing

Healthcare is expensive and the cost continues to escalate. The consumer must make choices based on financial considerations as well as medical need and can no longer afford to be passive in the process. The healthcare provider, such as the phlebotomist, in addition to being a consumer is also an employee of an institution that relies on third-party payers (health insurers) for a major portion of his or her income.

Third-Party Payers

A **third-party payer** can be an insurance company or government program that pays for healthcare services on behalf of a patient.

Third-party payers have greatly influenced the direction of medicine. In the past decade, major changes have come about in healthcare payments and third-party reimbursements.

Methods of Payment

Because of the rapid rise in healthcare costs, the government put into place the **prospective payment system (PPS).** The PPS, begun in 1983, attempted to limit and standardize the Medicare/Medicaid payments made to hospitals. This plan, originally designed by the American Hospital Association, reimburses hospitals a set amount for each patient procedure using established disease categories called **diagnostic-related groups (DRGs).** The DRG defines the amount of reimbursement the facility will receive for a particular admission. A new classification system implemented in 2000 for determining payment to hospitals for outpatient service is called **ambulatory patient classification (APCs).** The main factor that determines which DRG or APC grouping is assigned for the care provided is the code number that indicates the diagnosis at the time seen or admitted.

For coding of diagnoses, all major payers use **International Classification of Diseases, Ninth Revision, Clinical Modification (ICD-9-CM).** This coding system groups together similar diseases and operations for reimbursement. The **Center for Medicare and Medicaid Services (CMS),** formerly the Health Care Financing Administration, is in the process of developing a new procedure coding system called ICD-10 for the United States that is slated for adoption in the early part of 21st century. Another widely used coding system is the **CMS Common Procedure Coding System.** This system consists of three levels of codes. Level 1 is the **current procedural terminology (CPT),** level 2 is national codes, and level 3 is local codes. The CPT codes were originally developed in the1960s by the American Medical Association to provide a terminology and coding system for physician billing. Physician offices have continued to use it to report their services. Now all types of healthcare providers use CPT to classify, report, and bill for a variety of healthcare services.

Currently, ICD-9-CM procedure codes are used for inpatients and CPT procedure codes are used for patients seen in the ambulatory setting and for professional services in the inpatient setting. The lack of standardization and confusion in the diagnostic and procedural coding led to the passage in 1996 of the **Health Insurance Portability** and Accountability Act (HIPAA). This bill was designed to improve the efficiency of the healthcare system by establishing standards for electronic data exchange including coding systems. HIPAA regulations have as their goal to move to one universal procedural coding system as the future standard.

Reimbursement

The history of institutional reimbursement is tied to **entitlement programs** such as Medicare and public welfare in the form of Medicaid. Before 1983, hospitals were paid retrospectively and reimbursed for all services performed on Medicare and Medicaid patients. A comparison of Medicare and Medicaid Programs is listed in Box 1-4.

Box 1-4

MEDICARE AND MEDICAID PROGRAM COMPARISON

Medicare	Medicaid
First enacted in 1965	First enacted in 1965
Federally funded entitlement program for providing healthcare to people over the age of 65, regardless of their financial status, and to the disabled.	Federal and state program that provides medical assistance to the poor.
An entitlement program because it is a right earned by individuals through employment.	No entitlement features; recipients must prove their eligibility.
Financed through Social Security payroll deductions and copayments.	Funds come from federal grants and are administered by the state.
Benefits divided into two categories: Part A, called hospital services, and Part B, called supplementary medical insurance (SMI).	Benefits cover inpatient care, outpatient and diagnostic services, skilled nursing facilities, and home health and physician services.

Arizona is the only state that has devised its own system outside of Medicaid, called **Arizona Healthcare Cost Containment System (AHCCCS).** It differs in that the providers (private physician groups) must bid annually for contracts to serve this population and patients are able to choose their healthcare provider through annual open enrollment.

The Changing Healthcare System

Healthcare systems are currently undergoing major revisions. The driving force behind these changes is the perceived need to control the cost of healthcare. Government social programs and other managed healthcare plans continually negotiate discounts on the amount they will reimburse the hospitals, forcing the hospitals to cut costs and downsize operations.

Managed Care

Managed care is a generic term for a payment system that manages cost, quality, and access to healthcare. It is a system of controlling cost in healthcare by presetting reimbursement amounts and regulating patient access to participating physicians and healthcare institutions. Benefits or payments paid to the provider are made according to a set fee schedule, and enrollees must comply with managed care policies such as preauthorization for certain medical procedures and approved referral to specialists for claims to be paid.

Today's large managed care systems evolved from prepaid healthcare plans such as **health maintenance organizations (HMOs)** and **preferred provider organizations (PPOs).** HMOs are group practices reimbursed on a prepaid, negotiated, and discounted basis of admission. PPOs are independent groups of physicians or hospitals that offer services to employers at discounted rates in exchange for a steady supply of patients. Because managed care centers on the association of provider, payer, and consumer, several concepts have been developed to control this relationship, including gatekeepers and network services systems.

PRIMARY CARE GATEKEEPERS

One of the most important concepts in managed care is that of the primary care physician filling the role of **gatekeeper.** As the patient's advocate, this person has the responsibility to advise the patient on healthcare needs and coordinate responses to those needs. Gatekeeper responsibilities also include providing early detection and treatment for disease, which should reduce the total cost of care.

PROVIDER NETWORKS

Managed care organizations (MCO) contract with local providers to establish a complete network of services. Providers are reimbursed based on the number of enrollees served—not on the number of services delivered. The goal of the MCO is to reduce the total cost of care while maintaining patient satisfaction.

MEDICAL SPECIALTIES IN MANAGED CARE

In managed care, the primary physician is most often a family practitioner, a pediatrician, or an internist. The gatekeeper is expected to refer to the appropriate specialist as needed. Some of the many healthcare areas in which a doctor of medicine (MD) or doctor of osteopathy (DO) can specialize are listed in Table 1-5.

Table 1-5

Medical Specialties

Specialty	Area of Interest	Specialist Title
Anesthesiology	Partial or complete loss of sensation usually by injection or inhalation	Anesthesiologist
Cardiology	Diseases of the heart and blood vessels and cardiovascular surgery, a subspecialty of internal medicine	Cardiologist
Dermatology	Diseases and injuries of the skin; more recently, concerned with skin cancer prevention	Dermatologist
Endocrinology	Disorders of the endocrine glands, such as sterility, diabetes, and thyroid problems	Endocrinologist
Gastroenterology	Digestive tract and related structure diseases, a subspecialty of internal medicine	Gastroenterologist
Gerontology	Effects of aging and age-related disorders	Gerontologist
Hematology	Disorders of the blood and blood-forming organs	Hematologist
Internal Medicine	Diseases of internal organs and general medical condition, uses nonsurgical therapy	Internist
Nephrology	Diseases related to structure and function of the kidney	Nephrologist
Neurology	Disorders of the brain, spinal cord, and nerves	Neurologist
Obstetrics and Gynecology	Women through pregnancy, childbirth, disorders of the reproductive system, and menopause	Gynecologist
Oncology	Tumors, including benign and malignant conditions	Oncologist
Ophthalmology	Eye examinations, eye diseases, and surgery	Ophthalmologist
Orthopedics	Disorders of the musculoskeletal system, including preventing disorders and restoring function	Orthopedist
Otorhinolaryngology	Disorders of the eye, ear, nose, and throat	Otorhinolaryngologist
Pediatrics	Diseases of children from birth to adolescence; does wellness checks and gives vaccinations	Pediatrician
Psychiatry	Mental illness, clinical depression, and other behavioral and emotional disorders	Psychiatrist
Pulmonary Medicine	Function and disorders of the lungs and respiratory system	Pulmonologist
Rheumatology	Rheumatic diseases (acute and chronic conditions characterized by inflammation and joint disease)	Rheumatologist
Urology	Urinary tract disease and male reproductive organ disorders	Urologist

Departments Within the Healthcare Facility or Hospital

Hospitals are often large organizations with a complex internal structure. The healthcare delivery system in hospitals has traditionally been arranged by departments or medical specialties. People who do similar tasks are grouped into departments, the goal being to perform each task as efficiently and accurately as possible. This style of management segregates the departments and their processes (Fig. 1-7) for a typical hospital organization flow chart. Consequently, it is difficult to look at an institution-wide final outcome and judge patient satisfaction.

Managed care has led to a reduction in the number of healthcare personnel, whereas the number of services remains the same. This has resulted in the formation of teams of cross-trained personnel and the consolidation of services. Such reengineering, as it is called, is designed to make the healthcare delivery system more process-oriented by combining related groups of tasks into a system that is customer-focused. This management of process is reflected in a new type of hospital organization that blends former distinct departments into service or process areas. The intent is to create a "gentle hand off" for patients between service areas, instead of the abrupt "toss and catch" approach that can occur in traditional settings with distinct and separate departments. Although the lines between former departments are becoming blurred, Table 1-6 shows the services areas that are identified as essential.

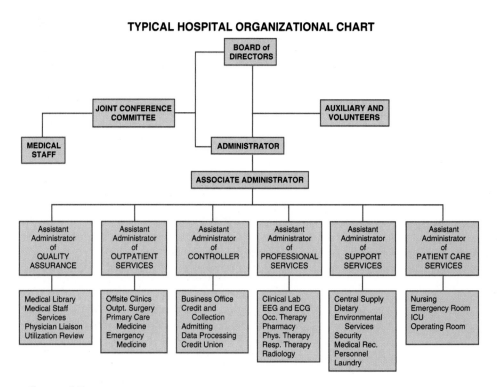

TYPICAL HOSPITAL ORGANIZATIONAL CHART

■ FIGURE 1-7 ■

Typical hospital organizational flow chart.

Table 1-6

Essential Service Areas of a Hospital

Service Area	Departments Within Area	Services Performed
PATIENT CARE SERVICES	Nursing Care	Direct patient care. Includes careful observation to assess conditions, administering medications and treatments prescribed by a physician, evaluation of patient care, and documentation in the health record that reflects this. Staffed by many types of nursing personnel including registered nurses (RNs), licensed practical nurses (LPNs), and certified nursing assistants (CNAs).
	Emergency Services	Around-the-clock service designed to handle medical emergencies that call for immediate assessment and management of injured or acutely ill patients. Staffed by specialists such as emergency medical technicians (EMTs) and MDs who specialize in emergency medicine.
	Intensive Care Units (ICUs)	Designed for increased bedside care of patients in fragile condition. Found in many areas of the hospital and named for the type of patient care they provide (e.g., trauma ICU, pediatric ICU, medical ICU).
	Surgery	Concerned with operative procedures to correct deformities and defects, repair injuries, and cure certain diseases. All work is performed by a licensed medical practitioner who specializes in surgery.
SUPPORT SERVICES	Central Supply	Prepares and dispenses all the necessary supplies required for patient care, including surgical packs for the operating room, intravenous pumps, bandages, syringes, and other inventory controlled by computer for close accounting.
	Dietary Services	Selects foods and supervises food services to coordinate diet with medical treatment.
	Environmental Services	Includes housekeeping and grounds keepers whose services maintain a clean, healthy, and attractive facility.
	Health Information Technology	Maintains accurate and orderly records for inpatient medical history, tests results and reports, and treatment plans and notes from doctors and nurses to be used for insurance claims, legal actions, and utilization reviews.
PROFESSIONAL SERVICES	Cardiodiagnostics (EKG or ECG)	Performs electrocardiograms (EKGs/ECGs, actual recordings of the electrical currents that are detectable from the heart), Holter monitoring, and stress testing for diagnosis and monitoring therapy in cardiovascular patients.

continued

Table 1-6

Essential Service Areas of a Hospital (continued)

Service Area	Departments Within Area	Services Performed
PROFESSIONAL SERVICES	Pathology and Clinical Laboratory	Performs highly automated and often complicated testing on blood and other body fluids to detect and diagnose disease, monitor treatments, and, more recently, assess health. There are several specialized areas of the laboratory called departments (see Departments in the Clinical Laboratory).
	Electroneurodiagnostic Technology (ENT) or electroencephalography (EEG)	Performs electroencephalograms (EEGs), tracings that measure electrical activity of the brain. Uses techniques, such as ambulatory EEG monitoring, evoked potential, polysomnography (sleep studies), and brain wave mapping to diagnose and monitor neurophysiologic disorders.
	Occupational Therapy (OT)	Uses techniques designed to develop or assist mentally, physically, or emotionally disabled patients to maintain daily living skills.
	Pharmacy	Prepares and dispenses drugs ordered by physicians; advises the medical staff on selection and harmful side effects of drugs, therapeutic drug monitoring, and drug use evaluation.
	Physical Therapy (PT)	Diagnoses physical impairment to determine the extent of disability and provides therapy to restore mobility through individually designed treatment plans.
	Respiratory Therapy (RT)	Diagnoses, treats, and manages patient's lung deficiencies (e.g., analyzes arterial blood gases [ABGs], tests capacity of the lungs, administers oxygen therapy).
	Diagnostic Radiology Services	Diagnoses medical conditions by taking x-ray films of various parts of the body. Uses latest procedures including powerful forms of imaging that do not involve radiation hazards, such as ultrasound machines, magnetic resonance (MR) scanners, and positron emission tomography (PET) scanners.

Clinical Laboratory Services

Clinical laboratory (lab) services perform tests on patient specimens. Results of testing are primarily used by physicians to confirm health or aid in the diagnosis, evaluation, and monitoring of patient medical conditions. Clinical labs are typically located in hospitals, outpatient clinics, and physicians' offices.

Traditional Laboratories

There are two major divisions in the clinical laboratory, the clinical analysis area and the anatomic and surgical pathology area. All laboratory testing is associated with either of these two areas. See Box 1-5.

Box 1-5

TWO MAJOR DIVISIONS IN THE CLINICAL LABORATORY

Clinical Analysis Areas
Specimen processing, hematology, chemistry, microbiology, blood bank/ immunohematology, immunology/ serology, and urinalysis testing

Anatomical and Surgical Pathology
Tissue analysis, cytologic examination, surgical biopsy, frozen sections, and performance of autopsies

---

CLINICAL ANALYSIS AREAS

Hematology

The hematology department performs laboratory tests that identify diseases associated with blood and the blood-forming tissues. The most commonly ordered hematology test is the complete blood count (CBC). The CBC is performed using automated instruments, such as the Coulter counter, that electronically count the cells and calculate results (Fig. 1-8). A complete blood count is actually a multi-part assay that is reported on a form called a hemogram (Tables 1-7 and 1-8).

Coagulation

Coagulation is the study of the ability of blood to form and dissolve clots. Coagulation tests are closely related to hematology tests and the department is often housed in the hematology area. Coagulation tests are used to discover, identify, and monitor defects in the blood clotting mechanism. They are also used to monitor patients who are taking medications called anticoagulants (chemicals that inhibit blood clotting) or "blood thinners." The two most common coagulation tests are the prothrombin time, used to monitor warfarin therapy, and the activated partial thromboplastin time for evaluating heparin therapy (Table 1-9).

Chemistry

The chemistry department performs the majority of laboratory tests. This department often has subsections such as toxicology and radioimmunoassay. Computerized instruments (Fig. 1-9, p. 31) used in this area are capable of performing discrete (individualized) tests or panels (multiple tests) from a single sample. Examples of panels frequently ordered to evaluate a single organ or specific body system are given in Table 1-10 (p. 31).

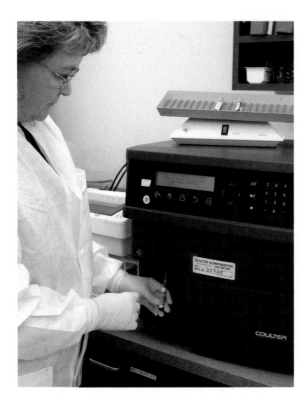

■ FIGURE 1-8 ■

Coulter MAXM automated hematology analyzer.

The most common chemistry specimen is serum; however, other types of specimens tested include plasma, whole blood, urine, and various other body fluids. Examples of tests normally performed in the automated clinical laboratory section are provided in Table 1-11 (p. 32).

Serology or immunology

Serology literally means the study of serum. Serology tests deal with the body's response to the presence of bacterial, viral, fungal, or parasitic diseases that stimulate antigen—antibody reactions that can easily be demonstrated in the laboratory (Table 1-12, p. 34). Autoimmune reactions, in which autoantibodies produced by B lymphocytes attack normal cells, are becoming more prevalent and can be detected by serologic tests. Testing is done by enzyme immunoassay (EIA), agglutination, complement fixation, or precipitation to determine the antibody or antigen present and to assess its concentration or titer.

Urinalysis

The urinalysis (UA) department may be housed in the hematology or chemistry area or may be a completely separate section. Urine specimens may be analyzed manually or using automated instruments. UA is a routine urine test that includes physical, chemical, and microscopic evaluations (Table 1-13, p. 35).The physical examination assesses the color, clarity, and specific gravity of the specimen. The chemical evaluation, performed using chemical reagent strips, screens for substances such as sugar and protein.

Table 1-7

Hemogram for Complete Blood Count (CBC) Assay

Name of Test	Abbreviation	Clinical Significance
Hematocrit	Hct	Values correspond to the red cell count and hemoglobin level; when decreased, indicate anemic conditions.
Hemoglobin	Hgb	Decreased values indicate anemic conditions; values normally differ with age, sex, altitude, and hydration.
Red blood cell count	RBC	Measure of erythropoietic activity; decrease in numbers related to anemic condition.
White blood cell count	WBC	Abnormal leukocyte response indicative of various conditions, such as infections and malignancies; when accompanied by WBC, differential test becomes more specific.
Platelet count	Plt Ct	Decreased number indicative of hemorrhagic diseases; values may be used to monitor chemotherapy or radiation treatments.
Differential white count	Diff	Changes in appearance or number of specific cell type signifies specific disease conditions; values also used to monitor chemotherapy or radiation treatments.
Indices		Changes in RBC size, weight, and Hgb content indicate certain types of anemias.
Mean corpuscular hemoglobin	MCH	Reveals the weight of the hemoglobin in the cell, regardless of the size. Decreased hemoglobin content indicative of iron deficiency anemia; increased hemoglobin content found in macrocytic anemia.
Mean corpuscular volume	MCV	Reveals the size of the cell. Decreased MCV associated with thalassemia and iron deficiency anemia; increased MCV because of folic acid or vitamin B12 deficiency and chronic emphysema.
Mean corpuscular hemoglobin concentration	MCHC	Reveals the hemoglobin concentration per unit volume of RBCs. Below-normal range means red cells are deficient in hemoglobin as in thalassemia, overhydration, or iron deficiency anemia; above-normal range will be seen in severe burns, prolonged dehydration, and hereditary spherocytosis.
Red blood cell distribution width	RDW	Reveals the size differences of the RBCs. An early predictor of anemia before other signs and symptoms.

Table 1-8

Other Common Hematology Tests

Bone marrow	Detects abnormal blood cells and evaluates blood cell formation and function
Cerebrospinal (CSF) and other body fluids	Presence or absence, number and type of cells Hematocrit on fluid indirectly measures fluid volume
Eosinophil count	Increased numbers in direct count indicate parasitic infections and allergies
Erythrocyte sedimentation rate (ESR)	Increased rate at which red blood cells settle out is indicative of inflammatory conditions or necrosis of tissue
Lupus erythematosus (LE prep)	Presence of typical LE cells is diagnostic of systemic LE
Osmotic fragility	Increased red cell fragility is indicative of hemolytic and autoimmune anemias; decreased fragility is indicative of sickle cell and thalassemia
Reticulocyte count (retic count)	Increased number of retics in circulating blood attest to bone marrow hyperactivity
Sickle cell	Sickling of red cells indicates presence of abnormal hemoglobin variant, Hgb S

Table 1-9

Common Coagulation Tests

Test	Clinical Significance
Activated partial thromboplastin time	Prolonged times may indicate stage one defects; values reflect adequacy of heparin therapy.
Bleeding time (BT)	Increased BT indicates hemorrhagic disorders associated with decreased platelet activity and lack of elasticity of capillary walls.
D-dimer test	Evaluates thrombin and plasmin activity and is very useful in testing for disseminated intravascular coagulation and used in monitoring thrombolytic therapy.
Fibrin degradation products (FDP)	High levels result in FDP fragments that interfere with platelet function and clotting.
Fibrinogen	Fibrinogen deficiency suggests hemorrhagic disorders and is used most frequently in obstetrics.
Prothrombin time (PT)	Prolonged times may indicate stage two and three defects; values used to monitor warfarin therapy.

A microscopic examination identifies the presence or absence of blood cells, bacteria, crystals, and other substances.

Microbiology

This department analyzes body fluids and tissues for the presence of microorganisms, primarily by means of culture and sensitivity (C & S) testing (Fig. 1-10, p. 36). Results of a C & S tell the physician the type of organisms present and the particular antibiotic

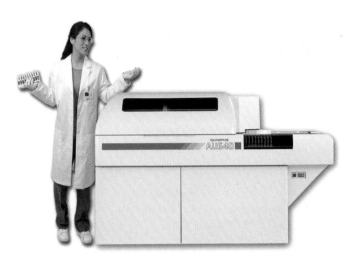

■ FIGURE 1-9 ■

Automated chemistry analyzer, Olympus AU640.
(Courtesy of Olympus America, Inc., Melville, NY)

Table 1-10

Disease- and Organ-Specific Chemistry Panels (CMS Approved)

Panel Grouping	Battery of Selected Diagnostic Tests
Basic metabolic panel (BMP)	Glucose, BUN, creatinine, sodium, potassium, chloride, CO_2, calcium
Comprehensive metabolic panel (CMP)	Glucose, BUN, creatinine, sodium, potassium, chloride, CO_2, AST, ALT, alkaline phosphatase, total protein, albumin, total bilirubin, calcium
Hepatic function panel A	AST, ALT, alkaline phosphatase, total protein, albumin, total bilirubin, direct bilirubin
Renal function panel	Glucose, BUN, creatinine, sodium, potassium, chloride, CO_2, calcium, albumin, phosphorus

ALT, alanine aminotransferase; AST, aspartate aminotransferase; BUN, blood urea nitrogen; CO_2, carbon dioxide.

that would be most effective for treatment. Collecting and transporting microbiology specimens is very important in the identification of microorganisms. Subsections of microbiology are bacteriology (study of bacteria), parasitology (study of parasites), mycology (study of fungi), and virology (study of viruses) (Table 1-14, p. 36).

Blood bank or immunohematology

This department of the laboratory prepares blood products to be used for patient transfusions. Blood components dispensed include whole blood, platelets, packed cells, fresh frozen plasma, and cryoprecipitates. Blood samples from all donors and the recipient must be carefully tested before transfusions can be administered so that incompatibility and transfusion reactions can be avoided (Table 1-15, p. 37). Transfusion services, offered by the blood bank department, collect, prepare, and store units of blood from donors or patients who wish to donate their own units for autologous transfusion, if necessary.

Table 1-11

Common Chemistry Tests

Common Chemistry Test	Associated Body System	Examples of Clinical Significance
Alanine amino-transferase (ALT)	Liver	Marked elevations point to liver disease; used for monitoring liver treatment.
Alpha-fetoprotein (AFP)	Liver	Increased values in hepatic carcinoma; elevation of AFP in prenatal screening indicates neural tube disorder.
Alkaline phosphatase (ALP)	Liver or bone	Elevated ALP levels because of biliary obstruction and bone disease.
Ammonia	Liver	Increased blood levels indicate cirrhosis and hepatitis.
Amylase	Pancreas and liver	Increased levels of this enzyme diagnostic of acute pancreatitis; decreased values associated with liver disease, cholecystitis, and advanced cystic fibrosis.
Aspartate amino-transferase (AST)	Liver or heart	Increase in enzyme indicative of liver dysfunction; significant increase following myocardial infarction.
Bilirubin	Liver	Increased levels in the blood stream point to red cell destruction and liver dysfunction.
Blood gases (ABG)	Kidneys, lungs	Measures pH, partial pressure of carbon dioxide (Pco_2), partial pressure of oxygen (Po_2) to evaluate the acid-base balance.
Blood urea nitrogen (BUN)	Kidney	Elevated values because of impaired renal function from toxins, inflammation, or obstruction.
Carcinoembryonic antigen (CEA)	Nonspecific	Increased in the cases of malignancy, effective in the early detection of colorectal cancer.
Calcium	Bone	Increased levels associated with diseases of the bone; used in monitoring effects of renal failure.
Cholesterol (total)	Heart	Indicative of high risk for cardiovascular disease.
Cortisol	Adrenals	Elevated levels signify adrenal hyper-function (Cushing's syndrome); decreased levels indicate adrenal hypofunction (Addison's disease).
Creatine kinase (CK)	Heart or muscle	Elevated values point to muscle damage (i.e., myocardial infarction, muscular dystrophy, or strenuous exercise).
Creatinine	Kidney	Increased levels indicate renal impairment; decreased levels associated with muscular dystrophy.
Drug analysis		Values monitored to maintain therapeutic range and avoid toxic levels for drugs such as barbiturates, digoxin, gentamicin, lithium, primidone, phenytoin, salicylates, theophylline, or tobramycin.

continued

Table 1-11

Common Chemistry Tests *(continued)*

Common Chemistry Test	Associated Body System	Examples of Clinical Significance
Electrolytes	Kidney, adrenals, heart	Sodium values (sodium, potassium, chloride) increased in disorders of the kidney and adrenals; decreased values of potassium seen in irregular heartbeat; chloride values are increased in kidney and adrenal disorders and decreased in diarrhea.
Glucose	Pancreas	Elevated levels signify diabetic problems; decreased values support liver disease and malnutrition.
Glycosylated hemoglobin	Pancreas	Glycohemoglobin level shows what type of diabetic control has occurred over the past several months.
Gamma-glutamyl transferase (GGT)	Liver	Elevated values assist in the diagnosis of liver problems, specific for hepatobiliary problems.
Lactic acid dehydrogenase (LD)	Heart, lungs, liver	Elevated levels confirm acute myocardial infarction; chronic lung, kidney, and liver dysfunction.
Lipase	Pancreas	Increased levels in acute pancreatitis, pancreatic carcinoma, and obstruction.
Prostate specific antigen	Prostate	Performed to screen patients for the presence of prostate cancer, monitor progression disease, and the response of the patient to treatment.
Total protein	Liver or kidney	Low levels point to liver and kidney disorders; elevated levels may occur with multiple myeloma and dehydration.
Triglycerides	Heart	Increased values indicate lipid metabolism disorders and serve as an index for evaluating atherosclerosis possibilities.
Uric acid	Kidney	Elevated values found in renal disorders and gout.
Vitamin B_{12} and folate	Liver	Decreased levels indicate anemias and disease of the small intestine.

ANATOMIC AND SURGICAL PATHOLOGY

Histology

Histology is literally defined as the study of the microscopic structure of tissues. In this department, pathologists evaluate samples of tissue from surgeries and autopsies under a microscope to determine if they are normal or pathologic (diseased). Histologic techniques include two of the most diagnostic tools found in the laboratory (1) biopsy, obtaining samples by removal of a plug (small piece) of tissue from an organ and examining it microscopically; and (2) frozen sections, obtaining tissue from surgery and freezing and examining it immediately to determine whether more extensive surgery is needed. Before tissues can be evaluated, they must be processed and stained. This is the role of a person called an histologist.

Table 1-12

Common Serology and Immunology Tests

Test	Examples of Clinical Significance
Bacterial Studies	
Antinuclear antibody (ANA)	Positive results in autoimmune disorders, specifically systemic lupus erythematosus
Antistreptolysin O (ASO) titer	To demonstrate infection from streptococcus bacteria
Cold agglutinins	Present in cases of atypical pneumonia
Febrile agglutinins	Presence of antibodies to specific organisms indicates disease condition (i.e., tularemia)
FTA-ABS	Fluorescent treponemal antibody absorption test, confirmatory test for syphilis
Rapid plasma reagin (RPR)	Positive screen indicates syphilis; positives need to be confirmed
Rheumatoid factor (RF)	Presence of antibody indicates rheumatoid arthritis
Viral Studies	
Anti-HIV	Human immunodeficiency virus is screened
Cytomegalovirus antibody (CMV)	Confirmation test
Epstein-Barr virus (EBV)	Presence of this heterophil antibody indicates infectious mononucleosis
Hepatitis B surface antigen (HBsAg)	Demonstrates the presence of hepatitis antigen on the surface of the red cells
General Studies	
C-reactive protein (CRP)	Increased levels in inflammatory conditions
Human chorionic gonadotropin (HCG)	Present in pregnancy (serum and urine)

Cytology

Cytology and histology are often confused. Whereas histology tests are concerned with the structure of tissue, cytology tests are concerned with the structure of cells. In this department, cells in body tissues and fluids are identified, counted, and studied to diagnose malignant and premalignant conditions. Histologists often process and prepare the specimens for evaluation by a pathologist or cytotechnologist. The Pap smear, a test for early detection of cancer cells, primarily of the cervix and vagina, is one of the most common examinations performed by this department.

 Key Point ➤ The Pap smear test is named after a staining technique used to detect malignant cells developed by Dr. George N. Papanicolaou.

Cytogenetics

An area found in larger labs is cytogenetics. In this section, samples are examined for chromosomal deficiencies that relate to genetic disease. Specimens used for chromosomal studies include tissue, blood, and amniotic fluid. The DNA probe analysis is the latest in testing for infectious pathogens, genetic and malignant disorders, and DNA fingerprinting for forensic medicine.

Table 1-13

Common Urinalysis Tests

Test	Clinical Significance
Physical Evaluation	
Color	Abnormal colors that are clinically significant result from blood, melanin, bilirubin, or urobilin in the sample.
Clarity	Turbidity may be the result of chyle, fat, bacteria, RBCs, WBCs, or precipitated crystals.
Specific gravity	Variation in this indicator of dissolved solids in the urine is normal; inconsistencies suggest renal tubule involvement or ADH deficiency.
Chemical Evaluation	
Blood	Hematuria may be the result of hemorrhage, infection, or trauma.
Bilirubin	Aids in differentiating obstructive jaundice from hemolytic jaundice, which will not cause increased bilirubin in the urine.
Glucose	Glucosuria could be the result of diabetes mellitus, renal impairment, or ingestion of a large amount of carbohydrates.
Ketones	Occurs in uncontrolled diabetes mellitus and starvation.
Leukocyte esterase	Certain white cells (neutrophils) in abundance indicate urinary tract infection.
pH	Variations in pH indicate changes in acid—base balance, which is normal; loss of ability to vary pH is indicative of tissue breakdown.
Protein	Proteinuria is indicator of renal disorders, such as injury and renal tube dysfunction.
Nitrite	Positive result suggests bacterial infection but is only significant on first-morning specimen or urine incubated in bladder for at least 4 hours.
Urobilinogen	Occurs in increased amounts when patient has hepatic problems or hemolytic disorders.
Microscopic Evaluation	Analysis of urinary sediment reveals status of the urinary tract; hematuria, pyuria, and presence of casts and tissue cells are pathologic indicators.

STAT Labs

In today's healthcare environment, laboratory services in many tertiary care facilities exist as STAT labs only. STAT means immediately. Consequently, tests performed are primarily those needed to respond to medical emergencies, along with some of the more frequently ordered tests. Specimens for all other laboratory tests are collected, processed, and sent to an offsite location or reference laboratory. This efficient way of performing lab work allows hospital laboratories to produce immediately needed test results without having to maintain the equipment and reagents necessary to do all routine testing.

Reference Laboratories

Reference laboratories are large, independent laboratories that receive specimens from many different facilities located in the same city, other cities in the same state, or even out of state. They provide routine and more specialized analysis of blood, urine, tis-

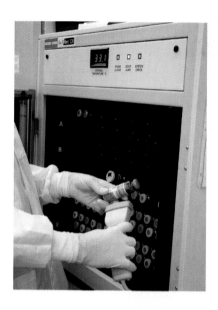

■ FIGURE 1-10 ■

Microbiologist reviews blood cultures processed by the BactALERT 3D.

sue, and other patient specimens. These laboratories offer fast **turnaround time (TAT)** and reduced costs because of the high volume of tests they perform. Specimens sent to offsite laboratories must be carefully packaged in special containers designed to protect the specimens and meet federal safety regulations for transportation of human specimens.

Table 1-14

Common Microbiology Tests	
Test	**Clinical Significance**
Acid fast bacilli (AFB)	Positive stain means pulmonary tuberculosis; used to monitor the treatment for TB.
Blood culture	Positive culture results (bacterial growth in media) indicate bacteremia or septicemia.
CLOtest	Presence of *Helicobacter pylori*.
Culture & sensitivity (C & S)	Growth of a pathogenic microorganism indicates infection (culture); in vitro inhibition by an antibiotic (sensitivity) allows the physician to select the correct treatment.
Fungus culture and identification	Positive culture detects the presence of fungi and determines the type.
Gram stain	Positive stain for specific types of pathogenic microorganisms permits antimicrobial therapy to begin before culture results are known.
Occult blood	Positive test indicates blood in the stool, which is associated with gastrointestinal bleeding from carcinoma.
Ova and parasites	Microscopic examination of stool sample showing ova and parasites solves many "etiology unknown" intestinal disorders.

Table 1-15

Common Blood Bank and Immunohematology Tests	
Test	**Clinical Significance**
Antibody (Ab) screen	Agglutination indicates abnormal antibodies present in patient's blood.
Direct antihuman globulin test (DAT)	Positive results point to autoimmune hemolytic anemia, hemolytic disease of the newborn (HDN), and transfusion incompatibility.
Type and Rh	Determination of blood group (ABO) and type (Rh) by identifying agglutinins present or absent.
Type and cross-match	Determination of blood group and general screening for antibodies of recipient's blood and then recipient and donor blood are checked against each other for compatibility.
Compatibility testing	Detection of unsuspected antibodies and antigens in recipient's and donor's blood that could cause severe reaction if transfused.

Clinical Laboratory Personnel

Laboratory Director/Pathologist

The pathologist is a physician who specializes in diagnosing disease, through the use of laboratory tests results, in tissues removed at operations and from postmortem examinations. It is his or her duty to direct laboratory services so they benefit the physician and patient. The laboratory director may be a pathologist or a clinical laboratory scientist with a doctorate degree. The laboratory director and the laboratory administrator share responsibilities for managing the laboratory.

Laboratory Administrator/Laboratory Manager

The lab administrator is usually a technologist with an advanced degree and several years of experience. Duties of the administrator include overseeing all operations involving physician and patient services. Today, the laboratory administrator may supervise several ancillary services, such as radiology and respiratory therapy, or all the laboratory functions in a healthcare system consisting of separate lab facilities across a large geographic area.

Technical Supervisors

For each laboratory section or subsection, there is a technical supervisor who is responsible for the administration of the area and who reports to the laboratory administrator. This person usually has additional education and experience in one or more of the clinical laboratory areas.

Medical Technologist/Clinical Laboratory Scientist

The medical technologist (MT) or clinical laboratory scientist generally has a bachelor's degree in chemistry or biology, with study in an MT program for 1 year or more. Some of the states require licensing for this level of personnel. The responsibilities of the MTs include performing all levels of testing in any area of the laboratory procedures, reporting results, performing quality control, evaluating new procedures, and conducting preventive maintenance and troubleshooting on instruments.

Medical Laboratory Technicians/Clinical Laboratory Technicians

The medical laboratory technician or clinical laboratory technician (CLT) is most often an individual with an associate degree from a 2-year program or certification from a military or proprietary (private) school. As with MTs, some states may require licensing for medical/clinical laboratory technicians. The technician is responsible for performing routine testing, operating all equipment, performing basic instrument maintenance and recognizing instrument problems, and assisting in problem solving.

Phlebotomist

The phlebotomist is trained to collect blood for laboratory tests that are necessary for diagnosis and care of patients. A number of facilities use phlebotomists as laboratory assistants or specimen processors (see Box 1-1, page 7, for duties). Formal phlebotomy programs in colleges and private schools usually require a high school diploma or the equivalent to enroll. After completing the program or acquiring 1 year of work experience, a phlebotomist can become certified by passing a national examination. A few states require licensing for this level of personnel.

Clinical Laboratory Assistants

Before the arrival of computerized instrumentation in the laboratory, the clinical laboratory assistant was a recognized position. Today, due to reduction in the laboratory staff, this category of personnel has been revived. A clinical laboratory assistant is a person with phlebotomy experience who has skills in specimen processing and basic laboratory testing. Clinical laboratory assistants are generalists, responsible for assisting the MT or MLT with the workload in any area.

Other Laboratory Personnel

Other laboratory personnel include programmers and laboratory information systems (LIS) operators, quality assurance managers, and point-of-care coordinators. Computer programmers and LIS operators are often laboratorians who, through additional training, have become experts in laboratory computer software. Quality assurance (QA) managers are detail-oriented MTs who collect statistics for QA purposes. Point-of-care coordinators are MTs who work closely with the nursing staff to assure the quality of point-of-care testing results. In some hospital settings, maintenance and QA checks on the POCT instruments has become the responsibility of the phlebotomy staff.

Clinical Laboratory Improvement Act

The Clinical Laboratory Improvement Amendments of 1988 **(CLIA '88)** were signed into law on October 31, 1988, and became effective in 1992. This public law mandates that all laboratories must be regulated using the same standards regardless of the loca-

STUDY & REVIEW QUESTIONS

1. Early equipment used for blood-letting includes all of the following *except* the
   a. hemostat.
   b. lancet.
   c. fleam.
   d. leech.

2. A factor that contributes to the phlebotomist's professional image is
   a. personal hygiene.
   b. national certification.
   c. a pleasant smile and a positive attitude.
   d. all of the above.

3. The initials for the title granted after successful completion of the National Credentialing Agency phlebotomy examination are
   a. CLPlb.
   b. CLT.
   c. CPT.
   d. PBT.

4. The principles of right and wrong conduct as they apply to professional problems are called
   a. certification.
   b. ethics.
   c. esteem.
   d. tort.

5. An example of a third-party payer is
   a. Medicare.
   b. DRG.
   c. OSHA.
   d. CPT.

6. Which of the following is a duty of a phlebotomist?
   a. Chart patient results
   b. Obtain blood pressures and temperatures of patients
   c. Analyze specimens for hematology
   d. Perform laboratory computer operations

7. Which of the following is an example of proxemics?
   a. Eye contact
   b. Zone of comfort
   c. Facial expressions
   d. Personal hygiene

8. Which of the following is proper telephone technique?
   a. Wait for the phone to ring three or four times so as not to appear anxious.
   b. Do not identify yourself in case there are problems later.
   c. Be careful of the tone of voice used and keep answers simple.
   d. Listen carefully; do not take notes because it takes too much time.

Continued

STUDY & REVIEW QUESTIONS *(CONTINUED)*

9. An institution that provides inpatient services is a
    a. clinic.
    b. doctor's office.
    c. hospital.
    d. day-surgery.

10. State and federally funded insurance is called
    a. HIPPA.
    b. PPO.
    c. ASCP.
    d. Medicaid.

11. The specialty that treats disorders of old age is called
    a. cardiology.
    b. gerontology.
    c. pathology.
    d. psychiatry.

12. The department in the hospital that records brain waves for diagnosis is
    a. electroneurodiagnostics.
    b. occupational therapy.
    c. physical therapy.
    d. radiology.

13. The microbiology department in the laboratory performs
    a. compatibility.
    b. enzyme-linked immunoassay.
    c. electrolyte monitoring.
    d. blood culture testing.

14. The abbreviation for the routine hematology test that includes hemoglobin, hematocrit, red blood count, and white blood count determinations is called
    a. CDC.
    b. CRP.
    c. CBC.
    d. CPK.

15. Which of the following laboratory professionals is specified by CLIA'88 as responsible for administration of a clinical area?
    a. Clinical laboratory scientist
    b. Clinical laboratory technician
    c. Laboratory manager
    d. Technical supervisor

tion, type, or size. The law requires that every clinical laboratory facility in the country obtain a certificate from the federal government assuring the customers that laboratory testing performed at that facility is reliable and accurate. Laboratories that fall under the CLIA regulations include those in hospitals, clinics, government facilities, independent laboratories, HMOs, and physician office laboratories. The regulations put into force by this law deal with, among other things, laboratory standards. The standards are designed for two types of laboratory facilities. The lab type is determined by the complexity of testing done at that facility; for example, moderately complex or highly complex. Personnel qualifications for each of the types are stated in the regulations.

Bibliography and Suggested Readings

Abdelhak, M., Grostick, S., Hanken, M., & Jacobs, E. (2001). *Health information: Management of a strategic resource* (2nd ed.). Philadelphia, PA: W. B. Saunders.

CLIA '88. (1992). Final standard is published. *Clinical Chemistry News,* March.

Cmiel, P. (1990). Postoperative management of the replant patient: Monitoring, complications, and education. *Critical Care Nursing Quarterly 13*(1), 47.

Davis, A., & Appel, T. (1979). *Bloodletting instruments in the National Museum of History and Technology.* Washington, DC: Smithsonian Institution Press.

Henry, J. B. (1996). *Clinical diagnosis and management by laboratory methods* (19th ed.). Philadelphia: W. B. Saunders.

National Center for Cultural Competence. *Policy Brief 1, Rationale for culture competence in primary healthcare.* Washington, DC: Georgetown University Child Development Center.

Simmers, L. (1998). *Diversified health occupations* (4th ed.). Albany, NY: Delmar Publishers.

Williams, S. J. (1995). *Essentials of health services.* New York: Delmar Publishers.

Wilson, D. (1999). *Nurses' guide to understanding laboratory and diagnostic tests.* Philadelphia, PA: Lippincott Williams & Wilkins.

2

QUALITY ASSURANCE AND LEGAL ISSUES

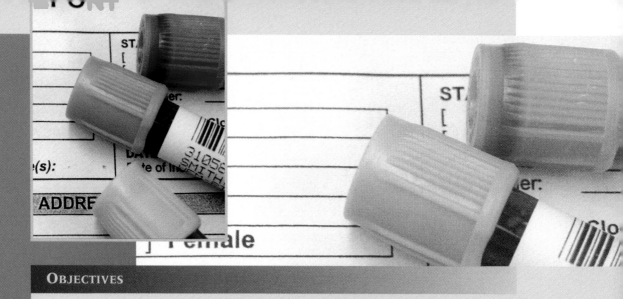

OBJECTIVES

Upon successful completion of this chapter, the reader will be able to:

1 Define the key terms and abbreviations listed at the beginning of this chapter.
2 Describe the evolution of quality assurance in healthcare.
3 Recognize national standards and regulatory agencies that require quality assurance in phlebotomy services.
4 Define quality and performance improvement measurements as they relate to phlebotomy.
5 List and describe the components of a quality assurance (QA) program and differentiate quality control (QC) from QA.
6 List areas in phlebotomy subject to QC and identify quality control procedures associated with each.
7 Demonstrate understanding of the legal implications associated with phlebotomy in the healthcare environment.
8 Define legal terminology associated with the healthcare setting and describe how a phlebotomist can avoid litigation.

QUALITY ASSURANCE IN HEALTHCARE

In the United States, an abundance of management tools and techniques have been offered for "getting the job done." All have promised to deliver more efficient and effective management. There were those that proved to be useful in the private, profit-making sector, whereas others were more successful in the not-for-profit, noncompetitive public sector. Very few were useful in both sectors. But beginning in 1988, **Total Quality Management (TQM)** made the jump from the private to the public sector. One of the leaders in TQM was Dr. W. Edwards Deming. As an engineer and physicist, Deming used statistics to analyze production processes and discover the source of product flaws. Deming's methods require that the workers actively participate in decisions to improve production continually; that is, a team effort with total involvement from all levels. Deming developed the idea that quality improvement reduces waste and leads to improved productivity, in turn reducing costs. This **quality improvement (QI)** process is now part of the accreditation requirements for all types of healthcare facilities and found in every aspect of healthcare, including phlebotomy procedures. One of the ways to improve quality is through the use of national standards and regulations.

National Standard and Regulatory Agencies

Joint Commission on Accreditation of Healthcare Organizations

One of the key players in bringing **QI** techniques to healthcare is the **Joint Commission on Accreditation of Healthcare Organizations (JCAHO).** JCAHO is a voluntary, nongovernmental agency charged with, among other things, establishing standards for the operation of hospitals and other health-related facilities and services. In 1994, JCAHO required healthcare facilities to have an institution-wide total quality management/continuous quality improvement (TQM/CQI) plan in place. This meant that all departments of a healthcare facility were required to have ongoing evaluations of their activities and customer expectations. Current standards from JCAHO stress performance improvement by requiring the facility to be directly accountable to their customer. To evaluate and track complaints about healthcare organizations relating to quality of care, the Office of Quality Monitoring was created. The office has a toll-free hot line and e-mail address that can be used to receive complaints. The Quality Incident Report Form is shown in Figure 2-1. Information and concerns often come from patients, their families, and many other sources. When a report is submitted, JCAHO reviews any past reports and the organization's most recent accreditation decision. Depending on the nature of the reported concern, JCAHO will:

- Request from the organization a written response to the reported concern.
- Conduct an onsite, unannounced assessment of the organization if the report raises serious concerns about a continuing threat to patient safety or continuing failure to comply with standards.
- Incorporate the concern into the performance improvement database that is used to identify trends or patterns in performance.
- Review the reported concern and compliance at the organization's next accreditation survey.

Quality Incident Report Form

Date: _____　　　　Time: _____

Name of person filing the report: _____

Relationship to patient:　Self _____　Family _____　Friend _____　Advocate _____

　　　　　　　　　　　　Attorney _____　　Employee _____　　Government _____

Telephone: (___) _____　　　　E-mail: _____

Address: _____　　　Fax: _____

Provider Information (Where did problem occur?)

Name of organization: _____

Address: _____

_____

Telephone: (___) _____

Type of organization (Provider):　Hospital _____　Ambulatory _____　Home Care _____

Laboratory _____　　　Long Term Care _____　　Psychiatric/Behavioral Health _____

Network, PPO, HMO _____

Quality Incident: (Please state your concern) _____

_____

_____

(Attach additional pages, if required. Please keep to no more than two pages.)

Confidentiality required: _____ Yes

Were concerns made known to provider?　　_____ Yes　_____ No

ACTIONS REQUIRED: (Office use only)

Referrals: _____

Quality Analyst: _____　　Analyst

Signature: _____

JCAHO incident report form.　(Copyright Joint Commission on Accreditation of Healthcare Organizations, 2002. Reprinted with permission.)

College of American Pathologists

Another agency that influences quality improvement in phlebotomy through standards is the **College of American Pathologists (CAP).** This national organization is an outgrowth of the American Society of Clinical Pathologists. The membership in this specialty organization is composed entirely of board-certified pathologists. CAP offers **proficiency testing** and a continuous form of laboratory inspection by a team made up of pathologists and laboratory managers. The CAP Inspection and Accreditation Program does not compete with the JCAHO accreditation for healthcare facilities because CAP is designed for pathology services only. A CAP-certified laboratory also meets Medicare/Medicaid standards because JCAHO grants reciprocity to CAP in the area of laboratory inspection.

Clinical Laboratory Improvement Amendments of 1988

The **Clinical Laboratory Improvement Amendments of 1988 (CLIA '88)** are federal regulations passed by Congress and administered by the Center for Medicare and Medicaid Services (CMS). These regulations establish quality standards that apply to all facilities, including clinics and physicians' office laboratories that test human specimens for the purpose of providing information used to diagnose, prevent, or treat disease, or to assess health status. The aim of the standards is to ensure the accuracy, reliability, and timeliness of patient test results, regardless of the location, type, or size of the laboratory. The standards address quality assurance, quality control, proficiency testing, laboratory records, and personnel qualifications.

All laboratory facilities subject to CLIA'88 regulations are required to obtain a certificate from the CMS according to the complexity of testing performed there. Three categories of testing are recognized: waived complexity, moderate complexity, (which includes a provider performed microscopy subcategory) and high complexity. Complexity of testing is based on the difficulty involved in performing the test and the degree of risk of harm to a patient if the test is performed incorrectly. CLIA requirements are more stringent for laboratories that perform moderate and high complexity testing and their facilities are subject to routine inspections.

Specimen collection is an important part of CLIA inspections, and laboratories are required to have written protocols for patient preparation, and specimen collection, labeling, preservation, and transportation.

National Committee for Clinical Laboratory Standards

The **National Committee for Clinical Laboratory Standards (NCCLS)** is an international, nonprofit, educational organization with representatives from the profession, industry, and government who use a consensus process to develop voluntary guidelines and standards for all areas of the laboratory. Phlebotomy program approval and certification examination questions are based on these important guidelines and standards.

National Accrediting Agency for Clinical Laboratory Sciences

The National Accrediting Agency for Clinical Laboratory Sciences (NAACLS), recognized by the United States Department of Education as an authority on educational quality, is a nonprofit organization that provides either accreditation or approval for clinical laboratory educational programs. The accreditation process involves an external peer review of the program, including an onsite evaluation, to determine whether the program meets certain established educational standards. The NAACLS approval process for phlebotomy programs requires that the program meet educational standards called **competencies** designed to improve student outcomes and maintain quality education.

Quality Improvement

An inexpensive and flexible approach for supporting CQI in JCAHO-accredited organizations is a new program designed to standardize measurements of performance nationally. Organizations will be expected to demonstrate, for each measurement, the ability to collect dependable data, conduct reliable analyses of the data, and initiate appropriate system and process improvements.

The principal intent of JCAHO is to identify, rather than develop, sound measurements that support the objectives of the organization's process improvement. In May 2001, JCAHO revealed the four initial core measurement areas for hospitals: acute myocardial infarction (heart attack); community-acquired pneumonia; pregnancy and related conditions; and heart failure. Beginning July 1, 2002, healthcare organizations will start to collect data in the core measurement areas on patients that have been discharged from their facilities.

Some of the recommended core measures directly relate to the quality and timeliness of phlebotomy. For example, the community-acquired pneumonia measure includes blood culture collection before administration of antibiotics as one of the standardized performance measures and how the collection, processing, and reporting affects patient outcome. A core measure for acute myocardial infarction includes time elapsed between the collection of specimens at specified times for tests whose results are used for critical decision-making, and the treatment or surgical intervention that is based on the results of those tests.

Quality Assurance in Phlebotomy

As members of the healthcare team, phlebotomists need to understand the significance of their role in providing quality patient care. Laboratory testing is an important part of patient diagnosis, and consequently a major part of patient care. Doctors rely on validity of test results. Preanalytical (before analysis) factors such as patient preparation, specimen collection procedures, and specimen handling can affect specimen quality and in turn affect validity of test results. Many of these factors fall under the responsibility of the phlebotomist. To ensure consistent quality, specimen collection and handling policies and procedures should be based on specific guidelines such as those established by NCCLS, and phlebotomists should strictly adhere to them. Established policies and procedures fall under an overall process called **quality assurance (QA).**

QA Defined

QA is defined as a program that guarantees quality patient care by tracking outcomes through scheduled reviews in which areas of the hospital look at the appropriateness, applicability, and timeliness of patient care. Guidelines are developed for all processes used, and when formally adopted, they become the QA program.

QA Indicators

One of the most important aspects of setting up a QA monitoring and evaluation process is establishing indicators to monitor all aspects of patient care. **QA indicators** must be measurable, well-defined, specific, objective, and clearly related to an important aspect of care. Indicators can measure quality, adequacy, accuracy, timeliness, effectiveness, customer satisfaction, and so on. They are designed to look at areas of care that tend to cause problems. For example, an indicator on the QA form shown in Figure 2-2 might be stated as follows: "The blood culture contamination rate will not exceed 3%." A contamination rate that increased beyond the pre-established threshold listed on the form would signify a problem.

Thresholds and Data

Threshold values must be established for all clinical indicators. A threshold value is a level of acceptable practice beyond which quality patient care cannot be assured. Exceeding this level of acceptable practice may trigger intensive evaluation to see if there is a problem that needs to be corrected. During the evaluation process, data are collected and organized. Data sources include such information as patient records, laboratory results, incident reports, patient satisfaction reports, and direct patient observation. A corrective action plan is established if the outcome of the data identifies a problem or opportunity for improvement. An action plan identifies what will change and when that change is expected to occur. Even when the problem appears to be corrected, monitoring and evaluation continue to ensure that care is consistent and that quality continually improves.

Process and Outcomes

QA must look at more than outcomes. Outcomes give us numbers only. For example, an outcome evaluation can give us the number of times that patients were redrawn because the improper tube was used for specimen collection. Although it is important to know how often this occurs, this does not tell us why it happened. If we wish to change an outcome, we need to look at the process. This means following the process from start to finish. In the previous example, that means looking at what the requester did at the time he or she decided the test was needed, how it was ordered, and how the laboratory processed the request until the time the results were on the patient's

#: _____

QUALITY ASSESSMENT AND IMPROVEMENT TRACKING
CONFIDENTIAL A.R.S. 36-445

STANDARD OF CARE/SERVICE: _____

IMPORTANT ASPECT OF CARE/SERVICE: LAB SVCS/BLOOD COLLECTION
SIGNATURES:
DIRECTOR:
MEDICAL DIRECTOR:
VICE PRESIDENT/ADMINISTRATOR:

DEPARTMENTS/POPULATION: LABORATORY-MICROBIOLOGY/ALL PATIENTS
DATA SOURCE(S): CULTURE WORKCARDS
DATA COLLECTOR: P. BABINA
FREQUENCY REVIEW: 3 MONTHS   100% SAMPLE
METHODOLOGY: RETROSPECTIVE
TYPE: OUTCOME
PERSON RESPONSIBLE FOR:
DATA ORGANIZATION: P. BABINA
ACTION PLAN: J. BENSON
FOLLOW-UP: J. BENSON
DATE MONITOR BEGAN: 1990
FOLLOW-UP: 3RD QTR.

INDICATORS		THRESHOLD			CRITICAL ANALYSIS/ EVALUATION	ACTION PLAN
		EXP.	ACT.	PREV.		
Blood culture contamination rate will not exceed 3% from three groups of drawing personnel.		3%			N= 1385	A communication has gone out to Nursing reminding to follow established protocols for drawing.
					Patient Centered Care draws a Nursing line draws are out of compliance but show improvement from January to March.	Microbiology has implemented new protocol disallowing a line draw unless two consecutive venipunctures have failed or protocol is overridden by physician order.
LAB	JAN	3%	1.1%			
	FEB		1.8%			PCC tecs have been reinserviced on proper technique.
	MAR		1.7%			
PCC	JAN	3%	5.6%			
	FEB		4.8%			
	MAR		3.2%			
LINE DRAWS	JAN	3%	5.6%			
	FEB		7.9%			
	MAR		0.0%			

QICONFID

■ FIGURE 2-2 ■

Quality assessment form.

chart and in the hands of the person that ordered them. To assure the same process is always followed, there must be controls and checks on quality along the way. The use of controls and checks is called **quality control (QC).**

QC Defined

QC is a component of a QA program and a form of procedure control. Consistently following national standards for phlebotomy procedures is a means of controlling the quality of results. A phlebotomy QC process involves checking all the operational procedures to make certain they are performed correctly. In phlebotomy, it is the responsibility of the person who supervises the phlebotomist to oversee QA and ensure that standards are being met. It is the responsibility of the phlebotomist to meet those standards at all times.

Areas of Phlebotomy Subject to QC

Patient Preparation Procedures

Quality control in laboratory testing actually starts before the specimen is collected, in the preanalytical stage of QA. To obtain a quality specimen, the patient must be prepared properly. In a hospital setting, the patient's nurse can find instructions on how to prepare a patient for testing by checking the laboratory **user manual** (Fig. 2-3), given to the nursing unit by the laboratory. The user manual describes patient preparation and other special instructions for specimen collection. The phlebotomist can carry a concise pocket version of this book to use in answering questions concerning unusual requests. It is important for the phlebotomist and others involved in specimen collection to stay informed and updated concerning testing protocol to be better able to answer inquiries.

Specimen Collection Procedures

IDENTIFICATION

Patient identification (as described in Chapter 8) is the most important aspect of specimen collection. Methods are being continually improved to ensure correct patient identification. An example is the use of barcode readers and accompanying labels (Fig. 2-4), which can substantially reduce human error.

EQUIPMENT

Puncture devices

Assuring the quality and sterility of every needle and lancet is essential for patient safety. All puncture devices come in sealed sterile containers and should be used only once. If the seal has been broken, the device should be put in a sharps container and a new one obtained. Manufacturing defects in needles, such as barbs and blunt tips, can be avoided before use by quickly inspecting the needle after unsheathing.

HEMATOLOGY

TEST	TEST VOLUME	VACUTAINER COLOR (TOP)	NORMAL VALUES	NOTES
APT test	1 mL feces or gastric fluid	Plastic container	Negative	Suitable for grossly bloody specimens only
Acid hemolysin	0.4 mL (RBC) 2.5 mL serum	Lavender and red (non-Corvac)	0%–5%	
Acid phosphatase stain	3 mL blood	Green		
Acid phosphatase w/tartrate stain (TRAP)	3 mL blood	Green		
Alpha naphthol butyrate stain (nonspecific esterase)	3 mL blood	Green		
Blood smear– differential	.03 mL blood	Lavender or fingerstick	See individual tests	See page 27
Body fluid HCT	1 mL	Fluid		
Bone marrow				Schedule in advance (4-6281)
Coulter count	1 mL blood	Lavender or lavender microtainer	See page 27	Includes WBC, RBC, HGB, HCT, MCV, MCH, MCHC
Differential	1 mL blood	Lavender		See page 28
Eosinophil count	0.5 mL blood	Lavender	150–350/uL	See page 28
Epinephrine/ endotoxin stimulation test				Schedule in advance (4-6281). Consultation form required
Fetal hemoglobin (APT) (qualitative)	1 mL feces or gastric fluid	Red Non-Corvac or plastic container	Negative	Suitable for grossly bloody specimens only

■ FIGURE 2-3 ■

User manual. (Courtesy University Medical Center, Tucson, AZ.)

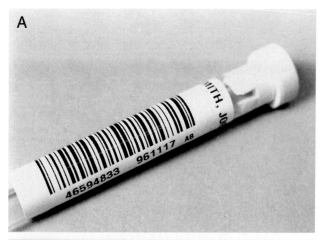

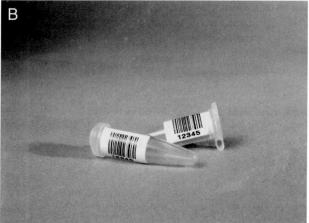

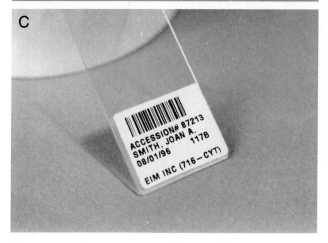

■ FIGURE 2-4 ■

(*A*) Specimen tube with barcode label. (*B*) Microcollection container with barcode label. (*C*) Slide with barcode label.   (Courtesy Electronic Imaging Materials, Inc., Keene, NH.)

Evacuated tubes

NCCLS has established standards for evacuated tubes to help assure specimen integrity. Manufacturers print expiration dates on each tube for quality assurance. Outdated tubes should not be used because they may not fill completely, causing dilution of the sample, distortion of the cell components, and erroneous results. In addition, anticoagulants in expired tubes may not work effectively, instead allowing small clots to form and thereby invalidating hematology and immunohematology test results. As part of QC, all new lots of evacuated tubes should be checked for adequate vacuum and additive, integrity of the stopper, ease of stopper removal, and tube strength during centrifugation. Results of these and other quality control checks should be documented.

LABELING

Labeling must be exact. Labeling requirements, as outlined in Chapter 8, should be strictly followed. Inaccuracies, such as transposed letters or missing information, will result in the specimen being discarded. With computer labels, the phlebotomist may be assured of correctly printed patient information; however, this correct label must still be placed on the correct patient's specimen.

TECHNIQUE

Proper phlebotomy technique must be carefully taught by a professional who understands the importance of following national standards and the reasons for using certain equipment or techniques. Incident reports, a form of QA documentation, are used to report inadequate technique or poor specimen quality.

 Key Point ➤ No matter how experienced phlebotomists may be, a periodic review of their techniques is necessary for quality assurance and performance improvement.

COLLECTION PRIORITIES

Specimen collection priorities must be stressed. The importance of knowing how to recognize which specimen request is the most critical or has special collection criteria (e.g., renins or therapeutic drug monitoring [TDM]) can save the patient unnecessary medication or additional testing. It may even shorten the patient's stay in the hospital, because in many instances therapy is based on test values that are assumed to have been collected at the right time and in the proper manner.

DELTA CHECKS

Delta checks help assure quality in testing. A **delta check** compares current results of a lab test with previous results for the same test on the same patient. Although some variation is to be expected, a major difference in results could indicate error and requires investigation.

Documentation

Documentation is a major component of a QA program. Different types of QA documents have been developed to standardize procedures, inform nursing personnel of the importance of patient preparation, and record problems. Documentation can be used for legal purposes as well. The majority of records kept in the process of providing healthcare can provide information for QA purposes. Easily the most important of these is the patient's medical record.

Medical Record

The medical record is a chronologic documentation of a patient's care. The law requires that medical records be kept on hospital patients but does not require physicians in their private practice to keep records on their patients, although most do in the form of a clinical record. Every notation in the patient's medical or clinical record should be legible, precise, and complete. The basic reasons for maintaining accurate, up-to-date medical records are as follows:

1. To provide an aid to practicing medicine. Through the use of a medical record, the physician can document treatment and give a written plan for continuation of the patient's care plan
2. To provide an aid to communications between the physician and others involved with the patient's care. It can also serve as a communications tool between past, present, and future physicians that care for the patient
3. To serve as a legal document that may be used in a court of law. It must be a factual, legible, and objective account of the patient, past and present
4. To serve as a very valuable tool for assisting the hospital in total quality management through utilization review because the medical records include such information as a history of examinations, laboratory, and other medical testing reports, prescriptions written, and supplies used

For confidentiality reasons, access to a patient's medical record is restricted to those who have a verifiable need to review the information.

The User Manual

The user manual (Fig. 2-3) is an example of a QA document found in the nursing units. It typically contains in chart form the type and minimum amount of specimen required, special handling desired, reference values for the test, the days testing is available, and the normal turnaround time (TAT). Refer to the Patient Preparation Procedures section discussed previously in this chapter for more information on the user manual.

Procedure Manual

A complete **procedure manual** must be made available to all employees of the laboratory for standardization purposes. Accrediting agencies such as CAP require that this manual be updated annually and that it be written in the NCCLS format. A procedure manual states the laboratory policy and procedures that apply to each test or practice performed in the lab. Box 2-1 lists typical information found in a procedure manual.

Box 2-1

INFORMATION FOUND IN PROCEDURE MANUAL

- Purpose of the procedure
- Specimen type and collection method
- Equipment and supplies required
- Detailed step-by-step procedure
- Limitations and variables of the method
- Corrective actions
- Method validation
- Normal values and references

The manual will also include updates to procedures and notification of these changes to the nursing staff (Fig. 2-5). The procedure manual is a QA document that shows the intent of the lab to adhere to the national standards of good practice.

QA Forms

Accreditation standards for agencies such as JCAHO require the facility to show documentation on all quality control checks and other QA activities. QA forms include equipment check forms and incident/occurrence report forms.

EQUIPMENT CHECK FORMS

Special forms for recording equipment checks on tube additives, vacuum strength, and expiration dates are available for verification of new lot numbers. Refrigerator temperatures, which must be recorded daily, are often the responsibility of the phlebotomist. Control checks on the centrifuge require periodic documentation of the tachometer readings and maintenance performed.

INTERNAL REPORTS

Confidential incident/occurrence reports must be filled out when a problem occurs. These forms identify the problem, state the consequence, and describe the corrective action (Fig. 2-6). Incident reports are not limited to situations in which an injury occurred. For example, an incident form would be filled out when a tube of blood was mislabeled. Incident reports should state facts and not feelings. It is not the function of an incident report to place blame, but only to identify what took place and the corrective action taken so that such an event does not happen again.

text continues on page 58

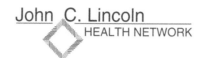

John C. Lincoln
HEALTH NETWORK

North Mountain Clinical Laboratory – C.D. Lambe, M.D., Medical Director

MEMO

Date: October 16, 2001

To: Physicians, Ordering Units, Unit Directors

From: Clinical Laboratory, Chemistry Department

Re: **Compliance Form for Sendout Tests to Reference Laboratories**

Effective immediately, Miscellaneous Laboratory tests not performed at JCLH-NM (Send Out tests) **may** require a completed Compliance Form prior to the sending of the procedure to the Reference Lab. The form requires diagnosis and ordering physician signature.

The laboratory will send the Compliance Form to the ordering unit (via tube system) or Physicians office (for outpatient orders only) when it is required. The completed form must be returned to the lab prior to processing of the order.

Situations in which this form **may** be required include:

1. Specimen and pricing are not available and Laboratory needs to research for information in order for specimen to be processed.
2. Test not performed by JCLH-NM Reference Lab (Quest) and will be sent elsewhere.
3. Test price exceeds $100.00
4. Pathologist Request

Thank you for your cooperation
Please contact Caren Creutzberger MT Laboratory Supervisor or Debbie Sazdoff CIS Systems Manager at Extension 1237 if you have any questions.

■ FIGURE 2-5 ■

Procedure manual update.

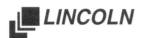 **LINCOLN**

EMPLOYEE ACTION RECORD

_____   _____   _____
     EMPLOYEE NAME   DEPARTMENT   DATE

This form is used to document discussion concerning a commendation or action taken to improve inappropriate performance by an employee. The information contained on this form will be included in the employee's personnel file.

( ) Commendation   ( ) Corrective Action   ( ) Other

I.   Describe issue or incident (provide dates and details):

_____
_____
_____
_____
_____

II.   Provide specific information discussed with the employee regarding Section I:

_____
_____
_____
_____
_____

III.   Provide the agreed-upon plan for taking corrective action, if applicable (include the date for follow-up and next action to be taken, if necessary):

_____
_____
_____
_____
_____

IV.   Employee comments:

_____
_____
_____
_____
_____

(Attach additional sheets if necessary)

_____ _____   _____ _____
DEPARTMENT MANAGER   DATE   EMPLOYEE (SIGNATURE DOES NOT   DATE
                                            NECESSARILY INDICATE AGREEMENT.)

_____ _____
VICE PRESIDENT   DATE

WHITE COPY: HUMAN RESOURCES   YELLOW COPY: DIRECTOR   PINK COPY: EMPLOYEE

JCL: 04/91 M-115

■ FIGURE 2-6 ■

Incident report. (Courtesy of John C. Lincoln Hospital, Phoenix, AZ.)

LEGAL ISSUES

Because of consumer awareness, lawsuits have increased in all areas of society. This is especially true in the healthcare industry, in which physicians and providers were once considered above reproach. As healthcare providers go about their daily activities, there are many practices that, if performed without reasonable care and skill, could result in a lawsuit. It has been proven in lawsuits that people performing phlebotomy can and will be held legally accountable for their actions.

Divisions of the Law

The legal system in the United States encompasses two areas of law: criminal and civil. Criminal cases involve crimes against the state, whereas civil cases involve crimes against a person.

 Key Point ➤ The same act may lead to both criminal and civil actions. For example, in assault and battery cases a guilty defendant can face imprisonment by the state, and also face civil action in which the injured party tries to collect monetary damages.

Criminal Law

Criminal law is concerned with laws that are designed to protect all members of society from injurious acts by others. Criminal acts are either felonies or misdemeanors. A felony is a crime punishable by death or imprisonment. The more serious crimes such as murder, assault, and rape are felonies. Misdemeanors are considered lesser offenses and usually carry a penalty of a fine or less than 1 year in jail.

Civil Law

Civil law is concerned with actions between two private parties, such as individuals, corporations, or organizations. They constitute the bulk of the legal actions dealt with in the medical office or other healthcare facilities. The most common civil actions in healthcare are based on **tort.**

TORT

A **tort** is a civil wrong, other than breach of contract, committed against a person or property for which damages may be awarded in a court of law. It is an act that is committed without just cause. The act may be intentional (willful) or unintentional (accidental). Examples of tort actions are as follows.

Assault

Assault is defined as the act (threat) of intentionally causing another to be in apprehension (fear) of immediate harm to his or her person (battery). Battery does not necessarily have to follow an assault for the assault to be a tort. To be called assault, the person that is committing the act must have the ability to carry out the threat or the person being assaulted must believe the ability is there.

Battery

Battery is the intentional harmful or offensive touching of another person without consent or legal justification. Legal justification would be, for example, when a mother gives permission to have her child examined or have blood drawn from the child. Intentional harm may range from permanent disfigurement to merely removing a person's hat without permission or grabbing something out of another person's hand.

 Key Point ➤ A phlebotomist who attempts to collect a blood specimen without the patient's consent can be charged with assault and battery.

Fraud

Fraud is a type of deceitful practice or willful plan resorted to to produce unlawful gain. An example includes billing for services that have not been provided.

Invasion of privacy

Invasion of privacy is the violation of one's right to be left alone. An individual's right to expect privacy while undergoing medical care must be respected by healthcare providers. Invasion of privacy can involve physical intrusion or the unauthorized publishing or releasing of private information. The latter of these can also be considered breach of confidentiality.

 Key Point ➤ In the medical field, invasion of privacy by physical intrusion may be no more than walking through a closed door into a patient's room without asking the patient for permission.

Breach of confidentiality

Breach of Confidentiality is failure to keep medical information confidential. Unauthorized release of laboratory results may cause great embarrassment to a patient or even greater consequences, such as loss of his or her job. Aside from being illegal, breaching confidentiality is unethical.

Negligence

Negligence involves doing something that a *reasonable* person would not do or not doing something that a *reasonable* person would do. In the majority of cases a person does not deliberately try to inflict harm on another person. If a medical procedure results in injury and there is no intent to injure, it is called negligence, and the injured person has the right to sue for damages. To claim negligence the following must be present:

- A legal duty or obligation owed by one person to another
- A breaking or breach of duty
- Harm done as a direct result of the action

Malpractice

Malpractice is defined as a type of negligence committed by a professional. The training and experience of the individual committing the act is taken into consideration, when deciding whether an act resulting in injury should be labeled negligence or malpractice. Malpractice is a term associated with any professional misconduct. A claim of malpractice implies that a greater standard of care was owed to the injured person than the reasonable person standard associated with negligence.

STANDARD OF CARE

Healthcare personnel have a duty to protect their clients from harm. This duty is established by standards of the profession and the expectations of society, and is termed **the standard of care.** This implies that all healthcare personnel perform their duties in the same fashion that any other reasonable and prudent person with the same experience and training would. Employers of healthcare personnel are ultimately liable for providing employees who possess the qualifications and training necessary to meet the standard of care.

RESPONDEAT SUPERIOR

An employer must conform to a specific standard of care to protect patients and must answer for damages an employee commits within the scope of employment. **Respondeat superior** is a Latin phrase that means "let the master respond." It is another way of saying that employers are liable for the actions of employees, even though the employee is the one at fault. This tort may be filed if a neglectful or intentional act of an employee results in some type of physical injury to a client. The key points in a claim of respondeat superior are that the employee is working within the scope of employment and has had the proper training to perform the required duties. An adult employee who is doing something that is outside of his or her scope of duties or training may be held solely responsible for that action because adults are legally responsible for their own acts.

VICARIOUS LIABILITY

In today's healthcare facilities, consultants and independent contractors perform some of the services once considered the responsibilities of the employees of the particular facility. Should injury occur as a result of a negligent act committed by an independent contractor, the healthcare facility that hired the person is liable. This is called **vicarious liability** and is based on the fact that the contractor is acting on behalf of the facility by virtue of the facility's allowing the contractor to practice within the confines of the facility or under the auspices of that particular healthcare organization. The hospital, as the employer, would be deceiving the public if it were to escape liability for a patient's injury by simply subcontracting out various services to other people and claiming it is not responsible because the party that caused the injury is not on its payroll.

MALPRACTICE INSURANCE

As a rule, individual healthcare personnel have not been targets for lawsuits because of respondeat superior or vicarious liability, which both involve the "deep pockets" theory (i.e., let the one with the most money pay.) Personnel can, however, be named as codefendants, in which case, the employer's malpractice insurance may not cover them. It is important for each individual to examine the possibility of a civil suit being brought against him or her, and consider carrying malpractice insurance.

The decision to purchase liability or malpractice insurance should be based on financial considerations and legal ones. From the legal point of view, it may be desirable to be covered by a separate professional liability policy because the employer may give his insurer the right to recover damages from an employee who is found to be negligent. Healthcare personnel may be able to purchase liability insurance from their professional organizations.

STATUTE OF LIMITATIONS

All malpractice actions have a limited amount of time after the alleged injury in which the injured person is permitted to file a lawsuit. The **statute of limitations** establishes the particular number of years within which one person can sue another. The time limit is specified in each state's medical malpractice law. The question for all parties involved is when the clock starts. Some of the most common occurrences given for when statute of limitations period begins are as follows.

- On the day the alleged negligent act was committed
- When the injury resulting from the alleged negligence was actually discovered, or should have been discovered, by a reasonably alert patient
- The day the physician–patient relationship ended, or the day of the last medical treatment in a series
- In the case of minors the statute may not begin to run until the minor reaches the age of majority

AVOIDING LAWSUITS

The best insurance against lawsuits is to take steps to avoid them. A good way to avoid lawsuits is to consistently apply the guidelines listed in Box 2-2.

Box 2-2

GUIDELINES TO AVOID LAWSUITS

- Acquire informed consent before collection of specimens.
- Respect a patient's right to confidentiality.
- Strictly adhere to accepted procedures and practices.

continued

- Use proper safety containers and devices.
- Listen and respond appropriately to the patient's requests.
- Accurately and legibly record all information concerning patients.
- Document incidents or occurrences.
- Participate in continuing education to maintain proficiency.
- Perform at the prevailing standard of care.
- Never perform procedures that you are not trained to do.

Patient Consent

Informed Consent

Informed consent implies voluntary and competent permission for a medical procedure, test, or medication and requires that a patient be given adequate information regarding the method, risks, and consequences involved before consenting to it. It is mandatory for the healthcare provider to explain the procedure and obtain the patient's permission or consent before initiating any medical procedure. Information must be given to the patient in non–technical terms and in his or her own language, if possible, meaning an interpreter may be necessary. Blood collection on minors requires consent of their parents or legal guardians.

Expressed Consent

Expressed consent may be given verbally or in writing. Expressed consent is necessary for proposed treatment that involves surgery, experimental drugs, or high-risk procedures. Written consent gives the best possible protection for both the person providing the treatment and the one receiving the treatment. Written consent must be signed by the person providing the treatment and the patient and should be witnessed by a third party. If consent is given verbally, the provider giving the treatment should make an entry in the patient's chart covering what was discussed with the patient. The consent should cover what procedures are going to be performed and should not be in a general form that allows the physician carte blanche to do whatever he or she wants to do. If such a general consent goes to court, the court generally takes the word of the patient as to what he or she understood was to take place.

Implied Consent

With **implied consent,** the patient need not make a verbal expression of consent. In the case of drawing blood from a patient, all that is needed is for the phlebotomist to explain what he or she is going to do. If after the explanation is given, the patient holds out an arm, that alone is consent. Implied consent may be necessary in emergency procedures such as cardiopulmonary resuscitation to save a person's life. Healthcare providers need to be aware that laws involving implied consent are enacted at the state level and may differ greatly from one state to another.

HIV Consent

Legislation governing informed consent for HIV testing has been enacted in most states. The laws specify exactly what type of information must be given to inform the client properly. Generally speaking, the client must be advised on (1) the test and its purpose, (2) how the test might be used, and (3) the meaning of the test and its limitations.

Consent for Minors

A minor is anyone who has not reached the age of majority. The age of majority is determined by state law and may be either 18 or 21 years of age. The general rule concerning the treatment of minors is that a minor cannot give consent for the administration of medical treatment; parental or guardian consent is required. Healthcare personnel who violate this rule are liable for assault and battery.

Refusal of Consent

An individual has a constitutional right to refuse a medical procedure such as venipuncture. The refusal may be based on religious or personal beliefs and preferences. A patient who refuses medical treatment is normally required to verify the refusal in writing on a special form.

The Litigation Process

Litigation is the process used to settle legal disputes. Approximately 10% of malpractice lawsuits actually go to court. The rest are settled out of court, which can happen any time before the final court decision. Malpractice litigation involves the following four phases:

- Phase one begins when an alleged patient incident occurs or the patient becomes aware of a prior possible injury.
- Phase two begins when the injured party or a family member consults an attorney. The attorney requests, obtains, and reviews copies of the medical records involved, and decides whether to take the case. If the attorney thinks that malpractice has occurred and takes the case, an attempt to negotiate a settlement is made. If not resolved by negotiation, a complaint is filed by the patient's attorney. After a complaint is filed, the injured party becomes the **plaintiff** and the person against whom the complaint is filed becomes the **defendant.** Both sides now conduct formal **discovery,** which involves taking depositions and interrogating parties involved. Giving a **deposition** is a process in which one party questions another under oath, whereas a court reporter records every word. The plaintiff, the defendant, and expert witnesses for both sides may give depositions. Expert witnesses are people who are asked to review medical records and give their opinion of whether or not the standard of care was met. A person who lies under oath while giving a deposition can be charged with perjury.

- Phase three is the trial phase, which is the process designed to settle a dispute before a judge and jury. Both sides present their versions of the facts and the jury determines which version appears to be correct. If the jury decides in the plaintiff's favor, damages may be awarded. At this point the lawsuit may proceed to phase four.
- Phase four begins with an appeal of the jury decision. Although either side has the right to an appeal, the losing party is usually the one to choose this option.

Risk Management

Risk is defined as "the chance of loss or injury" and is inherent in the healthcare environment. **Risk management** is an internal process focused on identifying and minimizing situations that pose risks to patients and employees. Risk is managed in two ways: controlling risk to avoid incidents and paying for occurrences after they have happened. Careful planning, in the form of objectives, will reduce risks and benefit the employee as well as the patient. Generic steps in risk management involve identification of the risk, treatment of the risk using policies and procedures already in place, education of employees and patients, and evaluation of what should be done in the future.

Risk factors can sometimes be identified by looking for trends in reporting tools such as incident or occurrence reports (Fig. 2-6). Proper investigation can be made if a situation is identified that deviates from the normal. As in any QI program, the objective is to reduce unfavorable outcomes continuously. As new procedures are instituted to reduce risk, employees must be informed immediately and instructed on what to do. Throughout the operation of a risk management program, evaluation of occurrences, trends, and outcomes is essential so that appropriate changes can be made.

Patient Safety and Sentinel Events

JCAHO is committed to improving safety for patients and residents in healthcare organizations. One of the ways this is demonstrated is through its sentinel event policy. The intent of this policy is to help healthcare organizations identify sentinel events and take steps to prevent them from happening again. A sentinel event is one that signals the need for immediate investigation and response and includes any unfavorable event that is unexpected and results in death or serious physical or psychologic injury, or any deviation from practice that increases the chance of adverse outcome should it reoccur. Loss of limb or its function is specifically included as a sentinel event. According to the policy, if a signal event occurs the healthcare organization is required to:

- Perform a thorough and credible analysis of the root cause
- Put improvements to reduce risk into practice
- Monitor improvements to determine if they are effective

Legal Cases Involving Phlebotomy Procedures

A Negligence Case Settled Through Binding Arbitration

A patient had a blood specimen collected at a physician's office. Blood had been collected from him at the same office on several prior occasions with no problem. The blood drawer, who was new to the patient and seemed to be in a hurry, inserted the needle deeper into the arm and at a much steeper angle than the patient was used to. She redirected the needle several times before hitting the vein. A hematoma began to form. Meanwhile the patient told the blood drawer that he felt great pain, but she told him it would be over soon and continued the draw. The pain continued after the draw and the patient's arm later became bruised and swollen. The patient suffered permanent nerve injury from compression of the nerve by the hematoma.

Jones Versus Rapides General Hospital

The plaintiff went to the hospital emergency room complaining of severe abdominal pain and headaches. The medical technician who drew a blood specimen had difficulty locating the vein and stuck the patient twice with the same needle before completing the draw. The patient was subsequently released, but returned to the hospital the next day complaining of pain and swelling in her forearm. A diagnosis was made of gas gangrene.

Key Point ➤ Gangrene is death of tissue resulting from deficient or absent blood supply. Gas gangrene is gangrene in a wound caused by infection with a microorganism such as *Clostridium perfringens*.

Congelton Versus Baton Rouge General Hospital

The plaintiff went to donate blood at a hospital. She complained of pain during the procedure and the technician repositioned the needle two times. The technician offered to remove the needle but the plaintiff chose to complete the procedure. After completing the donation she complained of numbness in her arm. Later evaluation by a neurologist indicated injury to the antebrachial cutaneous nerve.

Montgomery Versus Opelousas General Hospital

A patient had blood drawn for laboratory tests after gallbladder surgery. The venipuncture was painful despite the fact that the patient was under sedation from morphine. The technologist discontinued the venipuncture and performed a second one successfully. The patient continued to have pain after release from the hospital and subsequently sued for medical expenses, general damage, and loss of consortium.

Martin Versus Wentworth-Douglass Hospital

A phlebotomist performed venipuncture on a patient, during which the patient suffered an injury to the lateral antebrachial cutaneous nerve. The hospital was sued by the patient for failure to train the phlebotomist, failure to provide an appropriate chair, and for failure of the phlebotomist to exercise due care in performing the procedure.

STUDY & REVIEW QUESTIONS

1. QA programs are necessary
   a. because they are mandated by a regulatory agency.
   b. to receive third party reimbursements.
   c. for careful monitoring of patient care.
   d. all of the above.

2. A QA program monitors
   a. indicators.
   b. outcomes.
   c. procedures.
   d. threshold values.

3. What book describes in detail the steps to follow for specimen collection?
   a. Policy manual.
   b. QC manual.
   c. Safety manual.
   d. User manual.

4. Necessary elements of risk management are all of the following *except*
   a. education.
   b. evaluation.
   c. identification.
   d. obligation.

5. Informed consent means
   a. a phlebotomist tells the patient what is ordered and the implications of the test results.
   b. a patient agrees to a procedure after being told of the consequences associated with it.
   c. a patient has the right to look at all of his or her medical records.
   d. a nurse has the right to perform a procedure on a patient even if the patient refuses.

6. Quality improvement methods advocated by Dr. W. Edwards Deming accomplish all of the following except:
   a. improve productivity.
   b. monitor safety.
   c. reduce waste.
   d. reduce costs.

7. A national organization that develops guidelines and sets standards for laboratory procedures.
   a. CAP
   b. JCAHO
   c. NAACLS
   d. NCCLS

8. JCAHO will monitor quality improvement measures
   a. through the use of daily patient census records.
   b. by reviewing attendance records of employees.
   c. by checking the timeliness of phlebotomy collections.
   d. all the above.

9. The physician employer of a phlebotomist who injures a patient during a blood draw is sued for negligence. This is an example of
   a. assault and battery.
   b. fraud.
   c. respondeat superior.
   d. vicarious liability.

Continued

STUDY & REVIEW QUESTIONS *(CONTINUED)*

10. A young adult comes to an outpatient lab to have his blood drawn. What should the phlebotomist know before drawing this patient?
    a. Age of majority in the state
    b. Date of birth of the patient
    c. Name of the patient
    d. All of the above

■ CASE STUDY

A newly trained phlebotomist is sent to collect a blood specimen from a patient. The phlebotomist is an employee of a laboratory that contracts with the hospital to perform laboratory services, including specimen collection. The phlebotomist collects the specimen with no problems. Before the phlebotomist has a chance to leave the room, the patient asks for help to get to the bathroom. The patient is a very large woman, but the phlebotomist lends an arm to help her. On the way to the bathroom, the patient slips on some liquid on the floor. The phlebotomist tries but is unable to prevent her from falling. The patient fractures her arm in the fall.

QUESTIONS:

1. Was it wrong of the phlebotomist to try to help the patient? Explain why or why not.
2. Is the hospital liable for the patient's injury? Explain why or why not.
3. Can the phlebotomist be held liable for the patient's injuries? Explain why or why not.

Bibliography and Suggested Readings

British Deming Association. (1992). *A perspective on Dr. Deming's theory of profound knowledge* (booklet no. W1). Knoxville, TN: SPC Press.

Cowdrey, M. D., & Drew, D. (1995). *Basic law for the allied health professions* (2nd ed.). Boston: Jones and Bartlett Publishers.

Flight, M. (1998). *Law, liability, and ethics for medical office personnel* (3rd ed.). New York: Delmar Publishers.

Joint Commission on the Accreditation of Healthcare Organizations (JCAHO). (1996). *1996 Accreditation manual for hospitals.* Oakbrook Terrace, IL: JCAHO.

Judson, K., & Blesie, S. (1996). *Law and ethics for health occupations.* New York: Glencoe/McGraw-Hill.

Lipman, M. (1994). *Medical law and ethics.* Upper Saddle River, New Jersey, Prentice Hall.

Oran, D. (1991). *Dictionary of law.* Los Angeles: West Publishing.

Reitzel, J. D., Lyden, D. P., Roberts, N. J., & Severance, G. B. (1990). *Contemporary business law: Principles and cases* (4th ed.). New York: McGraw-Hill.

Veatch, R., & Flack, H., (1997). *Case studies in allied health ethics.* Upper Saddle River, New Jersey, Prentice Hall.

3

INFECTION CONTROL, SAFETY, FIRST AID, AND PERSONAL WELLNESS

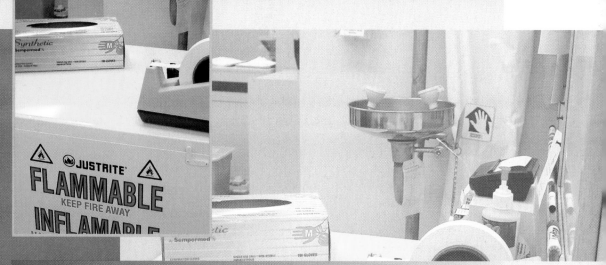

Upon successful completion of this chapter, the reader will be able to:

1 Define the key terms and abbreviations listed at the beginning of this chapter.

2 Identify the components of the chain of infection and give examples of each, describe infection control procedures used to break the chain, and identify four functions of infection control programs.

3 Describe proper procedures for handwashing, putting on and removing protective clothing, and entering the nursery or neonatal intensive care unit.

4 Describe standard and transmission-based precautions and identify the organizations that developed them.

5 State safety rules to follow when working in the laboratory or in patient areas.

6 List examples of bloodborne pathogens and describe their means of transmission in a healthcare setting.

7 Discuss the major points of the Bloodborne Pathogens Standard, including changes required by the Needlestick Safety and Prevention Act.

8 Describe hazards, identify warning symbols, list actions to take if incidents occur, and specify rules to follow for proper biologic, electrical, fire, radiation, and chemical safety.

9 Identify symptoms of shock, state first aid procedures for treating external hemorrhage, and shock, identify the main points of the international cardiopulmonary resuscitation and emergency cardiovascular care guidelines, and identify the links in the *American Heart Association Chain of Survival.*

10 Describe the role of personal hygiene, proper nutrition, rest, exercise, back protection, and stress management in personal wellness.

INFECTION CONTROL

Throughout history man has faced the spread of infection, pondering its causes and how to treat it or prevent it. Infections have been known to affect major segments of the population, as did the plague in the Middle Ages. Although important advances have been made in understanding and treating infection, the threat of infection looms as large as it ever has. Newer enemies in the battle of infection emerge such as HIV and hepatitis C virus (HCV). Once-conquered enemies become resistant to treatment, as in the case of *Mycobacterium tuberculosis* and methicillin-resistant *Staphylococcus aureus.* Healthcare personnel typically encounter numerous patients on a daily basis, many of whom may be harboring these or other agents of infection. Measures to prevent the spread of infection must be taken in the course of treating all patients. This chapter explains the infection process and describes infection control measures needed to protect healthcare patients, staff, visitors, and those who do business with healthcare facilities.

Infection

Our environment is full of microorganisms (microscopic organisms) referred to as **microbes.** Microbes include bacteria, fungi, protozoa, and viruses. The majority of microbes are **nonpathogenic,** meaning they do not cause disease under normal conditions. Microbes that are capable of causing disease (i.e., **pathogenic**) are called **pathogens.** If a pathogen invades the body and the conditions are favorable for it to multiply and cause injurious effects or disease, the resulting condition is called an **infection.** The pathogen responsible for causing the infection is referred to as the **infectious** or **causative agent.** Infection can be **local** (restricted to a small area of the body) or **systemic** (sis-tem′ik), in which the entire body is affected.

Communicable Infections

Some pathogenic microbes cause infections that can be spread from person to person. These infections are called **communicable infections** and the diseases that result are called **communicable diseases.** A division of the U.S. Public Health Service called the **Centers for Disease Control and Prevention (CDC)** is charged with the investigation and control of various diseases, especially those that are communicable and have epidemic potential. The CDC recommends safety precautions to protect healthcare workers and others from infection.

Nosocomial Infections

Approximately 5% of patients in the United States are exposed to and contract some sort of infection after admission to a hospital or other healthcare facility. These hospital or healthcare facility–acquired infections are called **nosocomial infections.** Nosocomial infections can result from contact with infected personnel, other patients, and visitors, or contaminated equipment. The most common nosocomial infection in the United States is urinary tract infection. The **Hospital Infection Control Practices Advisory Committee (HICPAC),** established in 1991, advises the CDC on updating guidelines regarding prevention of nosocomial infection.

The Chain of Infection

Infection transmission requires the presence of three main components, which make up what is referred to as the **chain of infection** (Fig. 3-1). This chain must be complete for an infection to occur. Components, or "links" in the chain of infection, are a **source** of pathogenic or infectious microbes, a **means of transmission** for the microbe, and a **susceptible host.** If the process of infection is stopped at any component or link in the chain, an infection is prevented. If a pathogen successfully enters a susceptible host the chain is completed, the host becomes a new source of infectious microorganisms and the process of infection continues.

 Key Point ➤ A phlebotomist, whose duties require coming in contact with many patients, must be fully aware of the infection process and take precautions to prevent the spread of infection.

Components of the Chain of Infection

SOURCE

The source is the origin of infectious microorganisms, also called the reservoir. Sources of infectious microbes include infected humans or animals and contaminated articles and equipment. In a healthcare setting, human sources of infectious microbes

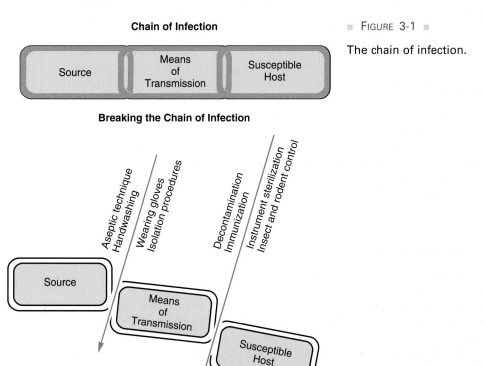

Chain of Infection

Source | Means of Transmission | Susceptible Host

Breaking the Chain of Infection

Aseptic technique
Handwashing
Wearing gloves
Isolation procedures
Decontamination
Immunization
Instrument sterilization
Insect and rodent control

Source

Means of Transmission

Susceptible Host

FIGURE 3-1

The chain of infection.

can be patients, personnel, or visitors, and can include those with active disease, those whose disease is in the incubation period, and those who are chronic carriers of a disease. Another potential source of infectious microbes is a person's own normal flora (microorganisms that normally live on the skin and other areas of the human body).

Inanimate objects such as contaminated equipment can be a major source of infection in a healthcare setting. Whether or not an inanimate source is capable of transmitting infection depends upon the amount of contamination, the **viability** or ability of the organism to survive on the source, the **virulence** or degree to which an organism is capable of causing disease, and the amount of time elapsed between when the source was contaminated and when it was contacted.

For example, the virus that causes hepatitis B is much more virulent, or capable of causing disease from a small amount of infective material, than HIV, the virus that causes AIDS. It is also more viable, meaning it is capable of surviving longer on surfaces than is HIV. However, if a long enough time elapses from the time of contamination until contact by a susceptible host, the microbe is no longer alive and is not capable of transmitting disease.

MODES OF TRANSMISSION

There are five basic modes or routes of infection transmission: **contact, droplet, airborne, vehicle,** and **vector.** The same microbe can be transmitted by more than one route.

Contact transmission

Contact transmission is the most frequent mode of infection transmission. There are two types of contact transmission, **direct transmission** and **indirect transmission.**

Direct contact transmission involves direct, physical transfer of a pathogenic microbe to a susceptible host through close or intimate contact such as touching or kissing.

Indirect contact transmission involves personal contact by a susceptible host with contaminated inanimate objects such as patient bed linens, clothing, dressings, and eating utensils. It includes contact with phlebotomy equipment such as gloves, needles, specimen tubes, and phlebotomy carts and trays. It also includes less obvious contaminated objects such as doorknobs and faucet handles. The transfer of infectious microbes from contaminated hands to a susceptible host is also considered indirect contact transmission.

 Key Point ➤ Inanimate objects or substances that are capable of harboring infectious material and transmitting infection are called **fomites** (fo'mi-tez). Fomites in the laboratory include computer terminals, countertops, pens or pencils, and telephones.

Droplet transmission

Droplet transmission involves the transfer of the infective microbe to the mucous membranes of the nose or mouth or the conjunctiva (mucous membranes) of the eyes of a susceptible individual through sneezing, coughing, or talking by an infected person. Droplet transmission can also occur during procedures such as suctioning and throat swab collection. It differs from airborne transmission in that droplets do not travel more than 3 feet, and do not remain suspended in air.

Airborne transmission

Airborne transmission involves dissemination of droplet nuclei. Droplet nuclei are the residue of evaporated droplets generated by sneezing, coughing, or talking. Infectious microbes within droplet nuclei can remain viable even though suspended in the air or in dust particles for long periods. Microbes carried in this manner can become widely dispersed before being inhaled by or deposited on a susceptible host. For this reason, special air handling and ventilation are required for rooms of patients having infections with airborne transmission. Persons entering the room must wear a snug-fitting mask with a special filter. *M. tuberculosis,* rubeola virus, and varicella virus are the most common microorganisms transmitted by the airborne route.

Vector transmission

Vector transmission involves the transfer of the microbe by an insect, arthropod, or animal. An example of vector transmission is the transmission of malaria by a mosquito or the plague by rodent fleas.

Vehicle transmission

Vehicle transmission involves the transmission of the infective microbe through contaminated food, water, or drugs. Examples of vehicle transmission are salmonella infection from handling contaminated chicken and shigella infection from drinking contaminated water. The transmission of hepatitis and HIV through blood transfusion is also considered vehicle transmission.

SUSCEPTIBLE HOST

A **susceptible host** is someone who has decreased ability to resist infection. Susceptibility is affected by age, health, and the immune status of the individual. For example, newborns whose immune systems are not yet developed and old people whose immune systems are no longer functioning properly are more susceptible to infections. In addition, disease, antibiotic treatment, and immunosuppressive drugs may compromise a person's resistance to infection. Procedures such as surgery, anesthesia, and insertion of catheters can also leave a patient more susceptible to infection. Recovery from a particular virus or vaccination against a virus also affects susceptibility. A healthy person who has received a vaccination against a disease-causing virus, or who has recovered from infection with a particular virus, has developed antibodies against that virus and is considered to be **immune,** or unlikely to develop the disease.

 Key Point ➤ Healthcare workers who are exposed to the hepatitis B virus (HBV) are unlikely to contract the disease if they have previously completed their HBV vaccination series.

Breaking the Chain of Infection

Breaking the chain of infection means stopping infections at the source, eliminating means of transmission, and reducing or eliminating the susceptibility of potential hosts. Ways to prevent transmission of infectious microbes are proper hand washing; use of gloves, gowns, masks, and other protective equipment when indicated; proper waste disposal; isolation procedures; insect and rodent control; and decontamination of surfaces and instruments. Susceptibility of potential hosts can be reduced through proper nutrition, reduction of stress, and immunization against common pathogens.

Infection Control Programs

Every healthcare institution is required by the Joint Commission on the Accreditation of Healthcare Organizations to have an infection control program responsible for implementing procedures designed to break the chain of infection. Such procedures are aimed at protecting not only patients, but also employees, visitors, and others. An infection control program is also responsible for monitoring and collecting data on all infections occurring within the healthcare institution and instituting special precautions in the event of outbreaks of particular infections.

Employee Screening and Immunization

One way infection control programs help prevent infections is through employee health programs that screen employees for infectious diseases before or upon employment and on a regular basis throughout employment. Screening commonly includes tuberculosis (TB) testing, also called PPD (purified protein derivative) testing. Employees with positive TB tests receive chest x-ray evaluations to determine their TB status. Screening may also include RPR (rapid plasma reagin) testing for syphilis and screening for diarrheal and skin diseases. In addition, most healthcare employers require employees to have current HBV, MMR (measles, mumps, rubella), diphtheria, and tetanus vaccinations. Most employers provide vaccinations free of charge. Employers are required to offer HBV vaccine free of charge to employees whose duties involve risk of exposure. Employees with certain conditions or infections may be subject to work restrictions. Conditions requiring work restrictions are listed in Appendix F.

Evaluation and Treatment

Infection control programs also provide evaluation and treatment for employees who are exposed to infections on the job. This includes Occupational Safety and Health Administration (OSHA)–mandated confidential medical evaluation, treatment, counseling, and follow-up as a result of exposure to bloodborne pathogens (see Safety).

Surveillance

Surveillance or monitoring is a major function of an infection control program. This involves monitoring patients and employees at risk of acquiring infections, as well as collecting and evaluating data on infections in patients and employees. Infection control measures are updated, and new policies are instituted based on this information.

Infection Control Methods

Hand Washing

Hand washing is the most important means of preventing the spread of infection, provided it is done properly and when required. There are different methods of hand washing, depending on the degree of contamination and the level of antimicrobial activity required. A routine hand wash procedure uses plain soap to mechanically remove soil and transient bacteria. Hand antisepsis requires the use of an antimicrobial soap to remove, kill, or inhibit transient microorganisms. A 2–minute surgical hand scrub uses an antimicrobial soap or equivalent to remove or destroy transient microorganisms and reduce levels of normal flora before surgical procedures. It is important that all healthcare personnel learn proper hand wash procedure and how to recognize situations when it should be performed. Box 3-1 lists situations when hand washing is required. Procedure Box 3-1 describes proper routine hand wash procedure.

Box 3-1

SITUATIONS THAT REQUIRE HAND WASHING

- Before and after each patient contact.
- Between different procedures on the same patient.
- Before putting on gloves and after taking them off.
- Before leaving the laboratory.
- Before going to lunch or break.
- Before and after going to the restroom.
- Whenever hands become visibly or knowingly contaminated.

PROCEDURES BOX 3-1

ROUTINE HAND WASH PROCEDURE

1. Remove rings and watch.
2. Stand back so that you do not touch the sink.
3. Turn on faucet with a clean paper towel.
4. Wet hands under warm, running water.
5. Apply soap and work up a lather.

---

continued

continued

6. Rub your hands together to create friction (friction loosens dead skin, dirt, and other debris).
7. Scrub everywhere, including between the fingers and around the knuckles.
8. Remove debris under fingernails with an orange stick or similar device. (Steps 4-8 should take at least 15 seconds.)
9. Rinse your hands in a downward motion from wrists to fingertips.
10. If hands are grossly contaminated, repeat steps 4 through 9.
11. Dry hands with a clean paper towel.
12. Turn faucet off with another clean paper towel.

Protective Attire

Protective clothing and other attire provide a barrier against infection. Used properly, it protects those wearing it. Disposed of properly, it prevents spread of infection to others. Protective clothing and other items worn by an individual are called **PPE,** which stands for **personal protective equipment.** PPE includes the following.

MASKS, GOGGLES, FACE SHIELDS, AND RESPIRATORS

A mask is worn to protect against droplets generated by coughing or sneezing. To put on a mask, place it over the nose and mouth. Adjust the metal band (if applicable) to fit snugly over the nose. For masks with ties, fasten the top ties around the upper portion of the head, then tie the lower ones at the back of the neck. If the mask has elastic fasteners, slip them around the ears.

A mask and goggles, or a face shield, are worn to protect the eyes, nose, and mouth from splashes or sprays of body fluids. If blood-drawing activities require goggles, they also require a mask. Some masks have plastic eye shields attached.

N95 (N category, 95% efficiency) respirators (Fig. 3-2) approved by the **National Institute for Occupational Safety and Health (NIOSH)** are required when entering rooms of patients with pulmonary tuberculosis and other diseases with airborne transmission. Respirators must fit snugly with no air leaks.

GOWNS

Clean, nonsterile, fluid-resistant gowns are worn by healthcare personnel to protect their skin and prevent soiling of their clothing during patient-care activities in which splashes or sprays of blood or body fluids are possible, or when entering isolation rooms (see Isolation Procedures in the following section). Sterile gowns are also worn to protect certain patients (e.g., newborns, patients with compromised immune systems) from contaminants on the healthcare worker's clothing. Most gowns are made

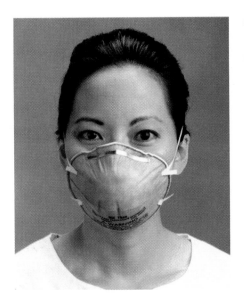

■ FIGURE 3-2 ■

N95 respirator.   (Courtesy 3M Occupational Health and Environmental Safety Division. St. Paul, MN.)

of disposable cloth or paper, are generous in size to adequately cover clothing, have long sleeves with knit cuffs, and fasten in the back.

Putting on/removing gowns

When putting on a gown, only inside surfaces of the gown should be touched. A properly worn gown has the sleeves pulled all the way to the wrist, the belt tied, and the gown overlapped, completely closed, and securely fastened. A gown is removed from the inside by sliding the arms out of the sleeves. The gown is then held away from the body and folded with the contaminated outside surface ending up inside.

LAB COATS

Lab coats, as with gowns, are worn to protect skin and prevent soiling of healthcare workers' clothing during patient-care activities in which splashes or sprays of blood or body fluids are possible. They are required attire for most phlebotomy situations. Lab coats used for specimen collection and handling are generally made of fluid resistant cotton or synthetic material, have long sleeves with knit cuffs, and come in both reusable and disposable styles.

GLOVES

Clean, nonsterile gloves are worn when collecting or handling blood and other body fluids, handling contaminated items, and when touching nonintact skin or mucous membranes. To provide adequate protection, gloves should be worn pulled over the cuffs of gowns or lab coats. The three main reasons for wearing gloves are as follows:

• To prevent contamination of the hands when handling blood or body fluids or when touching mucous membranes or nonintact skin.

- To reduce the chance of transmitting organisms on the hands of personnel to patients during invasive or other procedures that involve touching a patient's skin or mucous membranes.
- To minimize the possibility of transmitting infectious microorganisms from one patient to another.

Key Point ➤ Wearing gloves during most phlebotomy procedures is mandated by the OSHA Bloodborne Pathogens Standard.

Proper glove removal

After use, gloves should be removed promptly in an aseptic manner and discarded. To remove gloves properly (Fig. 3-3), grasp one glove at the wrist and pull it inside out and off of the hand, ending up with it in the palm of the still-gloved hand. Slip fingers of the ungloved hand under the second glove at the wrist and pull it off of the hand, ending with one glove inside the other with the contaminated surfaces inside. Hands should be washed immediately after glove removal and before going to another patient.

ORDER TO PUT ON AND REMOVE PROTECTIVE CLOTHING

When putting on complete protective clothing such as gown, mask, and gloves, the gown is put on first (Fig. 3-4A). The mask is put on next, making certain it covers the nose and mouth (Fig. 3-4B). Gloves are put on last and pulled over the cuffs of the gown (Fig. 3-4C).

Protective clothing is removed in the opposite order from which it was put on. It must be removed carefully in an aseptic manner to prevent contamination of the healthcare worker. Gloves are removed first, being careful not to touch contaminated surfaces with ungloved hands. The mask is removed next, touching only the strings. The gown is removed last. Hands must be washed promptly after removal of protective clothing.

Nursery and Neonatal Intensive Care Unit (ICU) Infection Control Technique

Newborns are more susceptible to infections than healthy older children and adults because their immune systems are not yet fully developed. For this reason, the phlebotomist as well as all other personnel who enter the nursery should use special infection control techniques. Most nurseries have a separate room just outside the nursery where hand washing, gowning, and so forth are performed before entering. Typical proper nursery infection control technique includes the following:

- Wash hands thoroughly with an antiseptic hand cleaner
- Put on clean gloves, gown, and mask
- Leave the blood collection tray in the washroom outside the nursery and take into the nursery only those items necessary to perform the specimen collection
- Remove gloves, wash hands, and put on new gloves after finishing with one patient and before going to the next

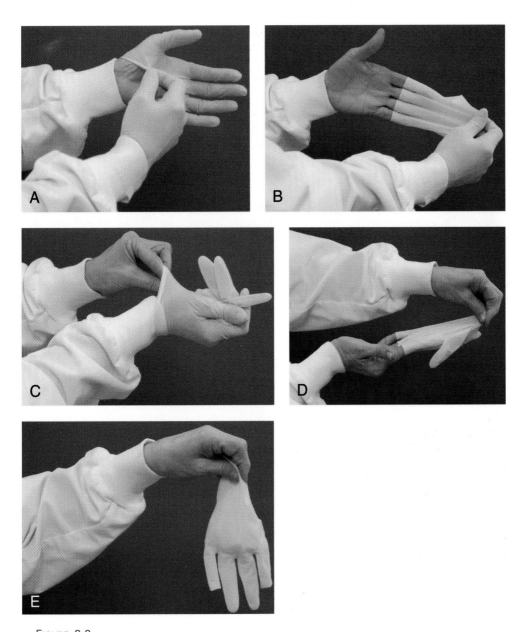

Glove removal. (*A*) The wrist of one glove is grasped with the opposite gloved hand. (*B*) The glove is pulled inside out over and off the hand. (*C*) With the first glove held in the gloved hand, the fingers of the nongloved hand are slipped under the wrist of the remaining glove without touching the exterior surfaces. (*D*) The glove is then pulled inside out over the hand so that the first glove ends up inside of the second glove; no exterior glove surfaces are exposed. (*E*) The contaminated gloves can then be dropped into the proper waste receptacle.

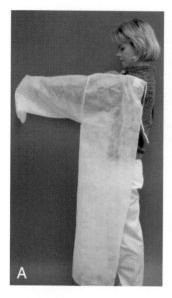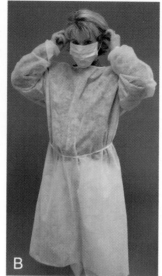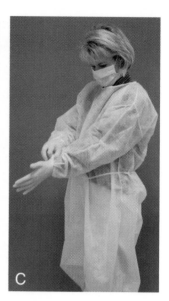

▪ FIGURE 3-4 ▪

Protective clothing. (*A*) Phlebotomist slips arms into a protective gown. (*B*) A mask is applied by slipping the elastic band over the ears. (*C*) Gloves are put on last and pulled over the gown cuffs.

Isolation Procedures

One way an infection control program minimizes spread of infection is through the establishment of **isolation procedures** designed to decrease the transmission of infectious microorganisms. Isolation procedures separate patients with certain transmissible infections or diseases from contact with other patients and limit their contact with hospital personnel and visitors. Isolating a patient requires a doctor's order and is implemented either to prevent the spread of infection from a patient who has or is suspected of having a contagious disease or to protect a patient whose immune system is compromised. Patients are most commonly isolated in a private room. The type of isolation, including a description of the precautions necessary, is generally posted on the patient's door. A cart containing all the supplies needed to enter the room and to care for the patient is placed outside the door.

Protective or Reverse Isolation

A special kind of isolation called **protective** or **reverse isolation** is used for patients who are highly susceptible to infections. In this type of isolation, protective measures are used to keep healthcare workers and others from transmitting infection to the patient rather than vice versa. Examples of patients requiring protective isolation include patients with suppressed immune systems such as organ transplant patients, patients with AIDS, some chemotherapy patients, neutropenic patients (patients with low neutrophil counts), and patients with burns.

Traditional Isolation Systems

At one time the CDC recommended either of two types of isolation systems: the **cate-gory-specific** system and the **disease-specific** system. The category-specific system had seven different isolation categories: strict, contact, respiratory, acid-fast bacillus or tuberculosis, enteric, drainage/secretion, and blood/body fluid precautions. Categories covered many diseases, which often resulted in over-isolation of patients, and needless extra costs. The disease-specific system was based on the mode of transmission of common diseases. A chart listed the diseases and identified specific isolation precautions recommended for each. A diagnosis or suspicion of the presence of a transmissible disease was needed to institute either system.

Universal Precautions

Isolation practices were altered dramatically in 1985, when the CDC introduced a strategy called **universal precautions (UP)** after reports of healthcare workers being infected with HIV through needlesticks and other exposures to HIV-contaminated blood. UP replaced blood/body fluid precautions and were followed for all isolation categories. Under UP, the blood and certain body fluids of *all* individuals were considered potentially infectious. With the introduction of UP, the focus of infection control turned from prevention of patient-to-patient transmission to prevention of patient-to-personnel transmission. The CDC required that UP be part of an overall infection control plan.

Body Substance Isolation

Because infection transmission can occur before a diagnosis is made, another system, **body substance isolation (BSI)** (Fig. 3-5), gained acceptance. BSI incorporated elements of disease-specific and category-specific precautions and was followed for *every* patient without needing a diagnosis or suspicion of a transmissible disease. BSI went beyond universal precautions by requiring that gloves be worn when contacting *any* moist body substance.

Revised Guideline for Isolation Precautions in Hospitals

In 1995, the CDC and HICPAC issued a new *Guideline for Isolation Precautions in Hospitals.* The concerns that led to development of the new guideline included widespread variation in the use of UP or BSI, confusion over which body fluids required precautions, lack of agreement about the importance of hand washing when gloves were used, and the need for additional precautions beyond BSI to prevent airborne, droplet, and contact transmission of other infectious agents and bloodborne pathogens.

This guideline, which is still in effect and supersedes previous CDC isolation recommendations, contains two tiers of precautions. The first tier, called **standard precautions,** identifies precautions to be used in caring for all hospital patients regardless of their diagnosis or presumed infection status. The second tier, called **transmission-based precautions,** identifies precautions to be used for patients either suspected or known to be infected with certain pathogens transmitted by airborne, droplet, or contact transmis-

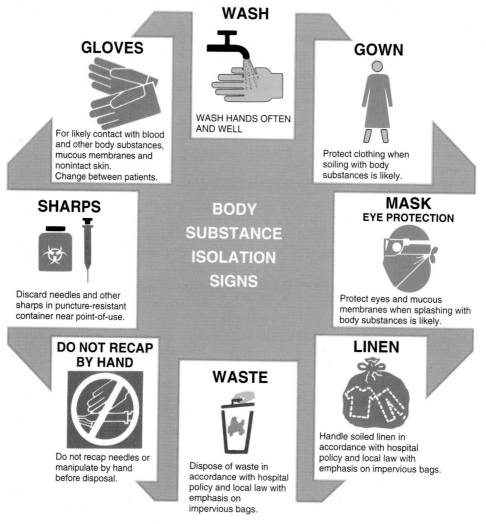

WASH

GLOVES

WASH HANDS OFTEN AND WELL

GOWN

For likely contact with blood and other body substances, mucous membranes and nonintact skin. Change between patients.

Protect clothing when soiling with body substances is likely.

SHARPS

BODY SUBSTANCE ISOLATION SIGNS

MASK
EYE PROTECTION

Discard needles and other sharps in puncture-resistant container near point-of-use.

Protect eyes and mucous membranes when splashing with body substances is likely.

DO NOT RECAP BY HAND

LINEN

WASTE

Do not recap needles or manipulate by hand before disposal.

Dispose of waste in accordance with hospital policy and local law with emphasis on impervious bags.

Handle soiled linen in accordance with hospital policy and local law with emphasis on impervious bags.

▩ FIGURE 3-5 ▩

Body substance isolation sign. (Adapted from Briggs Corp., Des Moines, IA.)

sion. The guideline also lists specific clinical syndromes or conditions that are highly suspicious for infection and identifies appropriate transmission-based precautions to use for each, in addition to standard precautions, until a diagnosis can be made.

STANDARD PRECAUTIONS

Standard precautions (Fig. 3-6) are intended to be the number one strategy for successful nosocomial infection control. Standard precautions combine the major features of UP and BSI. The intent of standard precautions is to minimize the risk of infection transmission from both recognized and unrecognized sources. Standard precautions

STANDARD PRECAUTIONS

FOR INFECTION CONTROL

Handwashing
Wash after touching **body fluids**, after **removing gloves**, and between **patient contacts**.

Gloves
Wear **Gloves** before touching **body fluids**, **mucous membranes**, and **nonintact skin**.

Mask & Eye Protection or Face Shield
Protect eyes, nose, mouth during procedures that cause **splashes** or **sprays** of **body fluids**.

Gown
Wear **Gown** during procedures that may cause **splashes** or **sprays** of **body fluids**.

Patient-Care Equipment
Handle soiled equipment so as to prevent personal contamination and transfer to other patients.

Environmental Control
Follow hospital procedures for cleaning beds, equipment, and frequently touched surfaces.

Linen
Handle linen soiled with **body fluids** so as to prevent personal contamination and transfer to other patients.

Occupational Health & Bloodborne Pathogens
Prevent injuries from needles, scalpels, and other sharp devices.
Never recap needles using both hands.
Place sharps in puncture-proof sharps containers.
Use **Resuscitation Devices** as an alternative to mouth-to-mouth resuscitation.

Patient Placement
Use a Private Room for a patient who contaminates the environment.

"Body Fluids" include **blood**, **secretions**, and **excretions**.

Form No. **SPR-C**   BREVIS CORP., 3310 S 2700 E, SLC, UT 84109   © 1996 Brevis Corp.

Condensed Version

■ FIGURE 3-6 ■

Standard precautions sign.   (Courtesy Brevis Corp., Salt Lake City, UT.)

apply to blood, *all* body fluids (including all secretions and excretions except sweat, whether or not they contain visible blood), nonintact skin, and mucous membranes. They are to be used for the care of all patients.

TRANSMISSION-BASED PRECAUTIONS

Transmission-based precautions are to be used for patients known or suspected to be infected or colonized with highly transmissible or epidemiologically (related to the study of epidemics) significant pathogens that require special precautions in addition to standard precautions. Table 3-1 lists clinical conditions that warrant transmission-based precautions pending diagnosis. Common diseases and conditions that require transmission-based precautions are listed in Table 3-2. Precautions may be combined for diseases that have more than one means of transmission. There are three types of transmission-based precautions:

- **Airborne precautions:** Airborne precautions (Fig. 3-7), or the equivalent, are used in addition to standard precautions for patients known or suspected to be infected with microorganisms transmitted by airborne droplet nuclei. An N95 respirator (see Fig. 3-2) must be worn when entering rooms of patients with airborne precautions.
- **Droplet precautions:** Droplet precautions (Fig. 3-8), or the equivalent, are used in addition to standard precautions for patients known or suspected to be infected with microorganisms transmitted by droplets (particles larger than 5 μm in size), generated when a patient talks, coughs, or sneezes, and during certain procedures.
- **Contact precautions:** Contact precautions (Fig. 3-9), or the equivalent, are used in addition to standard precautions when a patient is known or suspected to be infected or colonized with epidemiologically important microorganisms that can be transmitted by direct contact with the patient or indirect contact with surfaces or patient-care items. *text continues on page 88*

Table 3-1

Clinical Conditions Warranting Transmission-Based Precautions Pending Confirmation of Diagnosis

Condition	Potential Pathogen	Precaution
Diarrhea		
Acute diarrhea with a likely infectious cause in an incontinent or diapered patient	Enteric pathogen	Contact
Diarrhea in an adult with a history of broad-spectrum or long-term antibiotics	*Clostridium difficile*	Contact
Meningitis	*Neisseria meningitidis*	Droplet
Rash for inflamed skin eruptions		
Petechial/ecchymotic with fever	*Neisseria meningitidis*	Droplet
Vesicular	Varicella	Airborne & contact
Maculopapular	Rubeola (measles)	Airborne

continued

Table 3-1

Clinical Conditions Warranting Transmission-Based Precautions Pending Confirmation of Diagnosis (continued)

Condition	Potential Pathogen	Precaution
Respiratory infections		
Cough/fever/upper lobe pulmonary infiltrate in an HIV-negative patient and a patient at low risk for HIV infection	*Mycobacterium tuberculosis*	Airborne
Cough/fever/pulmonary infiltrate in any lung location in an HIV-infected patient and at high risk for HIV infection	*M. tuberculosis*	Airborne
Paroxysmal or severe persistent cough during periods of pertussis activity	*Bordetella pertussis*	Droplet
Respiratory infections, particularly bronchiolitis and croup, in infants and young children	Respiratory syncytial virus or parainfluenza virus	Contact
Risk of multidrug-resistant microorganisms		
History of infection or colonization with multidrug-resistant organisms	Resistant bacteria	Contact
Skin, wound, or urinary tract infection in a patient with a recent hospital or nursing home stay in a facility where multidrug-resistant organisms are prevalent	Resistant bacteria	Contact
Skin or wound infection		
Abscess or draining wound that cannot be covered	*Staphylococcus aureus* Group A streptococcus	Contact

Table 3-2

Transmission-Based Precautions for Common Diseases and Conditions

Airborne Precautions	Droplet Precautions	Contact Precautions
Herpes zoster (shingles)*	Adenovirus infection**	Adenovirus infection**
Measles (rubeola)	Diphtheria (pharyngeal)	Cellulitis (uncontrolled drainage)
Pulmonary tuberculosis	*Haemophilus influenzae* meningitis	*Clostridium difficile*
Varicella (chickenpox)	Influenza	Conjunctivitis (acute viral)
	Meningococcal pneumonia	Decubitus ulcer (infected, major)
	Meningococcal sepsis	Diphtheria (cutaneous)
	Mumps (infectious parotitis)	Enteroviral infections*
	Mycoplasma pneumoniae	Herpes zoster (shingles)*
	Neisseria meningitidis	Impetigo
	Parvovirus B19	Parainfluenza virus
	Pertussis (whooping cough)	Pediculosis (lice)
	Pneumonic plague	Respiratory syncytial virus
	Rubella (German measles)	Rubella (congenital)
	Scarlet fever**	Scabies
		Varicella (chickenpox)

*Widely disseminated or in immunocompromised patients
**Infants and children only

AIRBORNE PRECAUTIONS
(in addition to Standard Precautions)

VISITORS: Report to nurse before entering.

Patient Placement
Use **private room** that has:
  Monitored negative air pressure,
  6 to 12 air changes per hour,
  Discharge of air outdoors or HEPA filtration if recirculated.
Keep room door closed and patient in room.

Respiratory Protection
Wear an **N95 respirator** when entering the room of a patient with known or suspected infectious pulmonary **tuberculosis.**
Susceptible persons should not enter the room of patients known or suspected to have **measles** (rubeola) or **varicella** (chickenpox) if other immune caregivers are available. If susceptible persons must enter, they should wear an **N95 respirator.** (Respirator or surgical mask not required if immune to measles and varicella.)

Patient Transport
Limit transport of patient from room to essential purposes only.
Use **surgical mask** on patient during transport.

Form No. **APR**   BREVIS CORP., 3310 S 2700 E, SLC, UT 84109   © 1996 Brevis Corp.

■ FIGURE 3-7 ■

Airborne precautions sign.   (Courtesy Brevis Corp., Salt Lake City, UT.)

DROPLET PRECAUTIONS
(in addition to Standard Precautions)

VISITORS: Report to nurse before entering.

Patient Placement
Private room, if possible. Cohort or maintain spatial separation of **3 feet** from other patients or visitors if private room is not available.

Mask
Wear mask when working within **3 feet** of patient (or upon entering room).

Patient Transport
Limit transport of patient from room to essential purposes only.
Use **surgical mask** on patient during transport.

Form No. **DPR**   BREVIS CORP., 3310 S 2700 E, SLC, UT 84109   © 1996 Brevis Corp.

■ FIGURE 3-8 ■

Droplet precautions sign.   (Courtesy Brevis Corp., Salt Lake City, UT.)

CONTACT PRECAUTIONS
(in addition to Standard Precautions)

VISITORS: Report to nurse before entering.

Patient Placement
Private room, if possible. Cohort if private room is not available.

Gloves
Wear gloves when entering the room.
Change gloves after having contact with infective material that may contain high concentrations of microorganisms **(fecal** material and **wound drainage)**.
Remove gloves before leaving patient room.

Wash
Wash hands with an **antimicrobial** agent immediately after glove removal. After glove removal and handwashing, ensure that hands do not touch potentially contaminated environmental surfaces or items in the patient's room to avoid transfer of microorganisms to other patients or environments.

Gown
Wear gown when **entering** patient room if you anticipate that your clothing will have substantial contact with the patient, environmental surfaces, or items in the patient's room, or if the patient is **incontinent**, or has **diarrhea**, an **ileostomy**, a **colostomy**, or **wound drainage** not contained by a dressing. **Remove** gown before leaving the patient's environment and ensure that clothing does not contact potentially contaminated environmental surfaces to avoid transfer of microorganisms to other patients or environments.

Patient Transport
Limit transport of patient to essential purposes only. During transport, ensure that precautions are maintained to minimize the risk of transmission of microorganisms to other patients and contamination of environmental surfaces and equipment.

Patient–Care Equipment
Dedicate the use of noncritical patient–care equipment to a single patient. If common equipment is used, clean and disinfect between patients.

Form No. **CPR**   BREVIS CORP., 3310 S 2700 E, SLC, UT 84109   © 1996 Brevis Corp.

FIGURE 3-9

Contact precautions sign.   (Courtesy Brevis Corp., Salt Lake City, UT.)

SAFETY

Providing quality care in an environment that is safe for employees and patients is a concern that is foremost in the minds of healthcare providers. Safe working conditions must be ensured by employers as mandated by the Occupational Safety and Health Act of 1970 and enforced by **OSHA.** Even so, biologic, electrical, radiation, and chemical hazards are encountered in a healthcare setting, often on a daily basis. It is important for healthcare workers to be aware of the existence of hazards and to have knowledge of the safety precautions and rules necessary to eliminate or minimize them. General lab safety rules are listed in Box 3-2. Box 3-3 lists safety rules to follow when in patient rooms and other patient areas.

Box 3-2

GENERAL LABORATORY SAFETY RULES

- *Never* eat, drink, smoke, or chew gum in the laboratory. *Never* put pencils or pens in the mouth.
- *Never* place food or beverages in a refrigerator used for storing reagents or specimens.
- *Never* apply cosmetics, handle contact lenses, or rub eyes in the laboratory.
- *Never* wear long chains, large or dangling earrings, or loose bracelets.
- *Always* wear a fully buttoned lab coat when engaged in lab activities. *Never* wear a lab coat to lunch, on break, or when leaving the lab to go home. *Never* wear personal protective equipment outside the designated area for its use.
- *Always* tie back hair that is longer than shoulder length.
- *Always* keep fingernails short and well manicured. *Do not* wear nail polish or artificial nails. *Never* bite nails or cuticles.
- *Always* wear a face shield when performing specimen processing or any activity that might generate splashes or aerosol of body fluids.
- *Always* wear comfortable, sturdy shoes with nonslip soles. *Never* wear sandals, open-toed shoes, slippers, or high heels.
- *Always* wear gloves for phlebotomy procedures and when specimen processing.

Box 3-3

SAFETY RULES WHEN IN PATIENT ROOMS AND OTHER PATIENT AREAS

- Handle all specimens following standard precautions.
- Properly dispose of used and contaminated specimen collection supplies and return all other equipment to the specimen collection tray before leaving the patient's room. *Do not* recap needles!
- Replace bedrails that were let down during patient procedures.
- Do not touch electrical equipment in patient rooms, especially when in the process of drawing blood. Electrical shock could pass through the phlebotomist and the needle and shock the patient.
- Report infiltrated intravenous (IV) lines or other IV problems to nursing personnel.
- Report unresponsive patients to nursing personnel.
- Watch out for and report food, liquid, and other items spilled or dropped on the floor to nursing or housekeeping personnel.
- Report unusual odors to nursing personnel.
- Be careful when entering and exiting patient rooms. Watch out for housekeeping equipment, dietary carts, x-ray machines, and other pieces of equipment that are often left in the halls outside patient rooms.
- Avoid running. It is alarming to patients and visitors and may cause an accident.

Biologic Safety

A biologic hazard or **biohazard** is any material or substance harmful to health. Biohazards are identified by a special **biohazard symbol** (Fig. 3-10). Because the majority of laboratory specimens are blood and other body fluids and tissues with the potential to contain infectious agents that could be harmful to health, they are considered biohazards.

Biohazard Exposure Routes

There are many routes by which a healthcare worker can be exposed to biohazardous substances. Although ingestion into the digestive tract is probably the most easily recognized exposure route, **parenteral (par-en'ter-al)** routes, or routes other than the digestive tract are the most common routes of exposure for healthcare workers. The most common biohazard exposure routes are as follows.

■ FIGURE 3-10 ■

Biohazard symbol.

AIRBORNE

Biohazardous substances can be inhaled when splashes and aerosols are generated. Aerosols can be created during centrifugation of specimens and removal of stoppers, as well as when improperly aliquoting specimens. Dangerous fumes can be created when chemicals are improperly stored, mixed, or handled. Following proper procedures during handling and processing of specimens and when working with chemicals can minimize airborne exposure to biohazards. N95 respirators must be worn when entering rooms of patients with infections spread by airborne transmission.

INGESTION

Biohazardous substances can be ingested when healthcare workers neglect to wash contaminated hands and subsequently handle food, gum, candy, cigarettes, or drinks. Other activities such as covering the mouth with hands when coughing or sneezing, biting nails, chewing on pens or pencils, and licking fingers when turning pages in books or manuals can also lead to ingestion of biohazardous substances. Frequent handwashing is the best defense against accidental ingestion of biohazardous substances.

NONINTACT SKIN

Biohazardous substances can enter the body through both visible and invisible preexisting abrasions, burns, cuts, scratches, sores, dermatitis, and chapped skin. Defects in the skin should be covered with waterproof or nonpermeable tape or bandages to prevent contamination, even when gloves are worn.

PERCUTANEOUS

Percutaneous means through the skin. Infection with biohazardous microorganisms can result from direct inoculation with blood or body fluids by accidental needlesticks and injuries from other sharps including broken glass and specimen tubes. Human bites that break the skin and the transfusion of infected blood or blood products are also considered percutaneous inoculation.

Permucosal means through mucous membranes. Infectious microorganisms and other biohazards can enter the body through the mucous membranes of the mouth and nose and the conjunctiva of the eyes through droplets generated by sneezing and coughing, splashes, and aerosols, and by rubbing or touching the eyes, nose or mouth with contaminated hands. Procedures should be followed to prevent or minimize the generation of splashes and aerosols. Rubbing or touching the eyes, nose, or mouth should be avoided.

Bloodborne Pathogens

Bloodborne pathogen is a term applied to any infectious microorganism present in blood and other body fluids and tissues. Bloodborne pathogens are one of the most significant biohazards faced by healthcare workers. The most publicized bloodborne pathogens are HIV, HBV, and more recently hepatitis C virus (HCV). However, bloodborne pathogens include other hepatitis viruses; cytomegalovirus; the microorganisms that cause syphilis, malaria, and relapsing fever; and the as-yet unknown cause of Creutzfeldt-Jakob disease. Bloodborne pathogens can be present in a patient's body fluids even when there are no apparent symptoms of disease.

HBV AND HEPATITIS D VIRUS

Hepatitis B (formerly called serum hepatitis) is caused by **HBV,** a potentially life-threatening bloodborne pathogen that targets the liver. (Hepatitis means "inflammation of the liver.") It has been the most frequently occurring laboratory-associated infection and the major infectious occupational hazard in the healthcare industry. Anyone infected with HBV is at risk of also acquiring **hepatitis D (delta) virus (HDV),** which is a defective virus that can only multiply in the presence of HBV. A vaccine against HBV is available.

Hepatitis B vaccination

The best defense against HBV infection is vaccination. Vaccination consists of a series of three equal intramuscular injections of vaccine: an initial dose, a second dose 1 month after the first, and a third dose 6 months after the initial dose. Success of immunization can be confirmed by a blood test that detects the presence of the hepatitis B surface antibody in the person's serum. The most commonly used vaccine is derived from yeast culture and poses no risk of transmitting bloodborne pathogens, a problem of earlier vaccines. The vaccine also protects against HDV because HDV can only be contracted concurrently with HBV infection. OSHA requires employers to offer the vaccine free to employees within 10 days of being assigned to duties with possible exposure to bloodborne pathogens. Employees who decline the vaccination must sign a declination form.

HBV exposure hazards

HBV can be present in blood and other body fluids such as urine, semen, cerebrospinal fluid, and saliva. It can survive up to a week in dried blood on work surfaces, equipment, telephones, and other objects. In a healthcare setting, it can be transmitted through needlesticks and other sharps injuries; contact with contaminated equipment, objects, and surfaces; and contact with infectious material through aerosols, spills, and splashing. HBV can be transmitted through a single needlestick. In a nonmedical setting, it is transmitted primarily through sexual contact and sharing of dirty needles.

Symptoms of HBV infection

Symptoms of HBV infection resemble flu symptoms, but generally last longer. They include fatigue, loss of appetite, mild fever, muscle, joint and abdominal pain, nausea, and vomiting. Jaundice appears in about 25% of the cases. Approximately 50% of infected individuals show no symptoms. Some individuals become carriers with the ability to pass the disease on to others. Carriers have an increased risk of developing cirrhosis of the liver and liver cancer. Hepatitis B infection is confirmed if hepatitis B surface antigen is detected in a patient's serum.

HCV

Hepatitis C, caused by infection with **HCV,** has become the most widespread chronic bloodborne illness in the United States. The virus, discovered in 1988 by molecular cloning, was found to be the primary cause of non-A, non-B hepatitis. No vaccine is currently available.

HCV exposure hazards

HCV has been identified primarily in blood and serum. It is found less frequently in saliva, and seldom in urine and semen. HCV can enter the body in the same manner as HBV. However, HCV infection primarily occurs after large or multiple exposures. As with HBV, outside the healthcare setting it is transmitted primarily through sexual contact and sharing of dirty needles.

Symptoms of HCV infection

Symptoms are similar to HBV infection, although only 25% to 30% of infections even display symptoms. As with HBV, chronic and carrier states exist that can lead to cirrhosis of the liver and liver cancer. In fact, a leading indication for liver transplantation is HCV infection.

HIV

Human immunodeficiency virus (HIV) is the virus responsible for causing AIDS. The virus attacks the body's immune or "defense" system, leaving the host susceptible to opportunistic infections. Opportunistic infections are those that occur with organisms that would not ordinarily be considered pathogens to a normal healthy individual. Because HIV infection has a poor prognosis at best, it is of great concern to healthcare workers. Although the incidence of work-related infection with HIV is relatively low, studies by the CDC have shown that phlebotomy procedures are responsible for approximately 50% of the HIV exposures occurring so far in a healthcare setting.

HIV exposure hazards

HIV has been isolated from blood, semen, saliva, tears, urine, cerebrospinal fluid, amniotic fluid, breast milk, cervical secretions, and tissue of infected people. The major risk to healthcare workers, however, is primarily through exposure to blood. HIV can enter the body through all the same routes as the hepatitis viruses.

Symptoms of infection

The incubation period for HIV infection is thought to range from a few weeks up to a year or more. Initial symptoms are mild to severe flu-like symptoms. During this phase of infection the virus enters the T lymphocytes (T lymphs or helper T cells), triggering them to produce multiple copies of the virus. The T lymphs are inactivated or destroyed in the process.

Next the virus enters a seemingly inactive incubation phase in which it stays hidden in the T lymphs. Certain conditions reactivate the virus, which slowly destroys the T lymphs, eventually decreasing them to a point when the patient becomes prone to opportunistic infections.

If the T lymph count is reduced to 200 or less per milliliter of blood, the patient is officially diagnosed as having AIDS, the third and final phase of infection. In this phase the immune system deteriorates significantly, and opportunistic infections take hold. Two symptoms of AIDS are hairy leukoplakia, a white lesion on the tongue, and Kaposi's sarcoma, a cancer of the capillaries that produces bluish-red nodules on the skin. End stages of AIDS are characterized by deterioration of the nervous system leading to neurologic symptoms and dementia.

OSHA Bloodborne Pathogens Standard

OSHA promulgated (put into force) the **Occupational Exposure to Bloodborne Pathogens (BBP) Standard** when it was concluded that healthcare employees face a serious health risk as a result of occupational exposure to blood and other body fluids and tissues. Enforcement of this standard, which is mandated by federal law, is meant to minimize, if not eliminate, occupational exposure to bloodborne pathogens, particularly HBV, HCV, and HIV. The standard outlines necessary **engineering** and **work practice controls** that OSHA believes will help minimize or eliminate exposure of employees. In addition, the standard requires the availability and use of **personal protective equipment (PPE)** or clothing, special training, medical surveillance, and the availability of vaccination against HBV for all employees having contact with bloodborne pathogens. The standard was revised in 2001 to conform to the **Needlestick Safety and Prevention Act** passed by Congress and signed into law November 6, 2000. The act directed OSHA to revise the BBP standard in four key areas, which include:

- Revision and updating of the exposure control plan
- Solicitation of employee input in selecting engineering and work practice controls
- Modification of definitions relating to engineering controls
- New record-keeping requirements

The revised BBP standard went into effect on April 18, 2001.

Exposure Control Plan

To comply with the OSHA standard, employers must have a written exposure control plan. The plan must be reviewed and updated at least annually to document review and implementation of safer medical devices. Non–managerial employees with risk of exposure must be involved in the identification, review, and selection of engineering and work practice controls and their participation in the procedure must be documented. An exposure control plan includes:

1. An exposure determination: A list of all job classifications in which employees have or may have occupational exposure to bloodborne pathogens, and a list of tasks and procedures in which exposure may occur.
2. Methods of implementation and compliance including:

    Universal precautions statement: Requires all employees to observe UP or the equivalent.

    Engineering controls: **Engineering controls** means controls (e.g., sharps disposal containers, self–sheathing needles, safer medical devices, such as sharps with engineered sharps injury protections and needleless systems) that isolate or remove the bloodborne pathogen hazard from the workplace.

    Needleless systems indicate a device that does not use needles for:

    - Collection or withdrawal of body fluids after initial venous or arterial access is established.
    - Administration of medications or fluids
    - Any other procedure involving risk of percutaneous injury from contaminated sharps

    Sharps with engineered sharps injury protection means a nonneedle sharp or a needle device with a built–in safety feature or mechanism that effectively reduces the risk of an exposure incident.

    Work practice controls: Practices that alter the manner in which a task is performed to reduce the likelihood of exposure. Examples of work practice controls are prohibiting needle bending, breaking, or recapping; requiring hand washing after glove removal; and prohibiting eating, drinking, smoking, or applying cosmetics in work areas of the laboratory.

    PPE: PPE or barrier protection devices to minimize the risk of infection from bloodborne pathogens must be provided at no charge to all employees who have potential exposure. PPE includes gloves, gowns, lab coats, aprons, face shields, masks, and resuscitation mouthpieces. Laundry service for reusable protective outerwear such as gowns and lab coats must be provided by the employer.

    Housekeeping schedule and methods: Work surfaces must be cleaned at least once a day and after any contact with blood or other potentially infectious material. A 10% solution of household bleach (5.25% sodium hypochlorite) is an acceptable disinfectant.

3. Hepatitis B vaccine and postexposure follow-up: Hepatitis B vaccine series must be offered free of charge to employees within 10 days of assignment to duties with potential exposure. Confidential medical evaluation and follow-up must be available immediately to employees with exposure incidents.
4. Communication of hazards to employees:

    Warning labels and signs must be attached to containers of blood, contaminated waste, and other potentially infectious material. This includes refrigerators and freezers where infectious material may be stored. The labels should be predominantly fluorescent orange or orange-red, bearing the word "biohazard" and containing the biohazard symbol. Red bags or containers may be substituted for labels.

Training and information concerning bloodborne pathogens must be provided to employees at no cost and during working hours at the time of initial assignment to tasks involving occupational exposure. Employers should maintain an accessible copy of the Bloodborne Pathogen Standard as well as an explanation of its contents. Annual training is to be provided within 1 year of initial training.

5. Record keeping:

Medical records: Employers are required to maintain confidential medical records on each employee with occupational exposure. These records must include the employee's name, social security number, and HBV vaccination status.

Training records: Employers are required to maintain records of training sessions that include the content, the qualifications of persons conducting the session, and the names and titles of those attending.

Sharps injury log: Employers must establish and maintain a sharps injury log to record percutaneous injuries from contaminated sharps. Information recorded in the log must protect the confidentiality of the employee. Information in the log should identify the type and brand of device involved in the incident, where the incident occurred, and how it occurred.

Occupational Exposure to Bloodborne Pathogens

Occupational exposure to bloodborne pathogens can occur if any of the following occurs while a healthcare worker is performing his or her duties.

- The skin is pierced by a contaminated needle or sharp object
- Blood or other body fluid splashes into the eyes, nose, or mouth
- Blood or other body fluid comes in contact with a cut, scratch, or abrasion
- A human bite breaks the skin

Procedure for Needlesticks and Other Exposure Incidents

OSHA requires employers to provide free confidential medical evaluation and treatment to any employee in the event of an exposure incident. Initial response by the employee requires decontamination of a needlestick site with an appropriate antiseptic, such as povidone-iodine, for a minimum of 30 seconds. A mucous membrane exposure requires flushing the site with water for a minimum of 10 minutes. The employee must report the incident to his or her immediate supervisor. The employee is to then report directly to a licensed healthcare provider for a medical evaluation and counseling, as well as any treatment required. Medical evaluation involves the following:

1. The employee's blood is tested for HIV in an accredited laboratory
2. The source patient's blood is tested for HIV and HBV, with the patient's permission

3. If the source patient refuses testing or is HBV positive or in a high-risk category, the employee may be given immune globulin or HBV vaccination
4. If the source patient is HIV positive, the employee is counseled and tested for HIV infection immediately, and at periodic intervals—normally 6 weeks, 12 weeks, 6 months, and 1 year after exposure. The employee may be given azidothymidine (AZT) or other HIV therapy
5. The exposed employee is counseled to be alert for acute retroviral syndrome (acute viral symptoms) within 12 weeks of exposure

Decontamination of Surfaces

Specimen collection and processing areas should be decontaminated at the end of each shift with a 1:10 bleach solution or other **Environmental Protection Agency (EPA)**–approved disinfectant. Bleach solutions should be prepared daily. Gloves should be worn when cleaning.

Blood Spill Clean Up

Special EPA-approved chemical solutions are available for clean up of blood and body fluid spills and for disinfecting surfaces. Gloves must be worn during the cleaning process. Small spills of no more than a few drops can be absorbed carefully with a paper towel and the area cleaned with a disinfectant. Large blood or body fluid spills can be cleaned up using special clay or chlorine-based powder that absorbs or gels the liquid and allows it to be scooped or swept up for disposal in a biohazard waste bag. The area is then wiped with a disinfectant. Dried spills should be moistened with disinfectant before clean-up to avoid scraping, which could disperse infectious organisms into the air. Clean-up procedures should concentrate on absorbing the material and avoiding spread of the material over a wider area than that occupied by the original spill. Spills involving broken glass should be handled with heavy-duty utility gloves. Glass should be scooped or swept up and not handled with the hands. Reusable materials used for clean-up should be disinfected after use.

Biohazardous Waste Disposal

All discarded items contaminated with blood or body fluids are considered to be biohazardous waste and must be disposed of in special containers or bags marked with a biohazard symbol. Filled biohazardous waste containers require special handling in decontamination and disposal.

Electrical Safety

Fire and electrical shock are potential hazards associated with the use of electrical equipment. Knowledge of the proper use, maintenance, and servicing of electrical equipment such as centrifuges can minimize hazards associated with their use. Box 3-4 contains guidelines for electrical safety.

Box 3-4

GUIDELINES FOR ELECTRICAL SAFETY

- *Avoid* the use of extension cords.
- *Do not* overload electrical circuits.
- Inspect cords and plugs for breaks and fraying.
- Unplug equipment when servicing, including when replacing a light bulb.
- Unplug equipment that has had liquid spilled in it. Do not plug in again until the spill has been cleaned up and you are certain wiring is dry.
- Unplug and do not use equipment that is malfunctioning.
- *Do not* attempt to make repairs to equipment if you are not trained to do so.
- *Do not* handle electrical equipment with wet hands or when standing on a wet floor.
- Know the location of the circuit breaker box.
- *Do not* touch electrical equipment in patient rooms, especially when in the process of drawing blood. Electrical shock could pass through the phlebotomist and the needle and shock the patient.

Actions to Take if Electrical Shock Occurs

- Shut off the source of electricity
- If the source of electricity cannot be shut off, use nonconducting material (e.g., hand inside a glass beaker) to remove the source of electricity from a victim
- Call for medical assistance
- Start cardiopulmonary resuscitation if indicated
- Keep the victim warm

Fire Safety

All employees of any institution should be aware of procedures to follow in case of fire. They should know where fire extinguishers are located and be familiar with their use. They should also understand how to use fire blankets or heavy toweling to smother fires in clothing. In addition, they should be familiar with the location of emergency exits. Box 3-5 Lists "Do's and Don'ts if a Fire Occurs."

Box 3-5

DO'S AND DON'TS IF A FIRE OCCURS

- Do pull the nearest fire alarm.
- Do call the fire department.
- Do attempt to extinguish a small fire.
- Do close all doors and windows if leaving the area.
- Do smother a clothing fire with a fire blanket or have the person roll on the floor in an attempt to smother the fire.
- Do crawl to the nearest exit if there is heavy smoke present.
- Don't panic.
- Don't run.
- Don't use elevators.

Components of Fire

Four components, present at the same time, are necessary for fire to occur. Three of the components, **fuel** (combustible material), **heat** to raise the temperature of the material until it ignites or catches fire, and **oxygen** to maintain combustion or burning, have traditionally been referred to as the **fire triangle.** The fourth component, the **chemical reaction** that produces fire, actually creates a **fire tetrahedron** (Fig. 3-11), the latest way of looking at the chemistry of fire. Basic fire safety involves keeping the components apart to prevent fire or removing one or more of the components when there is a fire to extinguish it. Fire extinguishers put out fires by removing one or more components. There are different types of fire extinguishers, depending on the class of fire involved.

Classes of Fire

Four classes of fire are recognized by the **National Fire Protection Association (NFPA).** Classification is based on the fuel source of the fire. The four classes are as follows:

- Class A fires occur with ordinary combustible materials such as wood, papers, or clothing. Class A fires require water or water-based solutions to cool or quench the fire to extinguish it.

Memory Jogger ➤ To remember that Class **A** fires occur with ordinary combustible materials, emphasize the "a" when saying the word "ordinary."

Fire Tetrahedron

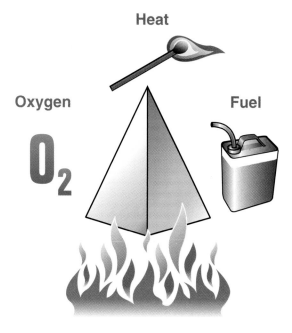

Heat

Oxygen

O_2

Fuel

Chemical Reaction

- Class B fires occur with flammable liquids and vapors such as paint, oil, grease, or gasoline. Class B fires require blocking the source of oxygen or smothering the fuel to extinguish the fire.

Memory Jogger ➤ To remember that Class **B** fires occur with flammable liquids, emphasize the "b" when saying the word "flammable."

- Class C fires occur with electrical equipment and require nonconducting agents to extinguish them.

Memory Jogger ➤ To remember that Class **C** fires are electrical fires, emphasize the "c" when saying the word "electrical."

- Class D fires occur with combustible or reactive metals such as sodium, potassium, magnesium, and lithium. Class D fires require dry powder agents or sand to extinguish. They are the most difficult fires to control and frequently lead to explosions.

Memory Jogger ➤   To remember Class **D** fires, remember that when you say the word "metal" quickly, it sounds almost like "medal," which has a "d" in it, and medals are commonly made of metal.

Fire Extinguishers

There is a fire extinguisher class (Fig. 3-12) to correspond with each class of fire, except class D. Class D fires present unique problems and are best left to firefighting personnel to extinguish.

- Class A extinguishers use soda and acid or water to cool the fire
- Class B extinguishers use foam, dry chemical, or carbon dioxide to smother the fire
- Class C extinguishers use dry chemical, carbon dioxide, halon, or other nonconducting agents to smother the fire
- Class ABC (multipurpose) extinguishers use dry chemical reagents to smother the fire. They can be used on Class A, B, and C fires, and eliminate the confusion of having several different types of extinguishers. Multipurpose extinguishers are the type most frequently used in healthcare institutions

Memory Jogger ➤   The NFPA code word for the order of action in the event of fire is RACE, in which the letters stand for the following:

R = *Rescue* individuals in danger.
A = *Alarm:* sound the alarm.
C = *Confine* the fire by closing all doors and windows.
E = *Extinguish* the fire with the nearest suitable fire extinguisher.

Radiation Safety

The principles involved in radiation exposure are **distance, shielding,** and **time.** This means that the amount of radiation you are exposed to depends upon how far you are from the source of radioactivity, what protection you have from it, and how long you are exposed to it. Exposure time is important because radiation effects are cumulative.

A clearly posted **radiation hazard symbol** (Fig. 3-13) is required in areas where radioactive materials are used and on cabinet or refrigerator doors where radioactive

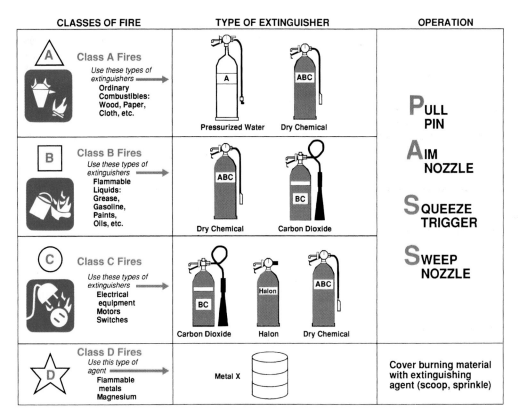

Classes of fire extinguishers. (Adapted with permission from the Environmental Health & Safety Department, The University of Texas, Houston, Health Science Center.)

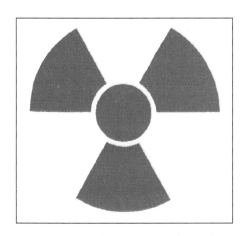

Radiation hazard symbol.

materials are stored. In addition, radioactive reagents and specimens must be labeled with a radiation hazard symbol. A radiation hazard symbol on a patient's door signifies that a patient has been treated with radioactive isotopes.

A phlebotomist may encounter radiation hazards when collecting specimens from patients who have been injected with radioactive dyes, when collecting specimens from patients in the radiology department or nuclear medicine, and when delivering specimens to radioimmunoassay sections of the laboratory. The phlebotomist should be aware of institution radiation safety procedures. In addition, the phlebotomist should recognize the radiation hazard symbol and be cautious when entering areas displaying it. Because radiation is particularly hazardous to a fetus, pregnant employees should avoid areas displaying the radiation symbol and patients who have recently been injected with radioactive dyes.

Chemical Safety

A phlebotomist may come in contact with hazardous chemicals when using cleaning reagents, adding preservatives to 24-hour urine containers, or delivering specimens to the laboratory. Inappropriate use of chemicals can have dangerous consequences. For example, mixing bleach with other cleaning compounds can release dangerous gases. In addition, many chemicals are acids (such as the hydrochloric acid [HCL] used as a urine preservative) and alkalis, both of which can cause severe burns. Container labels provide important information regarding the nature of the contents and should always be read carefully before use. See Box 3-6 for general rules for chemical safety.

Box 3-6

GENERAL RULES FOR CHEMICAL SAFETY

- Always wear proper protective clothing, including lab coat, apron, gloves, and safety goggles, when working with chemicals.
- Always use proper chemical clean-up materials when cleaning up chemical spills.
- Never store chemicals above eye level.
- Never add water to acid.
- Never indiscriminately mix chemicals together.
- Never store chemicals in unlabeled containers.
- Never pour chemicals into dirty containers, especially containers previously used to store other chemicals.
- Never use chemicals in ways other than their intended use.

OSHA Hazardous Communication Standard

OSHA developed the **Hazardous Communication (HazCom) Standard** to protect employees who may be exposed to hazardous chemicals. According to the law, all chemicals must be evaluated for health hazards, and all chemicals found to be hazardous must be labeled as such and the information communicated to employees. Because of this requirement the HazCom standard is also known as the "Right to Know Law."

HAZCOM LABELING REQUIREMENTS

Although labeling format may vary by company, all chemical manufacturers must comply with labeling requirements set by the Manufacturers Chemical Association. Labels for hazardous chemicals must contain a statement of warning such as "danger" or "poison," a statement of the hazard (e.g., toxic, flammable, combustible) and precautions to eliminate risk, and first aid measures in the event of a spill or other exposure.

MATERIAL SAFETY DATA SHEETS

The OSHA HazCom standard requires manufacturers to supply **material safety data sheets (MSDS)** for their products. An MSDS contains general information as well as precautionary and emergency information for the product. Every product with a hazardous warning on the label requires an MSDS to help assure that it will be used safely and as intended. Employers are required to obtain the MSDS for every hazardous chemical present in the workplace and make all MSDS readily accessible to employees.

Department of Transportation Labeling System

Hazardous materials may have additional labels of precaution, including a **Department of Transportation (DOT)** symbol incorporating a United Nations hazard classification number and symbol (Table 3-3).The DOT labeling system uses a diamond-shaped warning sign (Fig. 3-14) containing the United Nations hazard class number, the hazard class designation or four-digit identification number, and a symbol representing the hazard.

National Fire Protection Association Labeling System

Another hazardous material rating system was developed by the NFPA (Fig. 3-15) to label areas where hazardous chemicals and other materials are stored, thus alerting firefighters in the event of a fire. This system uses a diamond-shaped symbol divided into four quadrants. Health hazards are indicated in a blue diamond on the left, the level of fire hazard is indicated in the upper quadrant in a red diamond, stability or reactivity hazards are indicated in a yellow diamond on the right, and other specific hazards are indicated in a white quadrant on the bottom.

Safety Showers and Eye Wash Stations

The phlebotomist should know the location of and be instructed in the use of safety showers and eye wash stations (Fig. 3-16) in the event of a chemical spill or splash to the eyes or other body parts. The eyes or other body parts affected should be flushed

Table 3-3

Placard Recognition Information

United Nations Hazard Class	Symbol	Background Color	Examples
Class 1 Explosives	Bursting ball	Orange	Fireworks Ammunition Dynamite
Class 2 Gases (compressed, liquified, or dissolved under pressure)	Flame	*Flammable* Red	Flammable: Butane Propane
	Cylinder	*Nonflammable* Green	Nonflammable: Ammonia Chlorine
Class 3 Flammable liquids	Flame	Red	Brake fluid Camphor oil Glycol ethers Gasoline
Class 4 Flammable solids or substances	Flame	*Flammable Solid* Red and white vertical stripes	Lithium Magnesium Phosphorus Titanium
	Slashed W	*Water-Reactive Materials* Red and white vertical stripes with blue top quadrant	
Class 5 Division 5.1: oxidizing substances Division 5.2: organic peroxides	Circle with flame	Yellow	Ammonium nitrate Benzoyl peroxide Calcium chlorite
Class 6 Poisonous and infectious substances	Skull with crossbones	White	Chemical mace Pesticides Cyanide AIDS specimens
Class 7 Radioactive materials	Propeller	Yellow over white	Cobalt 14 Plutonium Radioactive waste Uranium 235

continued

Table 3-3

Placard Recognition Information *(continued)*

United Nations Hazard Class	Symbol	Background Color	Examples
Class 8 Corrosives	Test tube over hand Test tube over metal	White over black	Caustic potash Caustic soda Hydrochloric acid Sulfuric acid
Class 9 Miscellaneous dangerous substances	ORM-A ORM-B ORM-C ORM-D ORM-E	White	ORM-A: dry ice ORM-B: quick lime ORM-C: sawdust ORM-D: hair spray ORM-E: hazardous waste

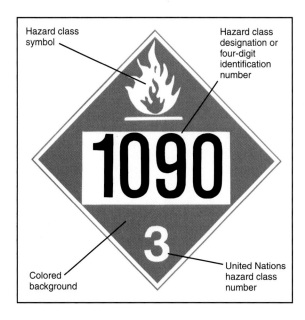

■ FIGURE 3-14 ■

Example of Department of Transportation hazardous materials labels (e.g., flammable, poison, corrosive). (Jones SA, Weigel A, White RD, McSwain NE, Breiter M., eds. Advanced Emergency Care for Paramedic Practice (1992). J.B. Lippincott.)

with water for a minimum of 15 minutes, followed by a visit to the emergency room for evaluation.

Chemical Spill Procedures

Chemical spills require clean-up using special kits (Fig. 3-17) containing absorbent and neutralizer materials. The type of materials used depends upon the type of chemical spilled. An indicator in the clean-up materials detects when the chemicals have been neutralized and are safe for disposal. The EPA regulates chemical disposal.

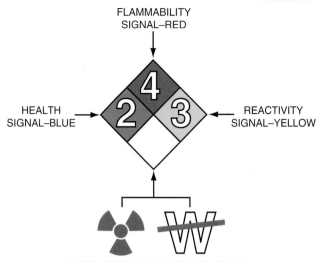

FLAMMABILITY
SIGNAL–RED

HEALTH
SIGNAL–BLUE

REACTIVITY
SIGNAL–YELLOW

RADIOACTIVE OR WATER REACTIVE

Identification of Health Hazard Color Code: **BLUE**		Identification of Flammability Color Code: **RED**		Identification of Reactivity (Stability) Color Code: **YELLOW**	
	Type of possible injury		Susceptibility of materials to burning		Susceptibility to release of energy
SIGNAL		SIGNAL		SIGNAL	
4	Materials that on very short exposure could cause death or major residual injury even though prompt medical treatment was given.	4	Materials that will rapidly or completely vaporize at atmospheric pressure and normal ambient temperature, or that are readily dispersed in air and that will burn readily.	4	Materials that in themselves are readily capable of detonation or of explosive decomposition or reaction at normal temperatures and pressures.
3	Materials that on short exposure could cause serious temporary or residual injury even though prompt medical treatment was given.	3	Liquids and solids that can be ignited under almost all ambient temperature conditions.	3	Materials that in themselves are capable of detonation or explosive reaction but require a strong initiating source or that must be heated under confinement before initiation or that react explosively with water.
2	Materials that on intense or continued exposure could cause temporary incapacitation or possible residual injury unless prompt medical treatment is given.	2	Materials that must be moderately heated or exposed to relatively high ambient temperatures before ignition can occur.	2	Materials that in themselves are normally unstable and readily undergo violent chemical change but do not detonate. Also materials that may react violently with water or that may form potentially explosive mixtures with water.
1	Materials that on exposure would cause irritation but only minor residual injury even if no treatment is given.	1	Materials that must be preheated before ignition can occur.	1	Materials that in themselves are normally stable, but that can become unstable at elevated temperatures and pressures or that may react with water with some release of energy, but not violently.
0	Materials that on exposure under fire conditions would offer no hazard beyond that of ordinary combustible material.	0	Materials that will not burn.	0	Materials that in themselves are normally stable, even under fire exposure conditions, and that are not reactive with water.

■ FIGURE 3-15 ■

National Fire Protection Association 704 marking system.

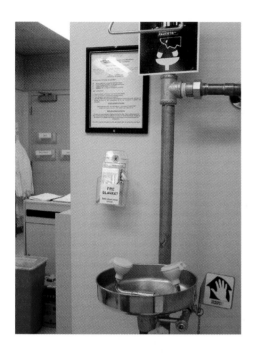

■ FIGURE 3-16 ■

Eyewash station.

First Aid Procedures

Ability to recognize and react quickly and skillfully to emergency situations may mean the difference between life and death for a victim.

External Hemorrhage

Control of hemorrhage (abnormal bleeding) from an obvious wound is most effectively accomplished by elevating the affected part above the level of the heart and applying direct pressure to the wound. However, do not attempt to elevate a broken extremity. Pressure should be applied using a clean cloth or compress. If the compress should become soaked with blood, a new compress should be placed over the original. The original compress should not be removed as removal may disrupt the clotting process.

If applying pressure over the site is ineffective in controlling bleeding, as may be the case with a very large injury, apply strong finger pressure over the pressure point of the main artery supplying the area. *Avoid* use of a tourniquet to control bleeding. A tourniquet should only be used as a last resort to save a patient's life after all other means to control bleeding are unsuccessful, such as may occur with an **avulsion** (amputation) or a severely mangled or crushed body part.

Shock

A state of shock results when there is insufficient return of blood flow to the heart, resulting in inadequate supply of oxygen to all organs and tissues of the body. Numerous conditions including hemorrhage, heart attack, trauma, and drug reactions can lead to

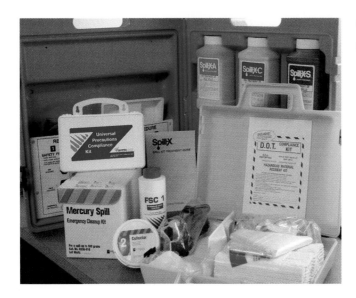

Spill cleanup kit.

some degree of shock. Because shock can be a life-threatening situation, it is important that the symptoms be recognized and dealt with immediately.

COMMON SYMPTOMS OF SHOCK

- Pale, cold, clammy skin
- Rapid, weak pulse
- Increased, shallow breathing rate
- Expressionless face and staring eyes

FIRST AID FOR SHOCK

1. Maintain an open airway for the victim
2. Call for assistance
3. Keep the victim lying down with the head lower than the rest of the body
4. Attempt to control bleeding or other cause of shock if known
5. Keep the victim warm until help arrives

Never give fluids if the patient is unconscious or semiconscious or has injuries likely to require surgery and anesthesia.

Cardiopulmonary Resuscitation and Emergency Cardiovascular Care

Most healthcare institutions require their personnel to be certified in **cardiopulmonary resuscitation (CPR).** Consequently, most phlebotomy programs require it as a prerequisite or corequisite or include it as part of the course. The American Heart Association recommends the 6- to 8-hour Basic Lifesaving Healthcare Provider Course for those in healthcare professions. The course includes instruction in how to perform CPR on victims of all ages, use of an automated external defibrillator (AED), and how to relieve foreign body airway obstruction. Certification is good for 2 years.

INTERNATIONAL CPR AND ECC GUIDELINES 2000

The American Heart Association unveiled important new recommendations for CPR and **Emergency Cardiovascular Care (ECC)** in August 2000. These guidelines, designed for both lay rescuers and healthcare providers, were developed by an international panel of experts and are called the *International CPR and ECC Guidelines 2000*. The aim of the 2000 guidelines is to simplify training by offering effective and easy-to-learn methods that focus on the most important aspects of resuscitation. Highlights of the new recommendation include:

- Deletion of the pulse check from layperson CPR training
- Standardizing the ratio of chest compressions to rescue breaths; performing 15:1 for both one- and two-rescuer CPR
- Requiring that CPR on unconscious adults be started without conducting abdominal thrusts or blind finger sweeps of the mouth.
- Advocating public access to and training in the use of AEDs

American Heart Association Chain of Survival

The **chain of survival** is a four-step course of action used to aid victims of sudden cardiac arrest, which can optimize their chance of survival and recovery. The links in the chain are:

1. Early access to care
2. Early CPR
3. Early defibrillation
4. Advanced care

Personal Wellness

"The doctor of the future will give no medicine but will interest his patients in the care of the human frame, in diet, and in the cause and prevention of disease."

THOMAS A. EDISON

Introduction

Today, many people are striving for personal wellness. A century ago, such a goal was unknown and people counted themselves lucky just to survive. For example, a person born in 1890 could expect to live only 40 years. Infectious disease took the lives of many, and environmental conditions contributed to the spread of disease. Today our most serious health threats are chronic illnesses such as heart disease or cancer—diseases that we have the power to prevent. Personal wellness requires a holistic approach, or one that meets the physical, emotional, social, spiritual, and economic needs. It is something almost everyone can have, but achieving it requires knowledge, self-awareness, motivation, and effort.

Personal Hygiene

Personal wellness starts with good personal hygiene. It is important to shower or bathe and use deodorant on a regular basis. Teeth should be brushed and mouthwash used more than once a day, if possible. Hair should be clean and neatly combed. Fingernails should be clean, short, and neatly trimmed. Personal hygiene communicates a strong impression about an individual. A fresh, clean appearance without heavily scented lotions or colognes portrays health and instills confidence in the employee and patients and employers as well.

 Key Point ➤ Phlebotomists should pay special attention to personal hygiene not only for optimal health but also because their job involves close patient contact.

Proper Nutrition

"Let thy food be they medicine, and they medicine be thy food."

Hippocrates, father of medicine, 500 BC

Nutrition has been defined as the "act or process of nourishing." In other words, a food is nutritious if it supplies the nutrients the body needs "to promote growth and repair and maintain vital processes." The basic purpose of nutrition is to keep us alive, but more importantly, good nutrition provides what the body needs for energy and day-to-day functioning.

Physical health requires eating well. In this fast-paced world, few of us receive the nutrition we need. Even though what we eat is described as the good American diet, in reality, what we eat is not always nutritious. Our food is often so highly processed and chemically altered that it no longer promotes healthy bodies. The American Institute for Cancer Research (AICR) recently published a recommended diet to reduce the risk of cancer. They suggested that a person choose a predominantly plant-based diet rich in a variety of vegetables, fruits, legumes, and minimally processed starchy staple foods. A healthy diet contains the widest possible variety of natural foods. It provides a good balance of carbohydrates, fat, protein, vitamins, minerals, and fiber. In general, the amount of food energy (calories) supplied by diet should not exceed the amount of energy expended, so that weight remains relatively constant over time.

Rest and Exercise

Personal wellness requires a nutritional diet, exercise, and getting the right amount of rest (Fig 3-18). Healthcare workers often complain of fatigue (physical or mental exhaustion). Fatigue brought on by physical causes is typically relieved by sleep. Lack of rest and sleep can lead to medical problems. The typical frantic pace in healthcare fa-

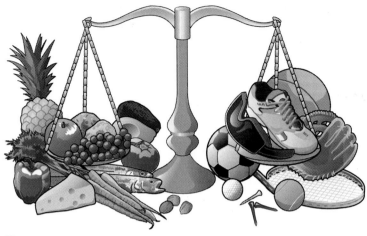

■ Figure 3-18 ■

Wellness through proper nutrition, exercise, and rest.

cilities today makes it especially important to get the required hours of sleep and to take breaks during the day to rest, refresh, and stay fit.

Studies show that being physically fit increases the chance of staying healthy and living longer. The most accurate measurements of fitness consist of evaluating three components—strength (the ability to carry, lift, push or pull a heavy load), flexibility (the ability to bend, stretch, and twist), and endurance (the ability to maintain effort for an extended period of time). No single measurement of performance classifies a person as fit or unfit. If a person becomes breathless after climbing a flight of stairs or hurrying to catch a bus but is otherwise healthy, clearly he or she could benefit from some form of conditioning or exercise.

Exercise contributes to improved quality of life on a day-to-day basis. It strengthens the immune system, increases energy, and reduces stress by releasing substances called endorphins that create a peaceful state. People who exercise tend to relax more completely, even when under stress. Regular physical activity also appears to reduce symptoms of depression and anxiety and increase ability to perform daily tasks.

Walking is a form of exercise that can be easily incorporated into almost anyone's life.

 Key Point ➤ If activity during work is low to moderate, AICR recommends that a person take an hour's brisk walk or similar exercise daily because there has been convincing evidence that physical activity helps prevent colon cancer.

Weight training is suggested as an excellent strength exercise. Studies have shown that using weights can build bone mass even in the very elderly. For flexibility, yoga and Pilates are two forms of exercise that emphasize bending, stretching, and twisting. When choosing an exercise activity, it is most important is to pick one that is enjoyable so you are more apt to do it routinely.

Back Protection

A healthy back is necessary to lead an active and healthy life. The spine is designed to withstand everyday movement, including the demands of exercise. Improper lifting and poor posture habits, however, can reveal weaknesses. It is estimated that back injuries account for approximately 20% of all workplace injuries and illnesses. Lower back pain is a costly health problem that affects both industry and society in general. Strategies to prevent back injuries include instruction concerning back mechanics and lifting techniques (Fig. 3-19), lumbar support, and exercise. Exercise promotes strong backs; it improves back support and directly benefits the discs in the spinal column. Stress can make a person vulnerable to back problems because of muscle spasms. Keeping back muscles flexible with exercises can alleviate this stress reaction.

Key Point ➤ Healthcare workers are at risk for back injury because of activities they are required to do (i.e., lift and move patients) and because of the stressful environment often associated with healthcare today.

Stress Management

Stress is a condition or state that results when physical, chemical, or emotional factors cause mental or bodily tension. It challenges our ability to cope or adapt. Stress is sometimes useful, keeping us alert and increasing our energy when we need it. Persistent or excessive stress, on the other hand, can be harmful.

Evidence suggests that "negative stress" (such as an emergency or an argument) has a damaging effect on personal wellness. Stressful situations are more likely to be damaging if they cannot be predicted or controlled. This fact is particularly apparent where job stress is concerned. Highly demanding jobs are much more stressful if an individual has no control over the workload, as is often the case in healthcare. Stress is more likely to have adverse effects on an individual if social support is lacking or there are personal or financial concerns. Although the signs of stress may not be immediately ap-

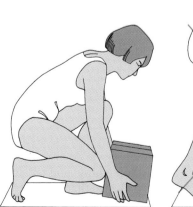
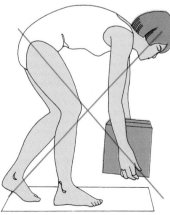

■ FIGURE 3-19 ■

Lifting techniques. (Used with permission from Smeltzer, S. C., Bare, B. G. (2000). *Brunner & Suddarth's textbook of medical-surgical nursing* (9th ed.). Philadelphia: Lippincott, p. 1810, Fig. 62-3)

parent, different organs and systems throughout the body are being affected. The immune system may be weakened, and other symptoms such as hypertension, ulcers, migraines, and nervous breakdowns may eventually result.

In the hectic healthcare environment of today, it is necessary to manage stress to maintain personal wellness. Box 3-7 lists ways to deal with stress.

Box 3-7

WAYS TO CONTROL STRESS

- Identify your problem and talk about it with a close friend, partner, or the person at the source of the problem.
- Learn to relax throughout the day—close your eyes, relax your body, and clear your mind.
- Exercise regularly—develop a consistent exercise routine that you can enjoy.
- Avoid making too many changes at once—plan for the future to avoid simultaneous major changes.
- Spend at least 15 minutes a day thoroughly planning the time you have.
- Set realistic goals—be practical about what you can accomplish.
- Avoid procrastination by tackling the most difficult job first.

STUDY & REVIEW QUESTIONS

1. Which of the following situations involves a nosocomial infection?
   a. A patient admitted to the hospital with a severe urinary tract infection
   b. An employee who contracts HBV from a needlestick
   c. A patient in ICU whose surgical wound becomes infected
   d. A baby in the nursery with congenital herpes infection

2. Reverse isolation may be used for
   a. a pediatric patient with measles.
   b. an adult patient with the flu.
   c. a patient with a urinary tract infection.
   d. a patient with severe burns.

3. The single most important means of preventing the spread of infection is
   a. proper hand washing.
   b. wearing a mask.
   c. wearing gloves.
   d. Nosocomial infections cannot be prevented.

4. Safe working conditions for employees are mandated by
   a. ASCP.
   b. CAP.
   c. CDC.
   d. OSHA.

5. The most frequently occurring lab-acquired infection is
   a. HBV infection.
   b. HIV infection.
   c. syphilis.
   d. tuberculosis.

6. To destroy transient microorganisms when washing hands, use
   a. antiseptic soap.
   b. bleach solution.
   c. plain soap.
   d. all the above.

7. Electrical safety involves
   a. distance, time, and shielding.
   b. knowing the circuit breaker box locations.
   c. knowing where the fire extinguishers are.
   d. none of the above.

Continued

STUDY & REVIEW QUESTIONS *(CONTINUED)*

8. In the event of a chemical splash in the eyes, the first thing the victim should do is

   a. call the paramedics.

   b. go to the emergency room.

   c. immediately flush eyes with water for 15 minutes.

   d. wipe the eyes with a tissue.

9. Which of the following items is PPE?

   a. Biohazard bag

   b. Countertop splash shield

   c. Nonlatex gloves

   d. Sharps container

10. Which of the following is an important difference between the new American Heart Association CPR recommendations and previous recommendations?

    a. Finger sweeps of the mouth must now be made before starting CPR

    b. The pulse check has been deleted

    c. The ratio of breaths to compressions is now 5:1

    d. Use of automated external defibrillators (AEDs) is now discouraged

11. All of the following examples of potential exposure to bloodborne pathogens involve a parenteral route of transmission except one. Which one is it?

    a. A phlebotomist cuts his hand on a broken tube of blood

    b. Blood leaks through the glove of a phlebotomist who has badly chapped hands

    c. Someone is chewing gum while collecting blood specimens

    d. The technician in specimen processing rubs her eye without washing her hands

12. Which of the following help prevent lower back pain?

    a. Exercise

    b. Lumbar support

    c. Proper lifting techniques

    d. All the above

■ CASE STUDY: AN ACCIDENT WAITING TO HAPPEN

A female phlebotomist works alone in an outpatient clinic. It is almost time to close for lunch when a patient arrives for a blood test. The phlebotomist is flustered because she has a special date for lunch. She is dressed up for the occasion, wearing a nice dress and high heels. She looks nice except for a large scratch on her left wrist that she got while playing with her cat this morning. She quickly draws the patient's blood. As she turns to put the specimen in a rack, she slips and falls. One of the tubes breaks. She does not get cut, but blood splashes everywhere, including her left wrist.

QUESTIONS:

1. What is the first thing the phlebotomist should do?
2. How did the phlebotomist's actions contribute to this accident?
3. What should she have done that might have prevented the exposure, despite the tube breaking?
4. What type of exposure did she receive?

Bibliography and Suggested Readings

American Heart Association. *Chain of survival and cardiac arrest.* (http://www.americanheart.org). Accessed March 18, 2002.

American Institute for Cancer Research—World Cancer Research Fund Report. (1998). *Food, nutrition and the prevention of cancer: A global perspective.* Washington, DC.

CDC. (1994). Guidelines for preventing the transmission of *Mycobacterium tuberculosis* in health-care facilities. *MMWR 43*(RR13); 1–132.

Dillingham, T.R. (1998). Lumbar supports for prevention of low back pain in the workplace. *Journal of the American Medical Association 279*(22), 1826–1827.

Dorling Kindersley, Ltd., and American Medical Association. (1991). *Monitoring your health.* Clayman, C. B., ed. Pleasantville, New York: Reader's Digest Association, Inc.

Garner, J. (1996). Guideline for isolation precautions in hospitals. *Infection Control and Hospital Epidemiology 17*(1), 53–80.

Hwang, M. Young (1998). Oh my aching back. *Journal of the American Medical Association 279*(22), 1846.

Larson, EL, APIC Guidelines Committee. (1995). APIC Guidelines for handwashing and hand antisepsis in the health care setting. *American Journal of Infection Control 23*, 251–269.

Linne, J., & Ringsrud, K. (1999). *Clinical laboratory science: the basics and routine techniques.* St. Louis: Mosby.

National Committee for Clinical Laboratory Standards, M29-A. (1997). *Protection of laboratory workers from instrument biohazards and infectious disease transmitted by blood, body fluids and tissue.* Approved Guideline. Villanova, PA: NCCLS.

Occupational Safety and Health Administration. (1991). *Occupational exposure to bloodborne pathogens: Final rule.* 29CFR Part 1910.1030.

Occupational Safety and Health Administration. (2001). *Occupational exposure to bloodborne pathogens: Needlestick and other sharps injuries: Final rule.* 29 CFR Part 1910, Docket No. H370A, RIN 1218-AB85.

OSHA Instruction. (2001). *Enforcement procedures for the occupational exposure to bloodborne pathogens.* Directives Number CPL 2-2.69. Effective date November 27, 2001.

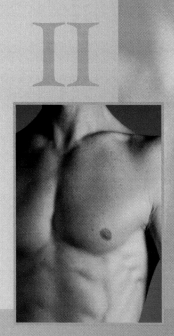

II

Overview of the Human Body

4

MEDICAL TERMINOLOGY

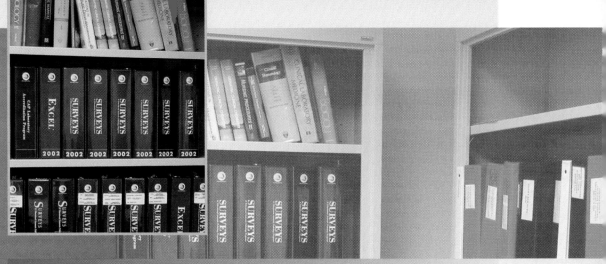

OBJECTIVES

Upon successful completion of this chapter, the reader will be able to:

1 Define the key terms and abbreviations listed at the beginning of this chapter.
2 Identify the basic word elements that make up medical terms.
3 State the meanings of common word roots, prefixes, and suffixes and identify unique plural endings.
4 State the meanings of medical terms composed of elements found in this chapter.
5 Demonstrate proper pronunciation of medical terms composed of word elements found in this chapter.
6 State the meanings of common medical abbreviations listed in this chapter.

INTRODUCTION

All professions have a special vocabulary of scientific or technical terms necessary to speak or write effectively and precisely. **Medical terminology** is the special vocabulary of the healthcare professions. It is based on an understanding of a few basic elements primarily derived from Greek and Latin words that are used to form most medical terms. These elements are word roots, prefixes, suffixes, and combining forms. After the meanings of the basic word elements are known, the general meaning of most medical terms can be established.

 Key Point ➤ To determine the meaning of a medical term start with the suffix, then the prefix, and identify the meaning of the word root or roots last.

WORD ROOTS

A **word root** establishes the basic meaning of a medical term. It is the foundation upon which the true meaning is built. The true meaning of a medical term is established by analyzing the other word elements such as prefixes and suffixes attached to the word root.

 Key Point ➤ A word root typically indicates a tissue, organ, body system, structure, substance, or condition. For example, the word root *phleb* means "vein," a body structure.

Some medical terms have more than one word root. The term *thrombophlebitis* is made up of the word root *phleb* and the word root *thromb*, meaning "clot." Occasionally both a Greek and Latin root mean the same thing. For example, the Greek root *nephr* and the Latin root *ren* both mean "kidney."

In a few instances, a root will have several very different meanings. For example, the root *ped* appears in words derived from both Greek and Latin words for "foot" and the Greek word for "child." In addition, some words containing the letters ped are derived from the Latin term *pediculus* meaning "lice." To establish the meaning of the root in these cases it is important to consider the context in which the word is used. Table 4-1 lists common medical word roots.

PREFIXES

The term **prefix** is derived from a Latin term that means "to fasten before." Accordingly, a prefix is a word element that comes before a word root. A prefix modifies the meaning of the word root by adding information such as presence or absence, location, number, or size. A term is never made up of a prefix alone.

Example: A /   NUCLEAR
             prefix   root
             (without)   (nucleus)

Table 4-1

Common Medical Word Roots

Root	Meaning	Example
aer	air	aerobic
angi	vessel	angiogram
arteri	artery	arteriosclerosis
arthr	joint	arthritis
bili	bile	bilirubin
bronch	bronchus	bronchitis
cardi	heart	electrocardiogram
cephal	head	cephalic
chondr	cartilage	osteochondritis
cry	cold	cryoglobulin
cyst	bladder	cystitis
cyt, cyte	cell	cytology
derm	skin	dermatitis
encephal	brain	encephalitis
esophag	esophagus	esophagitis
fibrin	fiber	fibrinolysis
gastr	stomach	gastrointestinal
glyc	glucose, sugar	glycolysis
hem	blood	hemolysis
hemat	blood	hematology
hepat	liver	hepatitis
lip	fat	lipemia
my	muscle	myalgia
nephr	kidney	nephritis
onc	tumor	oncologist
oste	bone	osteoporosis
path	disease	pathogen
phleb	vein	phlebotomy
pulmon	lung	pulmonary
ren	kidney	renal
scler	hard	sclerotic
thromb	clot	thrombosis
thorac	chest	thoracic
tox	poison	toxicology
vas	vessel	vascular
ven	vein	venipuncture

The prefix "a" means "without." The word root "nuclear" means nucleus. The word "anuclear" means "without a nucleus." Table 4-2 lists common medical prefixes.

SUFFIXES

The term **suffix** is derived from a Latin term that means "to fasten underneath or behind." Accordingly, a **suffix** is a word ending. It follows a word root and either changes or adds to the meaning of the word root. The best way to determine the meaning of a

Table 4-2

Common Medical Prefixes

Prefix	Meaning	Example
a-,an-,ar-	without	arrhythmia
aniso-	unequal	anisocytosis
anti-	against	antiseptic
bi-	two	bicuspid
brady-	slow	bradycardia
cyan-	blue	cyanotic
dys-	difficult	dyspnea
endo-	in, within	endothelium
epi-	on, over	epidermis
erythr-	red	erythrocyte
extra-	outside	extravascular
hetero-	different	heterosexual
homo-	same	homogeneous
homeo-	same	homeostasis
hyper-	too much, high	hypertension
hypo-	low, under	hypoglycemia
intra-	within	intramuscular
inter-	between	intercellular
iso-	equal, same	isothermal
macro-	large, long	macrocyte
mal-	poor	malnutrition
micro-	small	microcyte
mono-	one	mononuclear
neo-	new	neonatal
poly-	many, much	polyuria
post-	after	postprandial
pre-	before	prenatal
per-	through	percutaneous
semi-	half	semilunar
tachy-	rapid	tachycardia
tri-	three	tricuspid

medical term is to first identify the meaning of the suffix. As with a prefix, a suffix never stands alone.

Example: GASTR /   IC
         root   suffix
         (stomach)   (pertaining to)

The word root "gastr" means "stomach." The suffix "ic" means "pertaining to." The word gastric means "pertaining to the stomach." Table 4-3 lists common medical suffixes.

Key Point ➤ When a suffix begins with **rh,** the **r** is doubled, as in hemorrhage. When a suffix is added to a word ending in **x,** the **x** is changed to a **g** or **c** as in pharynx becoming pharyngeal and thorax becoming thoracic.

Table 4-3

Common Medical Suffixes

Suffix	Meaning	Example
-ac,-al,	pertaining to	cardiac, neural
-algia	pain	neuralgia
-ar,-ary	pertaining to	muscular, urinary
-centesis	surgical puncture to remove a fluid	thoracentesis
-emia	blood condition	anemia
-gram	recording, writing	electrocardiogram
-ic	pertaining to	thoracic
-ism	condition	hypothyroidism
-itis	inflammation	tonsillitis
-rhage	bursting forth	hemorrhage
-logist	specialist in the study of	cardiologist
-lysis	breakdown, separation	hemolysis
-megaly	enlargement	acromegaly
-meter	instrument that measures or counts	thermometer
-oma	tumor	hepatoma
-osis	condition	necrosis
-oxia	oxygen level	hypoxia
-pathy	disease	cardiomyopathy
-penia	deficiency	leukopenia
-pnea	breathing	dyspnea
-spasm	twitch, involuntary muscle movement	arteriospasm
-stasis	stopping, controlling, standing	hemostasis
-tomy	cutting, incision	phlebotomy

COMBINING VOWELS/FORMS

A **combining vowel** (frequently an "o") is added to make pronunciation easier when two word roots or a word root and a suffix are joined together. A word root combined with a vowel is called a **combining form.**

Key Point ➤ A combining vowel is not normally used when a suffix starts with a vowel. However, a combining vowel is kept between two word roots, even if the second root begins with a vowel.

Example #1: GASTR / O / ENTER / O / LOGY
word root + word root + suffix
  combining vowel   combining vowel
(combining form) (combining form)
(stomach) (intestines) (study of)

The two word roots are combined by the vowel "o" to ease pronunciation, even though the second root "enter" begins with a vowel. The vowel "o" is also used between the word root "enter" and the suffix "logy." The term gastroenterology means "study of the stomach and intestines." The combining forms created are "gastro" and "entero."

Example #2:   PHLEB /   ITIS
                  root   suffix
                    (vein)   (inflammation)

Because the suffix "itis" begins with a vowel, a combining vowel is not used after the word root "phleb." Phlebitis means "inflammation of a vein."

WORD ELEMENT CLASSIFICATION DISCREPANCIES

Medical terminology texts vary in the way they categorize medical term word elements. Also, some word elements may be categorized one way in one term and a different way in another term. For example, the word element *phasia,* which means "speech," is normally classified as a suffix. It functions as a word root, however, in the word *aphasia,* which means "without speech." Either way, the meaning is the same.

Key Point ➤ It is more important to be able to identify the meaning of a word element than to identify its category.

UNIQUE PLURAL ENDINGS

The plural forms of some medical terms follow English rules. Others have **unique plural endings** that follow the rules of the Greek or Latin languages from which they originated. It is important to evaluate medical terms individually to determine the correct plural form. Table 4-4 lists the unique plural forms of typical singular medical term endings.

PRONUNCIATION

It is important to pronounce medical terms correctly to convey the correct meaning. Even one mispronounced syllable can change a meaning. Most medical terms are pronounced by following the same basic rules used to pronounce English terms. However, some terms may have more than one acceptable pronunciation. For example hemophilia can be pronounced "he mo fil' e a" or "hem o fil' e a." In addition, some terms that are

Table 4-4

Unique Plural Endings			
Word Ending	**Plural Ending**	**Singular Example**	**Plural Example**
-a	-ae	vena cava	vena cavae (ka've)
-en	-ina	lumen	lumina (lu'min-a)
-ex, -ix	-ices	appendix	appendices (a-pen'di-sez)
-is	-es	crisis	crises (kri'sez)
-nx	-nges	phalanx	phalanges (fa-lan'-jez)
-on	-a	protozoon	protozoa (pro"to-zo'a)
-um	-a	ovum	ova (o'va)
-us	-i	nucleus	nuclei (nu'kle-i)

spelled differently have the same pronunciation. One example is *ilium,* which means "hip bone." It is pronounced the same as *ileum,* which means "small intestine." These terms can be confused when spoken rather than written. Verify the spelling of such terms to eliminate confusion. General pronunciation guidelines can be found in Table 4-5.

ABBREVIATIONS AND SYMBOLS

Abbreviation is a way of shortening words or phrases. Symbols are objects or signs that represent words or phrases. Use of abbreviations and symbols saves time, space, and paperwork and is common practice in the healthcare professions in which literally thousands of medical and scientific abbreviations and many symbols are used. Some of the most common abbreviations and symbols used in healthcare are listed in Table 4-6 and Table 4-7, respectively.

Table 4-5

General Pronunciation Guidelines

- **ae** is pronounced using only the second vowel as in chord**ae**.
- **c** before an "e," "i," or "y" in terms of Greek or Latin origin has the sound of "s," as in **c**ell, **c**irculation, and **c**ytology.
- **c** before other vowels has a hard sound as in **c**apillary, **c**olitis, and **c**ulture.
- **g** before an "e," "i," or "y" in terms of Greek or Latin origin has the sound of "j," as in **g**enetic, **G**iardia, and **g**yrate.
- **g** before other vowels has a hard sound as in **g**allbladder, **g**onad, and **g**ut.
- **ch** is often pronounced like a "k," as in **ch**loride and **ch**olesterol.
- **e** at the end of a term is sometimes pronounced separately, as in syncop**e** and diastol**e**.
- **es** at the end of a term is sometimes pronounced as a separate syllable, as in nar**es**.
- **i** at the end of the plural form of a term is pronounced "eye," as in fung**i** and nucle**i**.
- **ph** is pronounced with an "f" sound, as in the word **ph**armacy.
- **pn** at the start of a term is pronounced with the "n" sound only, as in **pn**eumonia.
- **pn** in the middle of a term is pronounced with a "p" and an "n" sound as in dys**pn**ea and a**pn**ea.
- **ps** is pronounced like "s," as in **ps**eudopod and **ps**ychology.

Table 4-6

Common Abbreviations

Abbreviation	Meaning	Abbreviation	Meaning
ABGs	arterial blood gases	ALL	acute lymphocytic leukemia
ABO	blood group system		
a.c.	before meals	ALT	alanine transaminase (see SGPT)
ACTH	adrenocorticotropic hormone		
		AML	acute myelocytic leukemia
ADH	antidiuretic hormone	aq	water (aqua)
ad lib	as desired	AST	aspartate aminotrans-ferase (see SGOT)
AIDS	acquired immunodefi-ciency syndrome		
		ASO	antistreptolysin O

continued

Table 4-6

Common Abbreviations *(continued)*

Abbreviation	Meaning	Abbreviation	Meaning
b.i.d.	twice a day (bis in die)	FBS	fasting blood sugar
bili	bilirubin	Fe	iron
BP	blood pressure	FSH	follicle stimulating hormone
BUN	blood urea nitrogen		
Bx	biopsy	FUO	fever of unknown origin
$\bar{c}$	with (cum)	gluc	glucose
Ca	calcium	GI	gastrointestinal
CAD	coronary artery disease	Gm, gm, g	gram
CBC	complete blood count	GTT	glucose tolerance test
cc	cubic centimeter	GYN	gynecology
CCU	coronary care unit	h	hour
chem	chemistry	Hb, Hgb	hemoglobin
chemo	chemotherapy	HbsAg	hepatitis B surface antigen
CK	creatine kinase	HBV	hepatitis B Virus
cm	centimeter	HCG	human chorionic gonadotropin
CML	chronic myelogenous leukemia	HCL	hydrochloric acid
CNS	central nervous system	Hct	hematocrit (see crit)
CO_2	carbon dioxide	HCV	Hepatitis C Virus
COPD	chronic obstructive pulmonary disease	HDL	high density lipoprotein
		Hg	mercury
CPR	cardiopulmonary resuscitation	HIV	human immunodeficiency virus
crit	hematocrit (see HCT)	h/o	history of
C-section	cesarean section	H_2O	water
CSF	cerebrospinal fluid	h.s.	at bedtime (hora somni)
CT scan	computed tomography scan	hx	history
		ICU	intensive care unit
CVA	cerebrovascular accident (stroke)	IM	intramuscular
		IV	intravenous
CXR	chest x-ray	IVP	intravenous pyelogram
DIC	disseminated intravascular coagulation	K^+	potassium
		Kg	kilogram
diff	differential count of white blood cells	L	liter
		L	left
dil	dilute	Lat	lateral
DNA	deoxyribonucleic acid	LD/LDH	lactic dehydrogenase
DOB	date of birth	LDL	low density lipoprotein
Dx	diagnosis	LE	lupus erythematosus (lupus)
EBV	Epstein-Barr virus		
ECG	electrocardiogram	lymphs	lymphocytes
EEG	electroencephalogram	lytes	electrolytes
EKG	electrocardiogram	m	meter
ENT	ear, nose, and throat	MCH	mean corpuscular hemoglobin
Eos	eosinophils		
ER	emergency room	MCHC	mean corpuscular hemoglobin concentration
ESR	erythrocyte sedimentation rate (sed rate)	MCV	mean corpuscular volume
exc	excision	mets	metastases

continued

Table 4-6

Common Abbreviations *(continued)*

Abbreviation	Meaning	Abbreviation	Meaning
mg	milligram	PVC	premature ventricular contraction
Mg^{++}	magnesium		
MI	myocardial infarction	QNS,	quantity not sufficient
mL	milliliter	q.n.s.	
mm	millimeter	R	right
mono	monocyte	RA	rheumatoid arthritis
MRI	magnetic resonance imaging	RBC	red blood cell or red blood count (also rbc)
MS	multiple sclerosis	req	requisition
Na^+	sodium	RIA	radioimmunoassay
neg	negative	R/O	rule out
NG	nasogastric	RPR	rapid plasma reagin
NPO	nothing by mouth (nulla per os)	RT	respiratory therapy
		RR	recovery room
O_2	oxygen	Rx	prescription
OB	obstetrics	$\bar{s}$	without
O&P	ova and parasite	Sed rate	erythrocyte sedimentation rate (ESR)
OR	operating room		
oz	ounce	segs	segmented white blood cells
P	pulse; phosphorus		
Path	pathology	SGOT	serum glutamic-oxaloacetic transaminase (see AST)
p.c.	after meals		
Pco_2	pressure of carbon dioxide in the blood		
		SGPT	serum glutamic-pyruvic transaminase (see ALT)
Peds	pediatrics		
pH	hydrogen ion concentration (measure of acidity or alkalinity)	SLE	systemic lupus erythematosus
		SMAC	sequential multiple analyzer computerized
PKU	phenylketonuria		
PMNs	polymorphonuclear leukocytes	sol	solution
		Staph	staphylococcus
PO_2	pressure of oxygen in the blood	STAT, stat	immediately (statum)
		STD	sexually transmitted disease
p/o	postoperative		
p.o.	orally (per os)	Strep	streptococcus
polys	polymorphonuclear leukocytes	Sx	symptoms
		T	temperature
pos	positive	T_3	triiodothyronine (a thyroid hormone)
post-op	after operation		
PP	after a meal (postprandial)	T_4	thyroxine (a thyroid hormone)
PPD	purified protein derivative (TB test)		
		TB	tuberculosis
pre-op	before operation	T cells	lymphocytes from the thymus
prep	prepare for		
PRN, prn	as necessary (pro re nata)	T & C	type and crossmatch (type & x)
PT	prothrombin time/protime		
PTT	partial thromboplastin time	TIBC	total iron binding capacity
		TPN	total parenteral nutrition (intravenous feeding)
pt	patient		

continued

Table 4-6

Common Abbreviations (continued)

Abbreviation	Meaning	Abbreviation	Meaning
TPR	temperature, pulse, and respiration	UV	ultraviolet
		VCU	voiding cystourethrogram
Trig	triglycerides	VD	venereal disease
TSH	thyroid stimulating hormone	VDRL	venereal disease research laboratory
Tx	treatment	W̶	water reactive
U	unit	WBC, wbc	white blood cell
UA, ua	urinalysis	wd	wound
URI	upper respiratory infection	WT, wt	weight
UTI	urinary tract infection	y/o	years old

Table 4-7

Common Symbols

Symbol	Meaning	Symbol	Meaning
α	alpha	$>$	greater than
β	beta	$\geq$	equal to or greater than
δ	delta	$\pm$	plus or minus, positive or negative
γ	gamma		
λ	lamda	®	registered trademark
∞	infinity	TM	trademark
μ	micro	#	number, pound
μm	micron	%	percent
μg	microgram	Δ	heat
+	plus, positive	♀	female
−	minus, negative	♂	male
=	equals	↑	increase
<	less than	↓	decrease
≤	equal to or less than		

STUDY & REVIEW QUESTIONS

1. Which part of gastr/o/enter/o/logy is the suffix?
   a. enter   b. gastr   √ c. logy   d. o

2. Of the following word parts, which is a prefix?
   a. arthro   b. emia   √ c. hyper   d. oste

3. To what part of the body does the word root "hepat" refer?
   a. Head   b. Heart   √ c. Liver   d. Stomach

4. What does the suffix "-algia" mean?
   a. Between   b. Condition   c. Disease   √ d. Pain

5. The pleural form of atrium is
   a. atri.   √ b. atria.   c. atrial.   d. atrices.

6. The singular form of the term phalanges is
   a. phalanis.   b. phalanum.   c. phalanus.   √ d. phalanx.

7. The medical term for red blood cell is
   √ a. erythrocyte.   b. hepatocyte.   c. leukocyte.   d. thrombocyte.

8. Which of the following means "inflammation of a vein?"
   a. Phlebectomy   √ b. Phlebitis   c. Phlebotomize   d. Phlebotomy

9. In which of the following terms is the "g" pronounced like a "j"?
   a. Gamete   b. Gastric   √ c. Genetic   d. Goiter

10. The "e" is pronounced separately in
    a. diastole.   b. syncope.   c. systole.   √ d. all the above.

11. The abbreviation CBC stands for
    a. calculated blood count.   c. chemical bilirubin concentration.
    b. cardiac basal calculation.   √ d. complete blood count.

12. The abbreviation NPO means
    a. negative patient outcome.   c. no parenteral output.
    b. new patients only .   √ d. nothing by mouth.

Bibliography and Suggested Readings

Cohen, B. J. (1997). *Medical terminology: An illustrated guide* (3rd ed.). Philadelphia: J. B. Lippincott.
Thomas, C. (1002). *Taber's cyclopedic medical dictionary* (19th ed.). Philadelphia: F. A. Davis.

5

HUMAN ANATOMY AND PHYSIOLOGY REVIEW

KEY TERMS

alveoli

anabolism

anatomic position

anatomy

anterior

avascular

body cavities

body plane

catabolism

diaphragm

distal

dorsal cavities

frontal plane

homeostasis

inferior

meninges

metabolism

mitosis

nephron

phalanges

physiology

prone/pronation

proximal

sagittal plane

superior

supine/supination

surfactant

transverse plane

ventral cavities

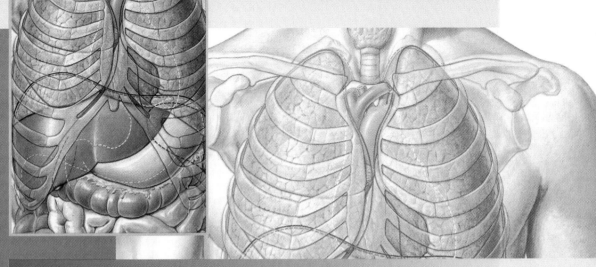

Upon successful completion of this chapter, the reader will be able to:

1 Define the key terms and abbreviations listed at the beginning of this chapter.
2 Identify and describe body positions, planes, cavities, and directional terms
3 Define homeostasis and the primary processes of metabolism.
4 Identify and describe structural components of cells and the four basic types of body tissue.
5 Describe the function and identify the components or major structures of each body system.
6 List disorders and diagnostic tests commonly associated with each body system.

INTRODUCTION

The human body is a wonder, consisting of more than 30 trillion cells, 206 bones, 700 muscles, approximately 5 liters of blood, and around 25 miles of blood vessels. To fully appreciate the workings of this wonder, it is necessary to have a basic understanding of human **anatomy** (structural composition) and **physiology** (function). Knowledge of human anatomy and physiology is also needed to understand fully the nature of the various disorders of the body and the rationale for the laboratory tests associated with them.

ANATOMIC POSITION

A person in the **anatomic position** is standing erect, arms at the side, with eyes and palms facing forward. When describing the direction or the location of a given point of the body, medical personnel normally refer to the body as if the patient is in the anatomic position, regardless of actual body position.

OTHER BODY POSITIONS

Two other body positions of particular importance to a blood drawer are **supine,** in which the patient is lying horizontal on the back with the face up, and **prone,** the opposite of supine, in which the patient is lying face down. The term prone also describes the hand with the palm facing down, a position sometimes used during blood collection.

 Key Point ➤ The act of turning the hand so that the palm faces down is called **pronation.** The act of turning the palm to face upward is called **supination.**

Memory Jogger ➤ A way to equate supine with lying down is to think of the *ine* as in *recline.* To remember that a person who is supine is *face up,* look for the word *up* in supine.

BODY PLANES

A **body plane** (Fig. 5-1) is a flat surface resulting from a real or imaginary cut through a body in the normal anatomic position. Areas of the body are often referred to according to their location with respect to one of the following body planes: frontal, sagittal, or transverse.

The **frontal** (or **coronal**) **plane** divides the body vertically into front and back portions.

The **sagittal plane** divides the body vertically into right and left portions. A vertical division resulting in equal right and left portions is called a **midsagittal** (or **medial**) **plane.**

The **transverse plane** divides the body horizontally into upper and lower portions. A procedure called **computerized axial tomography (CT** or **CAT scan)** produces an x-ray in a transverse plane of the body. **Magnetic resonance imaging (MRI)** can produce images of the body in all three planes using magnetic waves instead of x-rays.

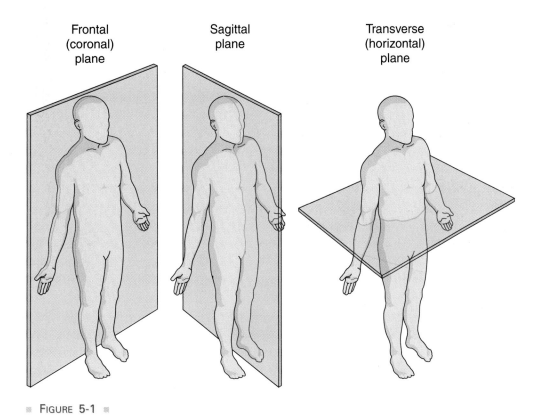

■ FIGURE 5-1 ■

Body planes. (Used with permission from Cohen, B. J. & Wood, D. L. (2000). *Memmler's structure and function of the human body* (7th ed.). Philadelphia: Lippincott Williams & Wilkins, p. 7.)

BODY DIRECTIONAL TERMS

Areas of the body are also identified using **directional terms** (Fig. 5-2). Directional terms describe the relationship of an area or part of the body with respect to the rest of the body or body part. Directional terms are often paired with a term that means the opposite. Table 5-1 lists common paired directional terms.

 Key Point ➤ Directional terms are relative positions in respect to other parts of the body. For example, the ankle can be described as distal to the knee and proximal to the foot.

BODY CAVITIES

Various organs of the body are housed in large, hollow spaces called **body cavities** (Fig. 5-3). Body cavities are divided into two groups, dorsal and ventral, according to their location within the body.

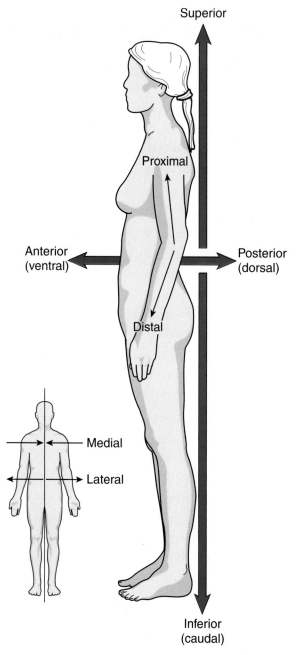

■ FIGURE 5-2 ■

Directional terms. (Used with permission from Cohen, B. J. & Wood, D. L. *Memmler's structure and function of the human body* (7th ed.). Philadelphia: Lippincott Williams & Wilkins, p. 6.)

Table 5-1

Common Paired Directional Terms

Anterior (ventral) refers to the front. **Posterior (dorsal)** refers to the back.
External (superficial) means on or near the surface of the body. **Internal (deep)** means
within or near the center of the body.
Medial means toward the midline or middle. **Lateral** means toward the side.
Palmar concerns the palm of the hand. **Plantar** concerns the sole of the foot.
Proximal means nearest to the center of the body, origin, or point of attachment. **Distal**
means farthest from the center of the body, origin, or point of attachment.
Superior (cranial) means higher, or above or toward the head. **Inferior (caudal)** means
beneath, or lower or away from the head.

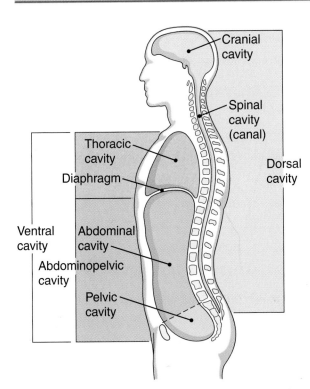

■ FIGURE 5-3 ■

Body cavities. (Used with permission
from Cohen, B. J. & Wood, D. L. *Memmler's
structure and function of the human body*
(7th ed.). Philadelphia: Lippincott Williams &
Wilkins, p. 8.)

Dorsal cavities are located in the back of the body and include the **cranial cavity,**
which houses the brain, and the **spinal cavity,** which encases the spinal cord.

Ventral cavities are located in the front of the body and include the **thoracic cavity,** which houses primarily the heart and lungs; the **abdominal cavity,** which houses
numerous organs including the stomach, liver, pancreas, gallbladder, spleen, and kidneys; and the **pelvic cavity,** which houses primarily the urinary bladder, and reproductive organs.

Key Point ➤ The thoracic cavity is separated from the abdominal cavity by a muscle called the **diaphragm.**

BODY FUNCTIONS

Homeostasis

The human body constantly strives to maintain its internal environment in a state of equilibrium or balance. This balanced or "steady state" condition is called **homeostasis** (ho'me-o-sta'sis), which literally translated means "standing the same." The body maintains homeostasis by compensating for changes in a process that involves feedback and regulation in response to internal and external changes.

Metabolism

Metabolism (me-tab'o-lizm) is the sum of all the physical and chemical reactions necessary to sustain life. There are two primary processes of metabolism: catabolism and anabolism.

Catabolism (kah-tab'o-lizm) is a destructive process by which complex substances are broken down into simple substances, usually with the release of energy. An example is the conversion of carbohydrates in food into the glucose needed by the cells, and the subsequent glycolysis or breakdown of glucose by the cell to produce energy.

Memory Jogger ➤ A way to equate catabolism with breakdown is to remember that it begins with *cat* just like *catastrophe*. When something (your car, for example) breaks down, you often think of it as a catastrophe.

Anabolism (ah-nab'o-lizm) is a constructive process by which the body converts simple compounds into complex substances needed to carry out the cellular activities of the body. An example is the body's ability use simple substances provided by the blood stream to synthesize or create a hormone.

BODY ORGANIZATION

Cells

The cell (Fig. 5-4) is the basic structural unit of all life. The human body consists of trillions of cells, responsible for all the activities of the body. There are many categories of cells, and each category is specialized to perform a unique function. No matter what their function, all cells have the same basic structural components.

All cells have an outer covering called a **cell membrane** that has the selective capability of allowing certain substances in and out of the cell. The fluid that fills the cell is called **cytoplasm.** Within the cytoplasm are structures called organelles. They are the **centrioles,** which function during cell division; **endoplasmic reticulum,** a network of tubules that transport proteins and synthesize lipids; **Golgi apparatus,**

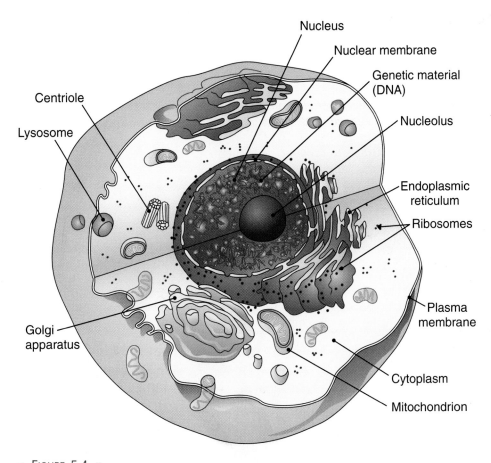

Nucleus

Nuclear membrane

Genetic material
(DNA)

Nucleolus

Endoplasmic
reticulum

Ribosomes

Plasma
membrane

Cytoplasm

Mitochondrion

Centriole

Lysosome

Golgi
apparatus

■ FIGURE 5-4 ■

Cell diagram. (Used with permission from Cohen, B. J. & Wood, D. L. *Memmler's structure and function of the human body* (7th ed.). Philadelphia: Lippincott Williams & Wilkins, p. 29.)

which is thought to play a role in storing protein substances such as secretory products; **lysosomes,** which contain enzymes that play a role in digestive processes that take place within the cell; **mitochondria,** which play a role in energy production; and **ribosomes,** which play a role in assembling proteins from amino acids. Most cells (red blood cells are a major exception) contain a nucleus surrounded by its own membrane. The **nucleus** is the command center of the cell. It contains the chromosomes or genetic material governing all the activities of the cell, including reproduction. Chromosomes are composed of long strands of DNA (deoxyribonucleic acid) organized into separate units called genes. Chromosomes occur in identical pairs. Humans have 23 pairs (46 individual) chromosomes. Most cells are able to duplicate themselves, which allows the body to grow, repair, and reproduce itself. When a cell duplicates itself, the DNA doubles and the cell divides by a process called **mitosis** (mi-to'sis).

Tissues

Tissues are groups of similar cells that work together to perform a special function. There are four basic tissue types:

1. **Connective** tissue supports and connects all parts of the body and includes adipose (fat) tissue, cartilage, bone, and blood.
2. **Epithelial** (ep-i-the'le-al) tissue covers and protects the body and lines organs, vessels, and cavities.
3. **Muscle** tissue contracts to produce movement.
4. **Nerve** tissue has the ability to transmit electrical impulses.

Organs

Organs are structures composed of tissues that function together for a common purpose.

BODY SYSTEMS

Body systems are structures and organs that are related to one another and function together. The following are 9 of 10 commonly recognized body systems. The tenth system, the circulatory system, is discussed in detail in Chapter 6.

Skeletal System

Functions

The skeletal system (Fig. 5-5) is the framework that gives the body shape and support, protects internal organs, and, along with the muscular system, provides movement and leverage. It is also responsible for calcium storage and **hemopoiesis** (he'mopoy-e'sis), also called **hematopoiesis** (hem'a-to-poy-e'sis), which is the production of blood cells that normally occurs in the bone marrow.

Structures

The skeletal system comprises all the bones (206) and joints of the body along with the connective tissue that form the body framework referred to as the skeleton. Skeletal bones are categorized by shape into four groups as shown in Table 5-2.

 Key Point ➤ Bones of particular importance in blood collection are the distal phalanx of the finger and the calcaneus or heel bone of the foot.

Skeletal System Disorders

- Arthritis (ar-thri'tis): a common joint disorder characterized by inflammation, usually accompanied by pain and swelling.
- Bursitis (bur-si'tis): inflammation of the fluid-filled sac (bursa) between muscle attachments and bone.

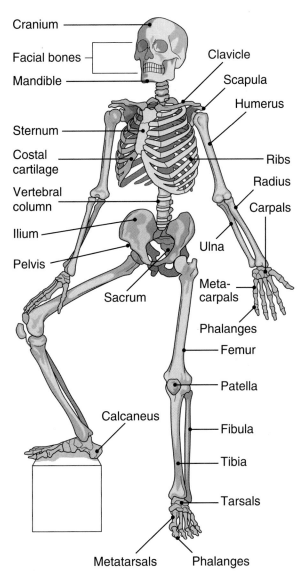

Cranium

Facial bones

Mandible

Sternum

Costal cartilage

Vertebral column

Ilium

Pelvis

Sacrum

Calcaneus

Metatarsals

Clavicle

Scapula

Humerus

Ribs

Radius

Carpals

Ulna

Meta-carpals

Phalanges

Femur

Patella

Fibula

Tibia

Tarsals

Phalanges

■ FIGURE 5-5 ■

Human skeleton. (Used with permission from Cohen, B. J. & Wood, D. L. *Memmler's structure and function of the human body* (7th ed.). Philadelphia: Lippincott Williams & Wilkins, p. 66.)

Table 5-2

Categories of Bones

Flat bones such as rib and most skull (cranial) bones
Irregular bones such as back bones (vertebrae) and some facial bones
Long bones such as leg (femur, tibia, fibula), arm (humerus, radius, ulna), and hand bones (metacarpals and phalanges)
Short bones such as wrist (carpals) and ankle bones (tarsals)

- Gout (gowt): a disorder of the joints (most commonly those of the feet), caused by faulty uric acid metabolism. It is a form of arthritis.
- Osteomyelitis (os'te-o-mi'el-i'tis): inflammation of the bone, especially the bone marrow, caused by bacterial infection.
- Osteochondritis (os'te-o-kon-dri'tis): inflammation of the bone and cartilage.
- Osteoporosis (os'te-o-por-o'sis): disorder involving loss of bone density.
- Rickets (rik'ets): abnormal bone formation indirectly resulting from lack of vitamin D, which is necessary for calcium absorption.
- Tumors: abnormal bone growth.

Diagnostic Tests

- Alkaline phosphatase
- Calcium
- Complete blood count (CBC)
- Erythrocyte sedimentation rate
- Phosphorus
- Synovial fluid analysis
- Uric acid
- Vitamin D

Muscular System

Functions

The muscular system gives the body the ability to move, maintain posture, and produce heat. It also plays a role in organ function and blood circulation.

 Key Point ➤ Skeletal muscle movement helps keep blood moving through your veins. For example, moving your arms helps move blood from your fingertips back to your heart.

Structures

The muscular system comprises all the muscles of the body. It includes not only those attached to the skeletal system, but also those that form the walls of the heart and those that line the walls of blood vessels and the digestive tract. Muscles are classified (Table 5-3) according to their location, their **histologic** (microscopic) structure, and how they are controlled.

Muscular System Disorders

- Atrophy (at'ro-fe): a decrease in size (wasting) of a muscle usually resulting from inactivity.
- Muscular dystrophy (dis'tro-fe): a genetic disease in which the muscles waste away or atrophy.

Table 5-3

Types of Muscles

Skeletal muscle is attached to bone, has **striated** (stri'a-ted) or banded muscle fibers, and is under **voluntary** (conscious) control.

Visceral (vis'er-al) **muscle** lines the walls of blood vessels and most internal organs, is **non-striated,** and is under **involuntary** or unconscious control. Visceral muscle is often called **smooth** muscle.

Cardiac muscle forms the wall of the heart, is a special kind of **striated** muscle, and is under **involuntary** control.

- Myalgia (mi-al'je-ah): painful muscle.
- Tendinitis (ten'di-ni'tis): inflammation of muscle tendons usually resulting from overexertion.

Diagnostic Tests

- Autoimmune antibodies
- Creatine phosphokinase (CPK/CK)
- CPK/CK isoenzymes
- Lactic acid
- Lactic dehydrogenase
- Myoglobin
- Electromyography

Reproductive System

Functions

The reproductive system (Fig. 5-6) produces the **gametes** (gam'eets), or **sex cells,** that are needed to form a new human being. In males, the gametes are called **spermatozoa** (sper'mat-o-zo'a), or sperm. In females, the gametes are called **ova** (o'va), or eggs. Reproduction occurs when an **ovum** (singular of ova) is fertilized by a sperm.

Structures

The reproductive system consists of glands called **gonads** (go'nads) and their associated structures and ducts. The gonads manufacture and store the gametes and produce hormones (see Endocrine System section in this chapter) that regulate the reproductive process.

Structures of the female reproductive system include the **ovaries** (female gonads), **fallopian** (fa-lo'pe-an) **tubes, uterus, cervix, vagina,** and **vulva.**

Key Point ➤ The PAP smear is a procedure used to diagnose cervical cancer. It is named after Dr. George Papanicolaou, who developed the technique.

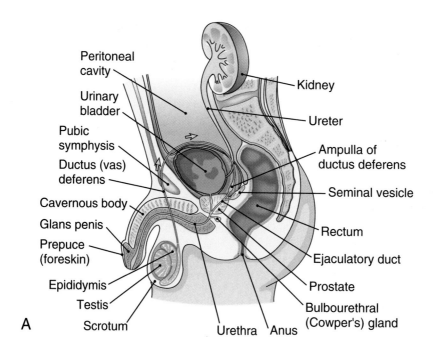

Peritoneal cavity
Kidney
Urinary bladder
Ureter
Pubic symphysis
Ampulla of ductus deferens
Ductus (vas) deferens
Seminal vesicle
Cavernous body
Glans penis
Rectum
Prepuce (foreskin)
Ejaculatory duct
Epididymis
Prostate
Testis
Bulbourethral (Cowper's) gland
Scrotum
Urethra Anus

A

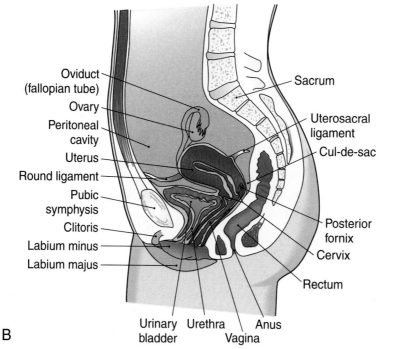

Oviduct (fallopian tube)
Sacrum
Ovary
Peritoneal cavity
Uterosacral ligament
Uterus
Cul-de-sac
Round ligament
Pubic symphysis
Clitoris
Posterior fornix
Labium minus
Cervix
Labium majus
Rectum

Urinary bladder Urethra Anus
Vagina

B

FIGURE 5-6

Reproductive system. (A) Male. (B) Female. (Used with permission from Cohen, B. J. & Wood, D. L. *Memmler's structure and function of the human body* (7th ed.). Philadelphia: Lippincott Williams & Wilkins, pp. 314, 321.)

Structures of the male reproductive system include the **testes** (male gonads), **seminal vesicles, prostate, epididymis** (ep'i-did'i-mis), **vas deferens** (vas def'er-enz), **seminal ducts, urethra, penis, spermatic cords,** and **scrotum.**

Reproductive System Disorders

- Cervical cancer: cancer of the cervix.
- Infertility: a lower than normal ability to reproduce.
- Ovarian cancer: cancer of the ovaries.
- Ovarian cyst: a usually nonmalignant growth in an ovary.
- Prostate cancer: cancer of the prostate gland.
- Sexually transmitted diseases (STDs), diseases such as syphilis, gonorrhea, and genital herpes, which are usually transmitted by sexual contact.
- Uterine cancer: cancer of the uterus.

Diagnostic Tests

- Acid phosphatase
- Estrogen
- Follicle-stimulating hormone (FSH)
- Human chorionic gonadotropin (HCG)
- Luteinizing hormone (LH)
- Microbiologic cultures
- PAP smear
- Prostate-specific antigen (PSA)
- Rapid plasmin reagin (RPR)
- Testosterone
- Viral tissue studies

Digestive System

Functions

The digestive system (Fig. 5-7) provides the means by which the body takes in food, breaks it down into usable components for absorption, and eliminates waste products.

Structures

The digestive system components form a continuous passageway called the **digestive tract** or **gastrointestinal (GI) tract** that extends from the mouth to the anus. GI tract components include the **mouth, pharynx, throat, esophagus, stomach,** and **small and large intestines.**

Key Point ➤ Some stomach ulcers are found to be caused by the *Helicobacter pylori* microorganism and are now treated with antibiotics in addition to antacids.

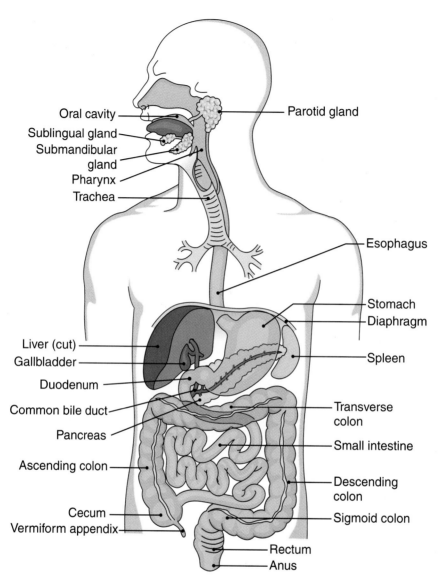

■ FIGURE 5-7 ■

Digestive system. (Used with permission from Cohen, B. J. & Wood, D. L. *Memmler's structure and function of the human body* (7th ed.). Philadelphia: Lippincott Williams & Wilkins, p. 265.)

Accessory Organs and Structures

The digestive system also includes and is assisted by a number of accessory organs and structures: **lips, teeth, tongue, salivary glands, liver, pancreas,** and **gallbladder.**

Accessory Organ Functions

Important digestive functions of the liver include glycogen storage, protein catabolism, the detoxification of harmful substances, and the secretion of bile necessary for the digestion of fat. Bile is concentrated and stored in the gallbladder. Digestive functions of the pancreas include the secretion of insulin and glucagon and the production of digestive enzymes, including amylase, lipase, and trypsin.

Digestive System Disorders

- Appendicitis (a-pen′di-si′tis): inflammation of the appendix.
- Cholecystitis (ko′le-sis-ti′tis): inflammation of the gallbladder.
- Colitis (ko-li′tis): inflammation of the colon.
- Diverticulosis (di′ver-tik′u-lo′sis): pouches in the walls of the colon.
- Gastritis (gas-tri′tis): inflammation of the stomach lining.
- Gastroenteritis (gas′tro-en-ter-i′tis): inflammation of the stomach and intestinal tract.
- Hepatitis (hep′a-ti′tis): inflammation of the liver.
- Pancreatitis (pan′kre-a-ti′tis): inflammation of the pancreas.
- Peritonitis (per′i-to-ni′tis): inflammation of the abdominal cavity lining.
- Ulcer: open sore or lesion.

Diagnostic Tests

Gastrointestinal

- Fecal fat
- Gastric analysis
- Occult blood
- Ova and parasites (O & P)
- Serum gastrin analysis
- Stool analysis

Accessory Organ

- Ammonia
- Amylase
- Bilirubin (bili)
- Carcinoembryonic antigen (CEA)
- Carotene
- Cholesterol
- CBC
- Glucose
- Glucose tolerance test (GTT)
- Lipase
- Triglycerides

Endocrine System

Functions

The word **endocrine** comes from the Greek words *endon,* meaning *"within"* and *"krinein,"* meaning *"to secrete."* The endocrine system (Fig. 5-8) consists of a group of ductless glands that secrete substances called hormones directly into the blood stream. Hormones are powerful chemical substances that have a profound effect on many body processes such as metabolism, growth and development, reproduction, personality, and the ability of the body to react to stress and resist disease.

Structures

Endocrine system structures include the various hormone-secreting glands and other organs and structures that have endocrine function. Table 5-4 lists the various hormone-secreting glands, organs and structures, their location in the body, the major hormones they secrete, and the principal function of each hormone.

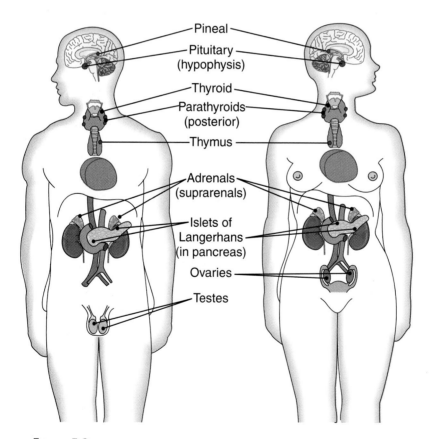

Pineal
Pituitary (hypophysis)
Thyroid
Parathyroids (posterior)
Thymus
Adrenals (suprarenals)
Islets of Langerhans (in pancreas)
Ovaries
Testes

■ FIGURE 5-8 ■

Endocrine glands. (Used with permission from Cohen, B. J. & Wood, D. L. *Memmler's structure and function of the human body* (7th ed.). Philadelphia: Lippincott Williams & Wilkins, p. 166.)

Table 5-4

Endocrine Glands

Gland	Location	Hormones Produced	Hormone Function
Pituitary (pi-tu′i-tar-ee)	Brain	Adrenocorticotropic (ad-re′no-kor′ti-ko-trop′ik) hormone (ACTH)	Stimulates the adrenal glands
		Antidiuretic (an′ti-di-u-ret′ik) hormone (ADH)	Decreases urine production
		Follicle-stimulating hormone (FSH)	Stimulates the development of ova and sperm and the secretion of estrogen in females.
		Growth hormone (GH)	Regulates growth
		Thyroid (thi′royd)-stimulating hormone (TSH)	Controls thyroid activity
Pineal (pin′eal)	In the brain, posterior to the pituitary	Melatonin	Helps set **diurnal** (daily) **rhythm** with levels lowest around noon and peaking at night
Thyroid (thi′royd)	In the throat near the larynx	Calcitonin (kal′si-to′nin)	Regulates the amount of calcium in the blood
		Triiodothyronine (tri-i-o-do-thi′ ro-nin) or T$_3$	Increases metabolic rate
		Thyroxine (thi-roks′in) or T$_4$	Increases metabolic rate
Parathyroid (par-a-thi′royd)	Behind the thyroid gland, two on each side	Parathyroid hormone (PTH)	Regulates calcium and phosphorous metabolism
Thymus (thi′mus)	Located in the chest behind the sternum (breastbone)	Thymosin (thi′mo-sin)	Necessary for the maturation of **T-lymphocytes** (specialized white blood cells) and the development of immunity
Adrenals	One located on top of each kidney	Epinephrine (ep-i-nef′rin) also called adrenalin (a-dren′a-lin)	Increases blood pressure, heart activity, metabolism, and release of glucose
		Norepinephrine, also called noradrenaline	Increases blood pressure, heart activity, metabolism, and release of glucose
		Cortisol (kor′ti-sol)	Suppresses inflammation
		Aldosterone (al-dos′ter-on)	Helps the kidneys regulate sodium and potassium in the blood stream

continued

Table 5-4

Endocrine Glands *(continued)*			
Gland	**Location**	**Hormones Produced**	**Hormone Function**
Islets (i'lets) of Langerhans (lahng'er-hanz)	Pancreas	Insulin	Necessary for the normal movement of glucose from the blood into the cells
		Glucagon (gloo'ka-gon)	Stimulates the liver to release glucose (stored as glycogen) into the blood stream
Testes	Scrotum	Testosterone (tes-tos'ter-on)	Growth and functioning of the male reproductive system and development of male sexual characteristics
Ovaries	Pelvic cavity	Estrogen (es'tro-jen) Progesterone (pro-jes'-ter-on)	Growth and functioning of the female reproductive system and development of female sexual characteristics. Prepares the body for pregnancy

ENDOCRINE GLANDS

The **pituitary** (pi-tu'i-tar-ee) gland is often called the master gland because it secretes hormones that stimulate other glands. Examples are **follicle** (fol'i-kle)**-stimulating hormone (FSH),** which affects the ovaries, and **thyroid** (thi'royd)**-stimulating hormone (TSH),** which affects thyroid activity.

The **pineal** (pin'e-al) function is not yet fully understood; however, it is known to play a role in biorhythms, seasonal affective disorder, and the sleep-wake cycle.

Key Point ➤ Travelers sometimes take melatonin (see Table 5-4) pills to help overcome the effects of jet lag brought on by crossing through different time zones.

The **thyroid** gland secretes hormones that increase metabolism and regulate the amount of calcium in the blood. Production of thyroid hormones requires the presence of adequate amounts of iodine in the blood.

Key Point ➤ Iodine was first added to salt to prevent goiter, an enlargement of the thyroid gland sometimes caused by a lack of iodine in the diet.

Four **parathyroid** (par-a-thi'royd) glands regulate calcium and phosphorous metabolism.

The **thymus** (thi'mus) gland secretes hormones that are necessary for the development of immunity and is most active before birth and during childhood.

Two **adrenal** (ad-re'nal) glands secrete numerous hormones. Some affect the body when under stress, some play a role in kidney function, and others have the ability to suppress inflammation.

 Key Point ➤ Adrenaline and noradrenaline are known as the "fight" or "flight" hormones because of their effects when the body is under stress. They act by increasing blood pressure, heart activity, metabolism, and release of glucose, permitting the body to do an extraordinary amount of work.

OTHER ORGANS AND STRUCTURES WITH ENDOCRINE FUNCTION

Other organs with endocrine function include the pancreas, the testes, and ovaries.

 Key Point ➤ **Islets** (i'lets) **of Langerhans** (lahng'er-hanz) in the pancreas secrete **insulin,** which is necessary for the normal movement of glucose from the blood into the cells. However, Islet cells also secrete **glucagon** (gloo'ka-gon), which counterbalances the effect of insulin by increasing blood glucose levels and preventing hypoglycemia (low blood sugar).

Other structures with endocrine function include the lining of the stomach, which secretes a hormone that stimulates digestion, the placenta, which secretes several hormones that function during pregnancy, and the kidneys, which secrete renin, which increases blood pressure, and erythropoietin (e-rith'ro-poy'e-tin), which stimulates red blood cell production.

 Key Point ➤ Pregnancy tests are based on a reaction with a hormone called **human chorionic** (ko-re-on'ik) **gonadotropin** (gon-ah-do-tro'pin) **(HCG)** secreted by embryonic cells that eventually give rise to the placenta.

Endocrine System Disorders

Endocrine disorders are most commonly caused by tumors, which can cause either **hypersecretion** (secreting too much) or **hyposecretion** (secreting too little) of the gland.

PITUITARY DISORDERS

- Acromegaly (ak'ro-meg'a-le): the overgrowth of the bones in the hands, feet, and face caused by excessive GH in adulthood.
- Diabetes insipidus (di'a-be'tez in-sip'id-us): a condition characterized by increased thirst and increased urine production caused by inadequate secretion of antidiuretic hormone (ADH), also called **vasopressin** (vas'o-pres'in).
- Dwarfism: the condition of being abnormally small, one cause of which is growth hormone (GH) deficiency in infancy.
- Gigantism: excessive development of the body or of a body part resulting from excessive GH.

THYROID DISORDERS

- Congenital hypothyroidism: insufficient thyroid activity in a newborn, either from a genetic deficiency or maternal factors such as lack of dietary iron during pregnancy.
- Cretinism: severe, untreated congenital hypothyroidism in which the development of the child is impaired, resulting in a short, disproportionate body, thick tongue and neck, and mental handicap.
- Goiter (goy'ter): an enlargement of the thyroid gland.
- Hyperthyroidism (Graves' disease): a condition characterized by weight loss, nervousness, and protruding eyeballs, resulting from an increased metabolic rate caused by excessive secretion of the thyroid gland.
- Hypothyroidism: a condition characterized by weight gain and lethargy resulting from a decreased metabolic rate caused by decreased thyroid secretion.
- Myxedema (hypothyroid syndrome): a condition characterized by anemia, slow speech, mental apathy, drowsiness, and sensitivity to cold resulting from decreased functioning of the thyroid gland.

PARATHYROID DISORDERS

Hypersecretion of the parathyroids can lead to kidney stones and bone destruction. Hyposecretion can cause muscle spasms and convulsions.

ADRENAL DISORDERS

- Addison's disease: a condition characterized by weight loss, dehydration, and hypotension (abnormally low blood pressure) caused by decreased glucose and sodium levels resulting from hyposecretion of the adrenal glands.
- Aldosteronism: a condition characterized by hypertension (high blood pressure) and edema caused by excessive sodium and water retention resulting from hypersecretion of aldosterone.
- Cushing's syndrome: a condition characterized by a swollen, "moon-shaped" face and redistribution of fat to the abdomen and back of the neck caused by an excess of cortisone.

PANCREATIC DISORDERS

- Diabetes mellitus: a condition in which there is impaired carbohydrate, fat, and protein metabolism resulting from a deficiency of insulin.
- Diabetes mellitus type I or insulin-dependent diabetes mellitus: a type of diabetes mellitus in which the body is totally unable to produce insulin. This type is often called juvenile-onset diabetes because it usually appears before 25 years of age.
- Diabetes mellitus type II or noninsulin-dependent diabetes mellitus: a type of diabetes mellitus in which the body is able to produce insulin, but either the amount produced is insufficient or there is impaired use of the insulin produced. This type of diabetes occurs predominantly in adults.
- Hyperinsulinism: a condition in which there is too much insulin in the blood resulting from excessive secretion of insulin or an overdose of insulin (insulin shock).
- Hypoglycemia (hi'po-gli-se'me-a): a condition in which the glucose (blood sugar) is abnormally low resulting from hyperinsulinism.

Diagnostic Tests

- Adrenocorticotropic hormone (ACTH)
- Aldosterone
- Antidiuretic hormone (ADH)
- Cortisol
- Erythropoietin
- Glucagon
- Glucose tolerance test (GTT)
- Glycosylated hemoglobin
- Growth hormone (GH)
- Insulin level
- Renin
- Thyroid function studies (triiodothyronine [T_3], thyroxine [T_4], thyroid stimulating hormone [TSH])

Nervous System

Functions

The nervous system (Fig. 5-9, *A*) controls and coordinates activities of the various body systems by means of electrical impulses and chemical substances sent to and received from all parts of the body.

Structures

The fundamental unit of the nervous system is the **nerve cell** or **neuron** (Fig. 5-9, *B*). Neurons are highly complex cells that are capable of conducting messages in the form of impulses that enable the body to interact with its internal and external environment. There are two main structural divisions of the nervous system, the **central nervous system (CNS)** and the **peripheral nervous system (PNS).**

CENTRAL NERVOUS SYSTEM

The **central nervous system** consists of the **brain** and **spinal cord,** both of which are completely enclosed and protected by three layers of connective tissue called the **meninges** (me-nin'jez). The brain and spinal cord are surrounded, cushioned, and separated from the meninges by a space filled with a clear, plasma-like fluid called **cerebrospinal** (ser'e-bro-spi'nal) **fluid (CSF).** A physician uses a procedure called **lumbar** (spinal) **puncture** to obtain CSF when needed for laboratory testing.

 Key Point ➤ CSF is collected by inserting a hollow needle into the space between the third and forth lumbar vertebrae. There is no danger of injuring the cord with the needle, because the spinal cord ends at the first lumbar vertebra.

The CNS functions as command center of the nervous system by interpreting information and dictating responses. Every part of the body is in direct communication with

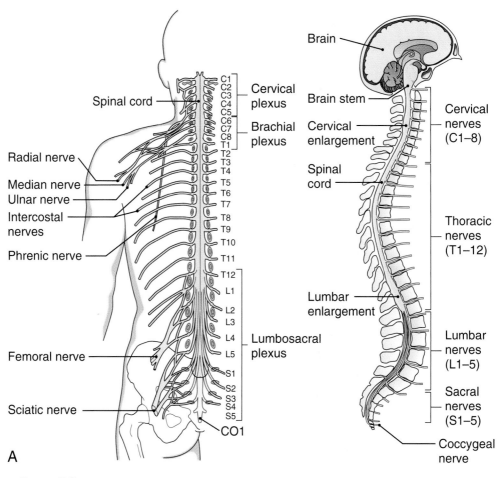

FIGURE 5-9

(*A*) Nervous system.

the CNS by means of its own set of nerves. All of these nerves come together in one large trunk that forms the spinal cord.

PERIPHERAL NERVOUS SYSTEM

The **PNS** consists of all the nerves that connect the CNS to every part of the body. Two functional divisions of the PNS are the **sensory** or **afferent** (a'fer-ent) **division** and the **motor** or **efferent** (ef'fer-ent) **division. Sensory nerves** carry impulses *to* the CNS from sensory receptors in various parts of the body. **Motor nerves** carry impulses *from* the CNS to organs, glands, and muscles.

The motor division can be further subdivided into the **somatic** (so-mat'ik) or **voluntary nervous system** and the **autonomic** (aw-to-nom'ik) or **involuntary ner-**

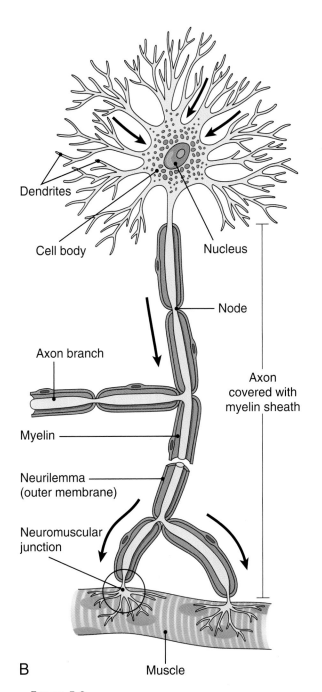

Dendrites

Cell body

Nucleus

Node

Axon branch

Axon
covered with
myelin sheath

Myelin

Neurilemma
(outer membrane)

Neuromuscular
junction

B

Muscle

■ FIGURE 5-9 ■

(*B*) Neuron. (Used with permission from Cohen, B. J. & Wood, D. L. *Memmler's structure and function of the human body* (7th ed.). Philadelphia: Lippincott Williams & Wilkins, pp. 114, 121.)

vous system (ANS). The somatic nervous system conducts impulses from the CNS that allow an individual to consciously control skeletal muscles. The ANS plays an important role in maintaining homeostasis by conducting impulses that affect involuntary activities of smooth muscle, cardiac muscle, and glands.

Disorders of the Nervous System

- Amyotrophic lateral sclerosis (ALS): a disease involving muscle weakness and atrophy resulting from degeneration of portions of the brain and spinal cord.
- Encephalitis: inflammation of the brain.
- Epilepsy: recurrent pattern of seizures.
- Hydrocephalus: accumulation of cerebrospinal fluid in the brain.
- Meningitis: inflammation of the membranes of the spinal cord or brain.
- Multiple sclerosis (MS): disease causing destruction of the myelin sheath (fat-like covering) of the nerves of the brain.
- Neuralgia (nu-ral'je-a): severe pain along a nerve.
- Parkinson's disease: chronic nervous disease characterized by fine muscle tremors and muscle weakness.
- Shingles: acute eruption of herpes blisters along the course of a peripheral nerve.

Diagnostic Tests

- Acetylcholine receptor antibody
- CSF analysis
    - Cell count
    - Glucose
    - Protein
    - Culture
- Cholinesterase
- Dilantin
- Electroencephalogram
- Serotonin

Urinary System

Functions

The urinary system (Fig. 5-10) filters waste products from the blood and eliminates them from the body. It also plays an important role in the regulation of body fluids. Activities of the urinary system result in the creation and elimination of urine.

Structures

The main structures of the urinary system are two kidneys, two ureters, a urinary bladder, and a urethra.

The **kidneys** are bean-shaped organs located at the back of the abdominal cavity, just above the waistline, one on each side of the body. The kidneys function to maintain water and electrolyte balance. **Electrolytes** include sodium, potassium, chloride, bicarbonate, and calcium ions and are essential to normal nerve, muscle, and heart activity. The

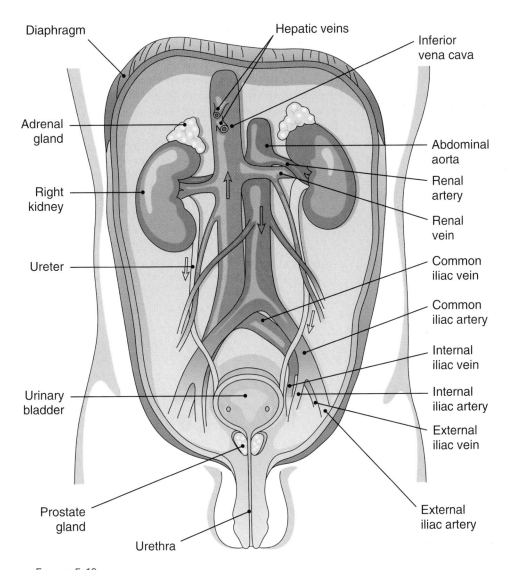

Diaphragm

Hepatic veins

Inferior
vena cava

Adrenal
gland

Abdominal
aorta

Renal
artery

Right
kidney

Renal
vein

Ureter

Common
iliac vein

Common
iliac artery

Internal
iliac vein

Urinary
bladder

Internal
iliac artery

External
iliac vein

Prostate
gland

External
iliac artery

Urethra

▣ FIGURE 5-10 ▣

Urinary system. (Used with permission from Cohen, B. J. & Wood, D. L. *Memmler's structure and function of the human body* (7th ed.). Philadelphia: Lippincott Williams & Wilkins, p. 294.)

kidneys also eliminate urea, a waste product of protein metabolism. In addition, the kidneys are responsible for the production of several hormones including erythropoietin.

The functional units of the kidneys are the **nephrons,** of which each kidney contains nearly a million. As blood travels through the nephrons, water and dissolved substances, including wastes, are filtered from the blood through a tuft of capillaries called the **glomerulus.** The resulting glomerular filtrate travels through other structures within the nephron, where water and essential amounts of substances such as sodium, potassium, and calcium are reabsorbed into the blood stream. The remaining filtrate is called urine.

A narrow, muscular tube called a **ureter** transports the urine from the kidney to the **urinary bladder.** The urinary bladder, located in the anterior portion of the pelvic cavity, is a muscular sac that acts as a reservoir for the urine. Urine is voided (emptied) from the bladder to the outside of the body through a single tube called the **urethra.**

 Key Point ➤ Blood creatinine is a measure of kidney function because creatinine is a waste product normally removed from the blood by the kidneys. If kidney function declines, creatinine accumulates in the blood.

Urinary System Disorders

- Renal failure: a sudden and severe impairment of renal function.
- Nephritis: inflammation of the kidneys.
- Uremia: impaired kidney function with a buildup of waste products in the blood.
- Kidney stones: uric acid, calcium phosphate, or oxalate stones in the kidneys, ureter, or bladder.
- Cystitis: bladder inflammation.
- Urinary tract infection (UTI): an infection involving the organs or ducts of the urinary system.

Diagnostic Tests

- Albumin
- Ammonia
- Blood urea nitrogen (BUN)
- Blood creatinine
- Creatinine clearance
- Electrolytes
- Osmolality
- Urinalysis
- Urine culture and sensitivity
- Intravenous pyelography
- Renal biopsy
- Nuclear magnetic resonance

Integumentary System

Functions

Integument (in-teg'u-ment) means "covering or "skin." The skin (Fig. 5-11), which is often referred to as the largest organ in the body, is a major part of the integumentary system and is the cover that protects the body from bacterial invasion, dehydration, and the harmful rays of the sun. It also functions in the regulation of body temperature, the elimination of small amounts of waste (through sweat), the reception of environmental stimuli (sensation of heat, cold, touch, and pain), and the manufacture of vitamin D from sunlight.

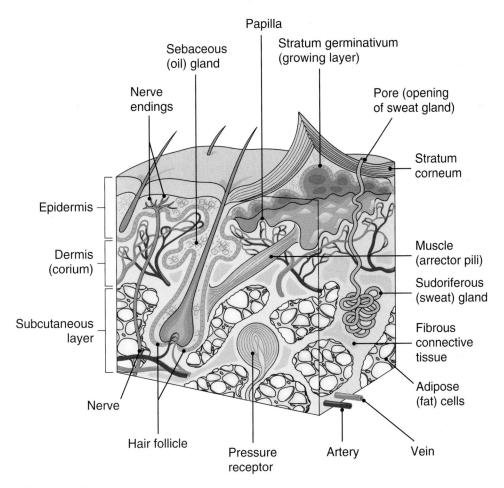

Papilla

Sebaceous
(oil) gland

Stratum germinativum
(growing layer)

Nerve
endings

Pore (opening
of sweat gland)

Stratum
corneum

Epidermis

Dermis
(corium)

Muscle
(arrector pili)

Sudoriferous
(sweat) gland

Subcutaneous
layer

Fibrous
connective
tissue

Adipose
(fat) cells

Nerve

Hair follicle

Pressure
receptor

Artery

Vein

FIGURE 5-11

Cross section of the skin. (Used with permission from Cohen, B. J. & Wood, D. L. *Memmler's structure and function of the human body* (7th ed.). Philadelphia: Lippincott Williams & Wilkins, p. 56.)

Structures

The integumentary system consists of the skin and associated structures referred to as appendages, which include oil and sweat glands, hair, and nails. It also includes blood vessels, nerves, and sensory organs within the skin.

Layers of the Skin

There are two main layers of the skin, the **epidermis** (ep′i-der′mis) and the **dermis.** They are connected to a layer of **subcutaneous tissue,** which connects the skin to surface muscles and bone.

EPIDERMIS

The epidermis is the outermost and thinnest layer of the skin. It is primarily made up of **stratified** (layered), **squamous** (scale-like) **epithelial** cells. The epidermis is **avascular,** meaning it contains no blood vessels. The only living cells of the epidermis are in its deepest layer, which is called the **stratum germinativum** (ger-mi-na-ti'vum). The stratum germinativum is the only layer of the skin where **mitosis** (cell division) occurs. It is also the layer where the skin pigment **melanin** is produced. The cells of the stratum germinativum are nourished by diffusion of nutrients from the dermis. As the cells divide they are pushed toward the surface where they gradually die from lack of nourishment and become **keratinized** (hardened), which helps thicken and protect the skin.

DERMIS

The **dermis,** also called **corium** or true skin, is the inner layer of the skin. It is much thicker than the epidermis and is composed of elastic and fibrous connective tissue.

Elevations called **papillae** (pa-pil'e) and resulting depressions in the dermis where it joins the epidermis give rise to the ridges and grooves that form fingerprints. This area is often referred to as the **papillary dermis.** The dermis contains blood and lymph vessels, nerves, **sebaceous** (se-ba'shus) and **sudoriferous** (su-dor-if'er-us) glands, and hair follicles. These structures can also extend into the subcutaneous layer.

SUBCUTANEOUS

The **subcutaneous** (under the skin) layer is composed of connective and adipose (fat) tissue that connects the skin to the surface of muscles.

Key Point ➤ Aging causes thinning of the epidermis, dermis, and subcutaneous. This makes the skin more translucent and fragile and leaves the blood vessels less well-protected. As a result the elderly bruise more easily.

Major Structures of the Skin

Hair follicles are the sheaths from which hair develops. Hair is nonliving and is primarily composed of **keratin** (ker'a-tin), a tough protein substance.

Nails are also nonliving and made of keratin. Nails grow continuously as new cells form from the nail root, located at the proximal end of the nail.

Sebaceous glands are connected to hair follicles. They are called oil glands because they secrete an oily substance called **sebum** (se'bum). Sebum helps lubricate the skin and hair and keeps them from drying out.

Sudoriferous glands, commonly called sweat glands, are coiled structures located in the dermis with ducts extending through the epidermis and ending in a pore on the surface of the skin. The sweat or perspiration produced by these glands is a mixture of water, salts, and waste.

Arrector pili are tiny, smooth muscles attached to hair follicles. These muscles are responsible for the formation of "goose bumps" as they react to pull the hair up straight when a person is cold or frightened. When the muscle contracts it also presses on the nearby sebaceous gland causing it to release sebum to help lubricate the skin.

Integumentary System Disorders

- Acne: inflammatory disease of the sebaceous gland and hair follicles.
- Cancer: basal cell, squamous, melanoma.
- Dermatitis: skin inflammation.
- Fungal infections: including tinea and ringworm.
- Herpes: including cold sore or viral infection.
- Impetigo: staph or strep infection.
- Keloid: fibrous tissue growth at scar area.
- Pediculosis: lice infestation.
- Pruritus: itching.
- Psoriasis: a chronic skin disease of unknown origin characterized by clearly defined red patches of scaly skin.

Diagnostic Tests

- Biopsy
- Microbiology cultures
- Skin scrapings for fungal culture
- Skin scrapings for KOH (potassium hydroxide) preparation
- Tissue cultures

Respiratory System

Functions

The function of the respiratory system (Fig. 5-12) is to deliver a constant supply of oxygen (O_2) to all the cells of the body and to remove carbon dioxide (CO_2), a waste product of cell metabolism. This is accomplished with the help of the circulatory system through **respiration.** Respiration permits the exchange of O_2 and CO_2 between the blood and the air and involves two processes, **external respiration** and **internal respiration.** During external respiration O_2 from the air enters the blood stream in the lungs and CO_2 leaves the blood stream and is breathed into the air from the lungs. During internal respiration, O_2 leaves the blood stream and enters the cells, and CO_2 from the cells enters the blood stream.

Structures

The major structures of the respiratory system form a continuous tract (pathway) for the flow of air to and from the lungs and include the nose, pharynx (throat), larynx (voice box), trachea, bronchi, and lungs.

Respiratory Tract

The **nose** provides the main airway for respiration. (Some air enters and leaves through the mouth.) The nose also warms, moistens, and filters entering air. In addition, the nose provides a resonance chamber for the voice and contains receptors for the sense of smell.

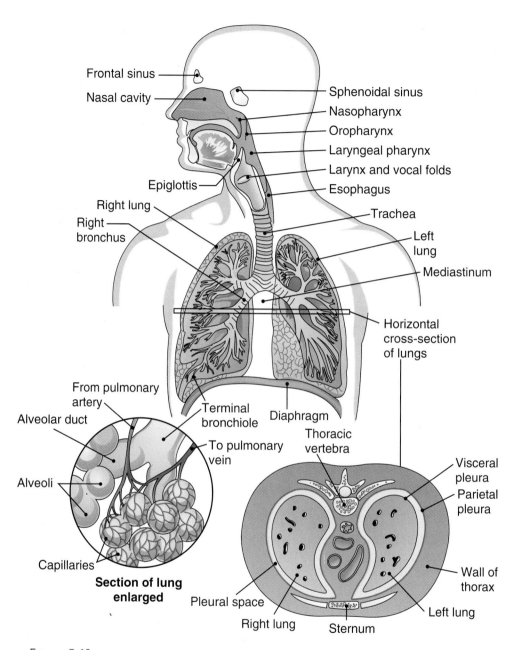

FIGURE 5-12

The respiratory system. (Used with permission from Cohen, B. J. & Wood, D. L. *Memmler's structure and function of the human body* (7th ed.). Philadelphia: Lippincott Williams & Wilkins, p. 248.)

From the nose the air moves into the **pharynx,** a funnel-shaped passageway for both food and air. The pharynx connects with the **larynx,** the enlarged upper end of the trachea leading to the **lungs,** and the esophagus, which leads to the stomach. A thin, leaf-shaped cartilage structure called the **epiglottis** covers the entrance of the larynx during swallowing and acts as a switching mechanism, routing food and air into the proper pathway. Vocal chords within the larynx produce the sounds of the voice. The end of the vocal chords marks the division between the upper and lower respiratory tract.

Air from the larynx moves into the lower trachea, which branches into two main airways called **bronchi,** which lead into the lungs.

The human body has two lungs, a right with three lobes and a left with only two lobes because of the space needed for the heart. The lungs are encased in a thin membrane consisting of several layers called pleura. An infinitely small space between the layer that covers the lungs and one that lines the inner thoracic cavity is called the pleural cavity. Fluid within this cavity helps keep the lungs expanded by reducing surface tension. It also helps prevent friction as the lungs expand and contract.

After the bronchi enter the lungs they divide into two branches, which in turn divide many more times into smaller and smaller branches until they reach the **terminal bronchioles.** The terminal bronchioles branch into **respiratory bronchioles,** which are attached to **alveolar** (al-ve'o-lar) **ducts.** The respiratory bronchioles, and the alveolar ducts, have cup-shaped outpouchings called **alveoli** (al-ve'o-li). The alveoli at the ends of the alveolar ducts are clustered together into **alveolar sacs.** Gas exchange between the air and the blood occurs across the walls of the alveoli.

The walls of the alveoli are composed of a singular layer of epithelium surrounded by a thin membrane. The thinness of the walls would ordinarily leave them prone to collapse. However, a coating of fluid called **surfactant** lowers the surface tension (or pull) on the walls and helps to stabilize them.

Key Point ➤ A deficiency of surfactant in premature infants causes their alveoli to collapse leading to a condition called **infant respiratory distress syndrome** or **IRDS.** Premature infants can be given surfactant through inhalation in an effort to treat this life-threatening condition.

Gas Exchange and Transport

During normal external respiration (Fig. 5-13), oxygen and carbon dioxide are able to diffuse (go from an area of higher concentration to an area of lower concentration) through the walls of the alveoli and the tiny, one-cell thick blood vessels (capillaries) of the lungs. Because the blood in lung capillaries is low in O_2 and high in CO_2, O_2 from the alveoli diffuses into the blood in the capillaries while CO_2 diffuses from the capillaries into the alveoli to be **expired** (breathed out).

The amount of oxygen that can be carried dissolved in the blood plasma is not enough to meet the needs of the body. Fortunately, hemoglobin (a protein found in red blood cells) has the ability to bind O_2, increasing the amount the blood can carry by more than 70%. Most of the O_2 that diffuses into the capillaries in the lungs binds to the iron-containing heme portion of hemoglobin molecules in the red blood cells. Very little is dissolved in the blood plasma. O_2 combined with hemoglobin is called **oxyhemoglobin.**

Hemoglobin also has the ability to bind with CO_2. Hemoglobin combined with CO_2 is called **carbaminohemoglobin.** However, only around 20% of the CO_2 from the tissues is carried to the lungs in this manner. Approximately 10% is carried as gas dissolved in the blood plasma. The remaining 70% is carried as a **bicarbonate ion** that was formed in the red blood cells and released into the blood plasma. In the lungs, the bicarbonate ion re-enters the red blood cells and is released as CO_2 to diffuse through the alveoli and be exhaled by the body.

CO_2 levels play a major role in acid-base (pH) balance of the blood. If CO_2 levels increase, blood pH decreases or becomes more acidic, which can lead to a dangerous condition called **acidosis.** The body responds by increasing the rate of respiration (hyperventilation) to increase O_2 levels. Prolonged hyperventilation causes a decrease in CO_2, resulting in an increase in pH and a condition called **alkalosis.**

Whether oxygen or hemoglobin **associates** (combines) with or **disassociates** (releases) from hemoglobin depends upon the **partial pressure** of each gas. Partial pres-

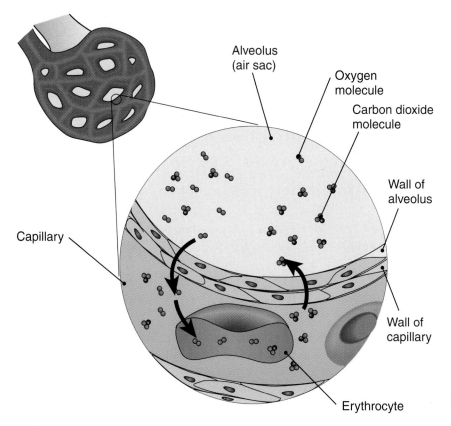

■ FIGURE 5-13 ■

External respiration. (Used with permission from Cohen, B. J. & Wood, D. L. *Memmler's structure and function of the human body* (7th ed.). Philadelphia: Lippincott Williams & Wilkins, p. 255.)

sure is defined as the pressure exerted by one gas in a mixture of gases. O_2 associates with hemoglobin in the lungs, where the partial pressure of O_2 (PO_2) is increased, and disassociates from hemoglobin in the tissues, where the PO_2 is decreased. CO_2 associates with hemoglobin in the tissues, where the partial pressure of CO_2 (PCO_2) is increased, and disassociates with hemoglobin in the lungs, where the PCO_2 is decreased.

Respiratory System Disorders

- Apnea (ap'ne-ah): a temporary cessation of breathing.
- Asthma: difficulty in breathing accompanied by wheezing caused by spasm or swelling of the bronchial tubes.
- Bronchitis: inflammation of the mucous membrane of the bronchial tubes.
- Cystic fibrosis: a genetic endocrine disease causing an excess production of mucus.
- Dyspnea (disp'ne-ah): difficult or labored breathing.
- Emphysema: chronic obstructive pulmonary disease.
- Hypoxia (hi-pok'se-ah): deficiency of oxygen.
- IRDS: severe impairment of respiratory function in the newborn resulting from a lack of a substance called surfactant in the baby's lungs.
- Pleurisy: inflammation of the pleural membrane.
- Pneumonia: inflammation of the lungs.
- Pulmonary edema: accumulation of fluid in the lungs.
- Tuberculosis (TB): infectious disease affecting the respiratory system caused by the bacteria *Mycobacterium tuberculosis.*
- Respiratory syncytial (sin-si'shal) virus (RSV): a virus that is a major cause of respiratory distress in infants and children.
- Rhinitis: inflammation of the nasal mucous membranes.
- Tonsillitis: infection of the tonsils.
- Upper respiratory infection (URI): an infection of the nose, throat, larynx, or upper trachea such as caused by a cold virus.

Diagnostic Tests

- Acid fast bacillus culture/smear
- Arterial blood gases (ABGs)
- Capillary blood gases
- CBC
- Cocci (immunoglobulin G/immunoglobulin M)
- Drug levels
- Electrolytes (lytes)
- Microbiology cultures
- Pleuracentesis
- Skin tests: Purified protein derivative (PPD) (tuberculin or TB test)(see page 393)
- Sputum culture
- Bronchial washings

STUDY & REVIEW QUESTIONS

1. The transverse plane divides the body
   a. diagonally into upper and lower portions.
   b. horizontally into upper and lower portions.
   c. vertically into front and back portions.
   d. vertically into right and left portions.

2. Proximal is defined as
   a. away from the middle.
   b. closest to the middle.
   c. farthest from the center.
   d. nearest to the point of attachment.

3. The lateral plantar surface of the foot is on the
   a. area of the arch.
   b. big toe side of the foot.
   c. little toe side of the foot.
   d. middle of the foot.

4. The process by which the body maintains a state of equilibrium is
   a. anabolism.
   b. catabolism.
   c. homeostasis.
   d. venostasis.

5. Which part of a cell contains the chromosomes or genetic material?
   a. cytoplasm
   b. Golgi apparatus
   c. nucleus
   d. organelles

6. The type of muscle that lines the walls of blood vessels.
   a. cardiac
   b. skeletal
   c. striated
   d. visceral

7. Which of the following is a test associated with the reproductive system?
   a. ABG
   b. BUN
   c. CK
   d. HCG

8. Which of the following is an accessory organ of the digestive system?
   a. heart
   b. liver
   c. lung
   d. ovary

9. Evaluation of the endocrine system involves
   a. blood gas studies.
   b. drug monitoring.
   c. hormone determinations.
   d. spinal fluid analysis.

Continued

STUDY & REVIEW QUESTIONS *(CONTINUED)*

10. The spinal cord and brain are covered by protective membranes called
    a. meninges.
    b. neurons.
    c. papillae.
    d. viscera.

11. Which statement is not true? Sebaceous glands
    a. are also called oil glands.
    b. help lubricate the skin.
    c. secrete sebum.
    d. are part of the endocrine system.

12. The majority of gas exchange between blood and tissue takes place in the
    a. arterioles.
    b. capillaries.
    c. pulmonary vein.
    d. venules.

Bibliography and Suggested Readings

Cohen, B. J., & Wood, D. L. (2000). *Memmler's structure and function of the human body* (7th ed.). Philadelphia: Lippincott Williams & Wilkins.

Cohen, B. J., & Wood, D. L. (2000). *Memmler's the human body in health and disease* (9th ed.). Philadelphia: Lippincott Williams & Wilkins.

Fischbach, F. (2000). *Laboratory diagnostic tests* (6th ed.). Philadelphia: Lippincott Williams & Wilkins.

Herlihy, B, & Maebius, N.K. (2000). *The human body in health and illness.* Philadelphia: W.B. Saunders

Mahon, C., Smith, L., & Burns, C. (1998) *An introduction to clinical laboratory science.* Philadelphia: W.B. Saunders

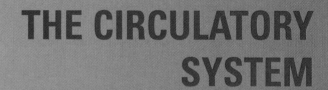

THE CIRCULATORY SYSTEM

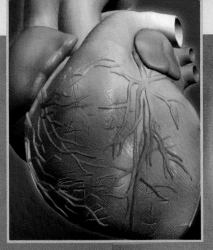
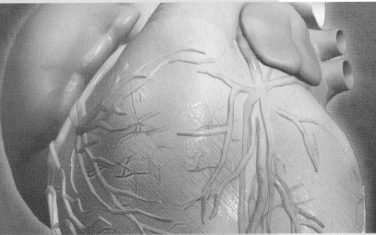

Upon successful completion of this chapter, the reader will be able to:

1 Define the key terms and abbreviations listed at the beginning of this chapter.

2 Identify the layers and structures of the heart.

3 Describe the cardiac cycle and how an ECG tracing relates to it; explain the origins of heart sounds and pulse rates.

4 Describe how to take blood pressure readings and what they represent.

5 Identify the two main divisions of the vascular system, describe the function of each, and trace the flow of blood throughout the system.

6 Identify the different types of blood vessels and describe the structure and function of each.

7 Name and locate major arm and leg veins and describe the suitability of each for venipuncture.

8 List the major constituents of blood, differentiate between serum and plasma, and describe the function of each of the formed elements.

9 Describe how ABO and Rh blood types are determined, and the importance of compatibility testing before transfusion.

10 Define hemostasis and describe basic coagulation and fibrinolysis processes.

11 Identify the structures and vessels and describe the function of the lymphatic system.

12 List the disorders and diagnostic tests of the circulatory system.

INTRODUCTION

The circulatory system consists of the cardiovascular system (heart, blood, and blood vessels) and the lymphatic system (lymph, lymph vessels, and nodes). The circulatory system is the means by which oxygen and food are carried to the cells of the body. It is also the means by which carbon dioxide and other wastes are carried away from the cells to the excretory organs: the kidneys, lungs, and skin. The circulatory system also aids in the coagulation process, assists in defending the body against disease, and plays an important role in the regulation of body temperature.

THE HEART

The **heart** (Fig. 6-1) is the major structure of the circulatory system. It is the "pump" that circulates blood throughout the body. It is located in the center of the thoracic cavity between the lungs with the apex (tip) pointing down and to the left of the body.

Heart Structure

The heart is a four-chambered, hollow, muscular organ, slightly larger than a man's closed fist. It has three layers and is surrounded by a thin, fluid-filled sac called the **pericardium** (per'i-kar'de-um). The heart has two sides, a right and a left, separated by a partition called the **septum.** Each side has two **chambers,** an upper and a lower. **Valves** between the chambers help prevent the back-flow of blood and keep it flowing through the heart in the right direction.

Layers of the Heart

The three layers of the heart are the epicardium, the myocardium, and the endocardium. The **epicardium** (ep'-i-kar'de-um) is the thin outer layer of the heart, continuous with the lining of the pericardium. The **myocardium** (mi-o-kar'de-um) is the middle layer and is the thick, muscle layer of the heart. The **endocardium** (en'do-kar'de-um), the inner layer, is the thin membrane lining the heart. It is continuous with the lining of the blood vessels.

Heart Chambers

The upper chambers on each side of the heart are called **atria** (a'tre-a), and the lower chambers are called **ventricles** (ven'trik-ls). The atria (singular is "atrium") are receiving chambers and the ventricles are pumping or delivering chambers.

The **right atrium** receives deoxygenated blood from the body via both the **superior (upper) vena cava** (ve'na ka'va) and **inferior (lower) vena cava** (plural is "vena cavae").

The **right ventricle** receives blood from the right atrium and pumps it to the lungs via the **pulmonary artery.**

The **left atrium** receives oxygenated blood from the lungs via the **pulmonary veins.**

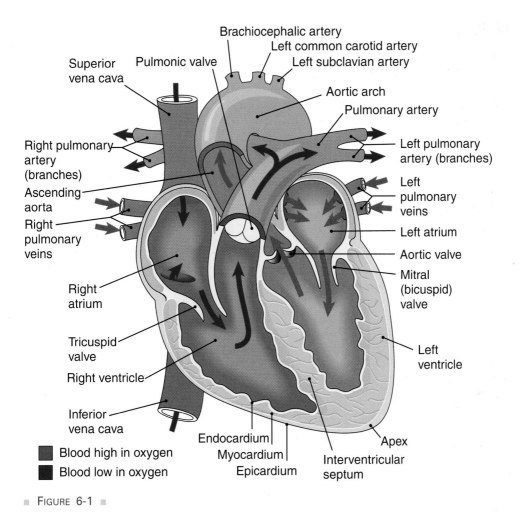

FIGURE 6-1

Heart and great vessels. (Used with permission from Cohen, B. J. & Wood, D. L. (2000). *Memmler's structure and function of the human body* (7th ed.). Philadelphia: Lippincott Williams & Wilkins, p. 196.)

The **left ventricle** receives blood from the left atrium and pumps it into the **aorta** (a-or'ta). The walls of the left ventricle are nearly three times as thick as the right ventricle because of the force required to pump the blood into the arterial system.

Valves

The valves at the entrance to the ventricles are called **atrioventricular** (a'tre-o-ven-trik'u-lar) **valves.** The valves that exit the ventricles are called **semilunar** (sem'e-lu'nar) **valves** because they are crescent-shaped, like the moon.

The right atrioventricular valve is called the **tricuspid** (tri-kus'pid) **valve** because it has three flaps or cusps. The left atrioventricular valve is called the **bicuspid** (bi-kus'pid) **valve** because it has two flaps. It is also called the **mitral** (mi'tral) **valve.**

Both of the atrioventricular valves are attached to the walls of the ventricles by thin threads of tissue called **chordae** (kor'de) **tendineae** (ten-din'e-e), which keep the valves from flipping back into the atria.

The right semilunar valve is called the **pulmonary** or **pulmonic semilunar valve** because blood passing through it goes into the pulmonary artery. The left semilunar valve is called the **aortic semilunar valve** because blood passing through it goes into the aorta.

Coronary Arteries

The heart does not receive nourishment or oxygen from the blood passing through it. The heart receives its blood supply via the right and left **coronary arteries** that branch off of the aorta, just beyond the aortic semilunar valve. Partial obstruction of a coronary artery or one of its branches causes an insufficient supply of blood to meet oxygen needs of the heart muscle and results in a condition called **myocardial ischemia** (is-kee'me-ah). Complete obstruction or prolonged ischemia leads to **myocardial** (mi'o-kar'de-al) **infarction (MI)** or "heart attack" resulting from necrosis (ne-kro'sis) or death of the surrounding tissue from lack of oxygen.

Key Point ➤ Fatty plaque buildup from a condition called atherosclerosis can lead to severe narrowing of coronary arteries. This condition is sometimes treated using a coronary bypass procedure. In this surgical procedure, a vein (commonly the saphenous vein from the leg) is grafted onto the artery to divert the blood around the affected area.

Heart Function

Cardiac Cycle

One complete contraction and subsequent relaxation of the heart is called a **cardiac cycle.** The contracting phase of the cardiac cycle is called **systole** (sis'to-le). The relaxing phase is called **diastole** (di-as'to-le).

Electrical Conduction System

Heart contraction is initiated by an electrical impulse generated from the **sino-atrial** (sin'o-a'tre-al) **node** or **SA node,** also called the **pacemaker,** located in the upper wall of the right atrium. The impulse causes both atria to contract simultaneously, pushing blood through the atrioventricular valves into the ventricles.

The impulse is picked up by the **atrioventricular (AV) node** located in the lower right atrium. As the atria relax, the pulse is relayed through the **AV bundle (bundle of His)** and along the **Purkinje** (pur-kin'jee) **fibers** throughout the ventricular muscle. This causes the ventricles to contract, forcing blood through the semilunar valves. Both atria and ventricles relax briefly before the entire cycle starts again. Each cycle lasts approximately 0.8 seconds. (See Fig. 6-2 for a diagram of the conduction system of the heart.)

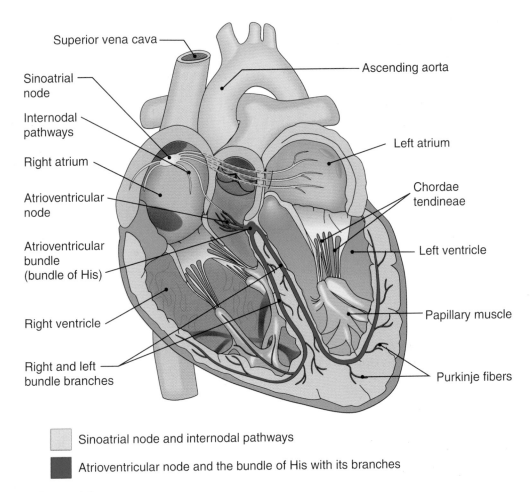

Superior vena cava

Sinoatrial node

Internodal pathways

Right atrium

Atrioventricular node

Atrioventricular bundle (bundle of His)

Right ventricle

Right and left bundle branches

Ascending aorta

Left atrium

Chordae tendineae

Left ventricle

Papillary muscle

Purkinje fibers

☐ Sinoatrial node and internodal pathways

■ Atrioventricular node and the bundle of His with its branches

■ FIGURE 6-2 ■

Electrical conduction system of the heart. (Used with permission from Cohen, B. J. & Wood, D. L. (2000). *Memmler's structure and function of the human body* (7th ed.). Philadelphia: Lippincott Williams & Wilkins, p. 201.).

Electrocardiogram

The cardiac cycle can be recorded by means of an **electrocardiogram (ECG, EKG),** an actual record of the electrical currents that correspond to each event in heart muscle contraction. The recording is called an ECG tracing (Fig. 6-3). The contractions are recorded as waves when electrodes (leads or wires) are placed on the skin. The P wave of the tracing represents the activity of the atria and is usually the first wave seen. The QRS complex (a collection of three waves), along with the T wave, represents the activity of the ventricles. An ECG is useful in diagnosing heart muscle damage and abnormalities in heart rate.

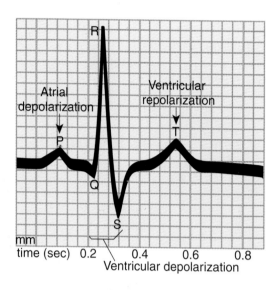

■ FIGURE 6-3 ■

Normal ECG tracing showing one cardiac cycle. (Used with permission from Cohen, B. J. & Wood, D. L. (2000). *Memmler's structure and function of the human body* (7th ed.). Philadelphia: Lippincott Williams & Wilkins, p. 205.)

Origin of the Heart Sounds (Heart Beat)

As the ventricles contract (systole), the atrioventricular valves close, resulting in the first heart sound: a long, low-pitched sound commonly described as a "lubb." The second heart sound comes at the beginning of ventricular relaxation (diastole) and is the result of the closing of the semilunar valves. It is shorter and sharper and described as a "dupp." Abnormal heart sounds are called **murmurs,** and are usually the result of faulty valve action.

Heart Rate and Cardiac Output

The **heart rate** is the number of heartbeats per minute. Normal adult heart rate is around 72 beats per minute. The volume of blood pumped by the heart in 1 minute is called the **cardiac output** and averages 5 liters per minute.

An irregularity in the heart rate, rhythm, or beat is called an **arrhythmia** (ah-rith'me-ah). A slow rate, less than 60 beats per minute, is called **bradycardia** (brad'e-kar'de-ah). A fast rate, more than 100 beats per minute, is called **tachycardia** (tak'e-kar'de-ah). Extra beats before the normal beat are called **extrasystoles.** Ventricular contractions before the normal time are called premature ventricular contractions (PVCs). Rapid, uncoordinated contractions are called **fibrillations** and can result in lack of pumping action.

Pulse

The **pulse** is caused by a wave of increased pressure created as the ventricles contract and blood is forced out of the heart and through the arteries. In normal individuals, the **pulse rate** is the same as the heart rate. The pulse is most easily felt by compressing the radial artery on the thumb side of the wrist.

Blood Pressure

Blood pressure is a measure of the force (pressure) exerted by the blood on the walls of blood vessels. It is commonly measured in a large artery (such as the brachial artery in the upper arm), using a **sphygmomanometer** (sfig′mo-mah-nom′e-ter), more commonly known as a "blood pressure cuff." Blood pressure results are expressed in millimeters of mercury (mm Hg) and are read from a manometer that is either a gauge or a mercury column, depending upon the type of blood pressure cuff used. Two components of blood pressure are measured: the systolic (sis-tol′ik) pressure and the diastolic (di-as-tol′ik) pressure.

Systolic pressure is the pressure in the arteries during contraction of the ventricles, and averages 120 mm Hg for adults.

Diastolic pressure is the pressure during relaxation of the ventricles, and averages 80 mm Hg.

Key Point ➤ A blood pressure reading is expressed as the systolic pressure over the diastolic pressure. Average normal blood pressure is verbally expressed as 120 over 80, and is written 120/80.

A brachial blood pressure reading is taken by placing a blood pressure cuff around the upper arm and a stethoscope over the brachial artery. The cuff is inflated until the brachial artery is compressed and the blood flow is cut off. Then the cuff is slowly deflated until the first heart sounds are heard with the stethoscope. The pressure reading at this time is the systolic pressure. The cuff is then slowly deflated until a muffled sound is heard. The pressure at this time is the diastolic pressure.

Heart Disorders

- Angina pectoris (an′-ji′na pek′to-ris): also called **ischemic heart disease;** pain on exertion caused by decreased blood flow to the myocardium from the coronary artery.
- Aortic stenosis (a-or′tik ste-no′sis): narrowing of the aorta or its opening.
- Bacterial endocarditis (en′do-kar-di′tis): an infection of the lining of the heart, most commonly caused by streptococci.
- Congestive heart failure: impaired circulation caused by inadequate pumping of a diseased heart, resulting in fluid buildup (edema) in the lungs or other tissues.
- MI: heart attack or death of heart muscle resulting from obstruction (occlusion) of a coronary artery.
- Pericarditis (per-i-kar-di′tis): inflammation of the pericardium.

Diagnostic Tests

- Arterial blood gas (ABGs)
- Aspartate aminotransferase (AST) (serum glutamic-oxaloacetic transaminase [SGOT])

- Cholesterol
- Creatine kinase (CK)
- Creatine kinase-MB isoenzyme
- Digoxin
- ECG (EKG)
- Lactate dehydrogenase (LD) isoenzyme
- Microbial cultures
- Myoglobin
- Potassium
- Triglycerides
- Troponin T

Key Point ➤ When a person has a heart attack the heart muscle is damaged, releasing the enzymes CK and AST into the blood stream. A sample of blood can be tested for these enzymes. If the results are elevated, a heart attack is suspected.

THE VASCULAR SYSTEM

Functions

The vascular system is a closed system by which blood is circulated to all parts of the body. There are two divisions to this system, the pulmonary circulation and the systemic circulation.

The Pulmonary Circulation

The **pulmonary circulation** carries blood from the heart to the lungs to remove carbon dioxide and pick up oxygen. It then returns the oxygenated blood to the heart to be pumped throughout the body.

The Systemic Circulation

The **systemic circulation** carries oxygenated blood from the heart, along with nutrients from the digestive system, to all the cells of the body. The systemic circulation is also responsible for carrying carbon dioxide and other waste products of metabolism away from the cells for disposal.

Structures

The structures of the vascular system are the various blood vessels that, along with the heart, form the closed system for the flow of blood. Blood vessels are tube-like structures capable of expanding and contracting. There are three types of blood vessels—arteries, veins, and capillaries.

Blood Vessels

ARTERIES

Arteries (Fig. 6-4) carry blood away from the heart. They have thick walls because the blood is under pressure from the contraction of the ventricles. This pressure creates a pulse that can be felt, distinguishing them from veins.

 Key Point ➤ When arterial blood is collected by syringe, the pressure normally causes the blood to "pump" or pulse into the syringe under its own power.

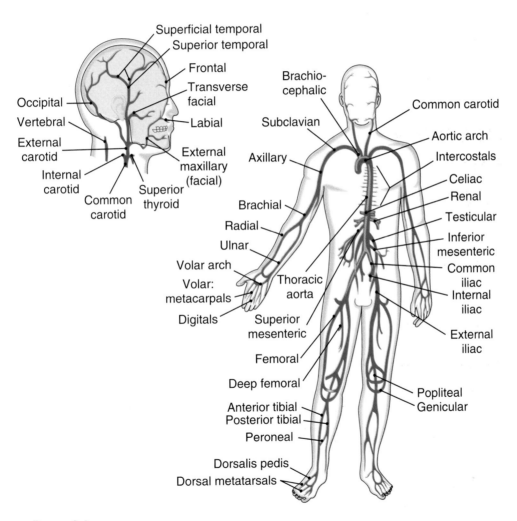

■ FIGURE 6-4 ■

Principal arteries of the body. (Used with permission from Cohen, B. J. & Wood, D. L. (2000). *Memmler's structure and function of the human body* (7th ed.). Philadelphia: Lippincott Williams & Wilkins, p. 215.)

Systemic arteries carry blood that is oxygenated (oxygen rich). Because it is oxygen rich or full of oxygen, normal systemic arterial blood is bright, cherry red in color.

 Key Point ➤ The pulmonary artery is the only artery that carries deoxygenated or oxygen poor blood. It is part of the pulmonary circulation and carries deoxygenated blood to the lungs. It is classified as an artery because it carries blood away from the heart.

The smallest branches of arteries that join with the capillaries are called **arterioles** (ar-te're-olz). The largest artery in the body is the **aorta.** It is approximately 1 inch (2.5 cm) wide.

VEINS

Veins (Fig. 6-5) return blood to the heart. Veins carry blood that is low in oxygen (deoxygenated), except for the pulmonary vein, which carries oxygenated blood from the lungs back to the heart. Because systemic venous blood is oxygen poor, it is much darker and more bluish-red in color than is normal arterial blood.

The walls of veins are thinner than arteries because the blood is under less pressure than arterial blood. Because the walls are thinner, veins can collapse more easily than arteries. Blood is kept moving through veins primarily as a result of skeletal muscle movement.

 Key Point ➤ Most veins have **valves** to prevent the backflow of blood and keep it moving along despite the fact that most of the venous system is flowing against the pull of gravity.

The smallest veins at the junction of the capillaries are called **venules** (ven'ulz). The largest vein in the body is the vena cava. The longest vein in the body is the **great saphenous** (sa-fe'nus) vein in the leg.

CAPILLARIES

Capillaries are microscopic, one-cell-thick vessels that connect the arterioles and venules. Blood in the capillaries is a mixture of both venous and arterial blood. In the systemic circulation, arterial blood delivers oxygen and nutrients to the capillaries. The thin capillary walls allow the exchange of oxygen for carbon dioxide and of nutrients for wastes to take place between the cells and the blood. Carbon dioxide and wastes are carried away in the venous blood. In the pulmonary circulation, carbon dioxide is delivered to the capillaries in the lungs and exchanged for oxygen.

Blood Vessel Structure

Arteries and veins are composed of three main layers. The thickness of the layers varies with the size and type of blood vessel. Figure 6-6 shows a cross section of an artery and a vein as seen through a microscope. Capillaries are composed of a single layer of en-

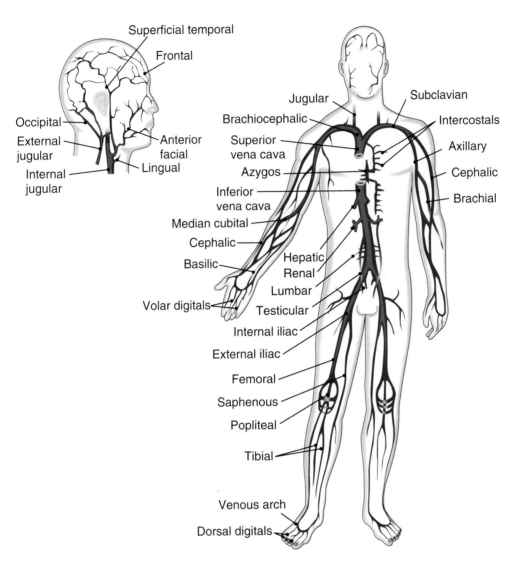

■ FIGURE 6-5 ■

Principal veins of the body. (Used with permission from Cohen, B. J. & Wood, D. L. (2000). *Memmler's structure and function of the human body* (7th ed.). Philadelphia: Lippincott Williams & Wilkins, p. 218.)

dothelial cells enclosed in a basement membrane. (See Figure 6-7 for a comparison diagram of arteries, veins, and capillaries.)

LAYERS

• **Tunica** (tu'ni-ka) **adventitia** (ad'ven-tish'e-a): the outer layer of a blood vessel, sometimes called the tunica externa. It is made up of connective tissue and is thicker in arteries than veins.

Smooth muscle

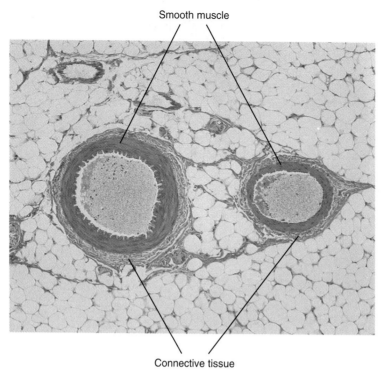

Connective tissue

■ FIGURE 6-6 ■

Cross-section of an artery and a vein as seen through a microscope. (Cormac, D. H. (1993). *Essential histology.* Philadelphia: JB Lippincott, Plate 11-1.)

- **Tunica media:** the middle layer of a blood vessel. It is made up of smooth muscle tissue and some elastic fibers. It is much thicker in arteries than in veins.
- **Tunica intima** (in'ti-ma): the inner layer or lining of a blood vessel, sometimes called the tunica interna. It is made up of a single layer of endothelial cells with an underlining basement membrane, a connective tissue layer, and an elastic internal membrane.

Lumen

The internal space of a blood vessel through which the blood flows is called the **lumen** (lu'men).

VALVES

The presence of valves within veins is a major structural difference between arteries and veins. Venous blood is often flowing against gravity. As blood moves through veins, valves, similar to the semilunar valves of the heart, open and close momentarily, helping to keep the blood flowing toward the heart.

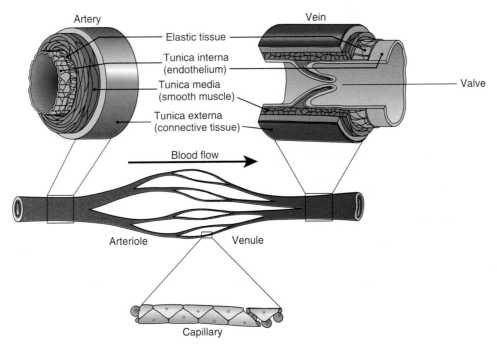

■ FIGURE 6-7 ■

Artery, vein, and capillary structure. (Used with permission from Cohen, B. J. & Wood, D. L. (2000). *Memmler's structure and function of the human body* (7th ed.). Philadelphia: Lippincott Williams & Wilkins, p. 211.)

The Flow of Blood

1. Oxygen-poor blood is returned to the heart via the superior and inferior (upper and lower) vena cavae and enters the right atrium of the heart.
2. Contraction of the right atrium forces the blood through the tricuspid valve into the right ventricle.
3. Contraction of the right ventricle forces the blood through the pulmonary semilunar valve into the pulmonary artery.
4. Blood flows through the pulmonary artery to the capillaries of the lungs where carbon dioxide is released from the red blood cells and exchanged for oxygen through the walls of the alveoli.
5. Oxygen-rich blood flows back to the heart by way of the pulmonary veins and enters the left atrium.
6. Contraction of the left atrium forces the blood through the bicuspid valve into the left ventricle.
7. Contraction of the left ventricle forces the blood through the aortic semilunar valve into the aorta.
8. The blood travels throughout the body by way of the arteries, which branch into smaller and smaller arteries, the smallest of which are the arterioles.
9. The arterioles connect with the capillaries where oxygen, water, and nutrients from the blood diffuse through the capillary walls to the cells. At the same

time, carbon dioxide and other end products of metabolism enter the blood stream (Fig. 6-8).

10. The capillaries connect with the smallest branches of veins (venules).

11. The venules merge into larger and larger veins until the blood returns to the heart again by way of the superior or inferior vena cava and the cycle starts again (Fig. 6-9).

Vascular and Related Anatomy of the Arm and Leg

Antecubital Fossa

The major veins for venipuncture are located in what is referred to as the **antecubital** (an'te-ku'bi-tal) **fossa.** This is the area of the arm that is anterior to (in front of) and below the bend of the elbow. Several major arm veins lie close to the surface in this area, making them easier to locate and penetrate with a needle. These major superficial veins are referred to as **antecubital veins** (Fig.6-10, *A*).

Antecubital Veins Subject to Venipuncture

- **Median cubital vein:** the first-choice vein for venipuncture; it is usually large and well-anchored, making it the easiest and least painful to puncture and also the least likely to bruise.

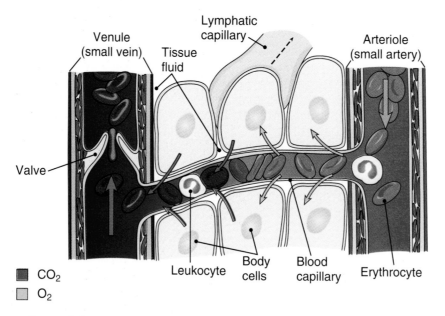

■ FIGURE 6-8 ■

Oxygen and carbon dioxide exchange at the capillaries. (Used with permission from Cohen, B. J. & Wood, D. L. (2000). *Memmler's structure and function of the human body* (7th ed.). Philadelphia: Lippincott Williams & Wilkins, p. 222.)

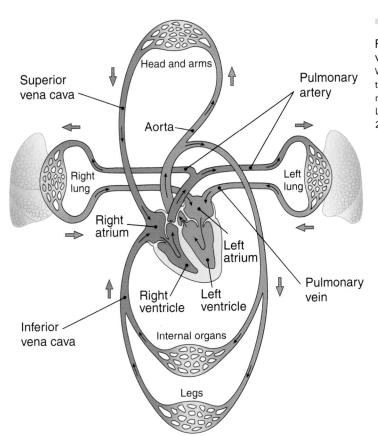

■ FIGURE 6-9 ■

Representation of the vascular flow. (Cohen BJ, Wood DL: Memmler's Structure and Function of the Human Body, 7th edition. Phila., Lippincott Williams & Wilkins, 2000, p. 197.)

- **Cephalic vein:** the second-choice vein for venipuncture; it is often harder to palpate than the median cubital, but is fairly well-anchored. It is often the only vein that can be palpated (felt) in obese patients.
- **Basilic vein:** The basilic vein is the third-choice vein for venipuncture. The basilic is generally easy to palpate, but it is not as well-anchored and rolls and bruises more easily. Venipuncture of this vein tends to be more painful to the patient. There is also the possibility of accidental puncture of the median nerve, located in this area, or the brachial artery, which lies close to the skin surface in this area.

Key Point ➤ Vein location may differ somewhat from person to person. Though you may not see the exact textbook pattern, the cephalic vein extends almost the entire length of the arm and the median cubital vein connects the cephalic and the basilic vein.

Other Arm and Hand Veins Subject to Venipuncture

When antecubital veins are unsuitable or unavailable, other veins subject to venipuncture include, dorsal hand and wrist veins and forearm veins (Fig. 6-10, *B*).

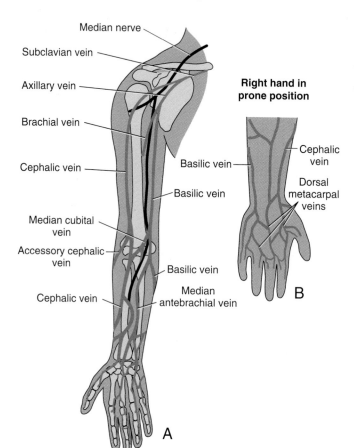

Right arm in anatomic position

Median nerve

Subclavian vein

Axillary vein

Brachial vein

Cephalic vein

Median cubital vein

Accessory cephalic vein

Cephalic vein

Right hand in prone position

Basilic vein

Basilic vein

Basilic vein

Median antebrachial vein

Cephalic vein

Dorsal metacarpal veins

A

B

■ FIGURE 6-10 ■

(*A*) Principal veins of the arm, including major antecubital veins subject to venipuncture. (*B*) Forearm, wrist, and hand veins subject to venipuncture.

Leg, Ankle, and Foot Veins Subject to Venipuncture

Leg, ankle, and foot veins (Fig. 6-11) are sometimes used for venipuncture when no other sites are available but only with permission of the patient's physician. Puncture of the femoral vein is performed only by physicians or specially trained personnel.

Arteries Subject to Puncture

Arterial puncture requires special training to perform, is more painful and hazardous to the patient, and is generally limited to the collection of ABG specimens for evaluating respiratory function. Arteries of the arm subject to puncture are the **radial** and the **brachial arteries.** Puncture of the **femoral artery** of the leg may be performed during emergency situations or when no other arterial site is available. Puncture of the femoral artery is performed only by physicians and specially trained emergency room personnel. Arterial puncture is explained further in Chapter 12.

Median Cutaneous Nerve

Cutaneous nerves convey impulses for stimuli to the skin. The median cutaneous nerve is a major arm nerve that lies along the path of the brachial artery and in the vicinity of the basilic vein.

 Key Point ➤ Lawsuits have been filed over damage to major nerves as a result of improper venipuncture procedures.

Vascular System Disorders

- Aneurysm (an'u-rizm): a localized dilation or bulging in the wall of a blood vessel, usually an artery.
- Arteriosclerosis (ar-te're-o-skle-ro'sis): thickening, hardening, and loss of elasticity of artery walls.
- Atherosclerosis (ath'er-o'skle-ro'sis): a form of arteriosclerosis involving changes in the intima of the artery resulting from an accumulation of lipids and so on.
- Embolism: obstruction of a blood vessel by an embolus.

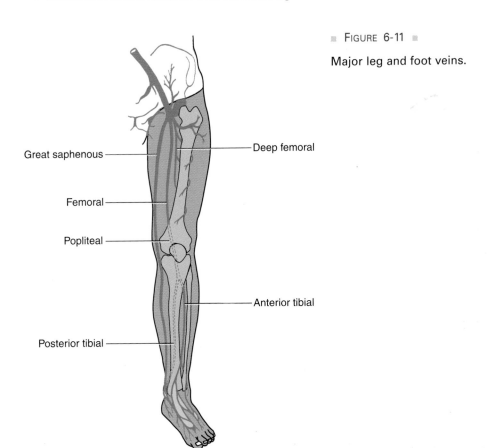

■ FIGURE 6-11 ■

Major leg and foot veins.

- Embolus (em'bo-lus): a blood clot, part of a blood clot, or other mass of undissolved matter circulating in the blood stream.
- Hemorrhoids: varicose veins in the rectal area.
- Phlebitis (fle-bi'tis): inflammation of a vein.
- Thrombophlebitis (throm'bo-fle-bi'tis): inflammation of a vein along with thrombus (blood clot) formation.
- Thrombus: a blood clot in a blood vessel.
- Varicose veins (varices): swollen, knotted superficial veins.

Diagnostic Tests

- Disseminated intravascular coagulation (DIC) screen
- Lipoproteins
- Prothrombin time (PT)
- Partial thromboplastin time (PTT/APTT)
- Triglycerides

THE BLOOD

Blood has been referred to as "the river of life." It flows throughout the circulatory system delivering nutrients, oxygen, and other substances to the cells and transporting waste products away from the cells for elimination.

Blood Composition

Blood is a mixture of fluid and cells that is about five times thicker than water, salty to the taste, and with a slightly alkaline pH of about 7.4 (pH is the degree of acidity or alkalinity on a scale of 1 to 14, with 7 being neutral). In vivo (in the living body), the fluid portion of the blood is called plasma and the cellular portion is referred to as the **formed elements** (Fig. 6-12, *A*). The average adult weighing 70 kg (approximately 154 pounds) has a blood volume of about 5 L (5.3 quarts), of which approximately 55% is plasma and 45% is formed elements.

Plasma

Normal plasma is a clear, pale yellow fluid that is nearly 90% water and 10% solutes (dissolved substances). Composition of the solutes includes the following:

- Proteins, such as **albumin,** which is manufactured by the liver and functions to help regulate osmotic pressure or the tendency of blood to attract water; **antibodies,** which combat infection; and **fibrinogen,** which is also manufactured by the liver and functions in the clotting process.
- Nutrients, which supply energy. Plasma nutrients include **carbohydrates,** such as **glucose,** and **lipids (fats)** such as **triglycerides** and **cholesterol.**
- Minerals such as **sodium (Na), potassium (K), calcium (Ca),** and **magnesium (Ma).** Sodium helps maintain fluid balance, pH, and calcium and potassium balance necessary for normal heart action.

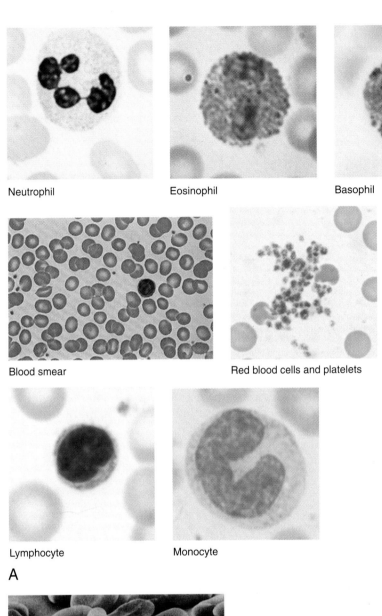

Neutrophil

Eosinophil

Basophil

Blood smear

Red blood cells and platelets

Lymphocyte

Monocyte

A

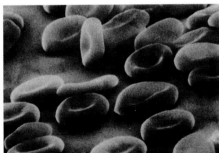

B

■ FIGURE 6-12 ■

(A) Normal blood smear and close-up view of individual blood cells. (B) Red blood cells as seen by scanning electron microscopy. (Used with permission from Cohen, B. J. & Wood, D. L. (2000). *Memmler's structure and function of the human body* (7th ed.). Philadelphia: Lippincott Williams & Wilkins, p. 184.)

Key Point ➤ Potassium is essential for normal muscle activity and the conduction of nerve impulses. Calcium is needed for proper bone and teeth formation, nerve conduction, and muscle contraction. In addition, calcium is essential to the clotting process.

- Gases, such as oxygen, carbon dioxide, and nitrogen.
- Other substances, including vitamins, hormones, and waste products of metabolism such as urea, creatinine, and uric acid.

Formed Elements

ERYTHROCYTES

Erythrocytes (e-rith'ro-sites), or red blood cells (RBCs) (Fig. 6-12, *B*), are the most numerous cells in the blood, averaging 4.5 to 5 million per cubic millimeter of blood. Their main function is to carry oxygen from the lungs to the cells. They also carry carbon dioxide from the cells back to the lungs to be exhaled. RBCs are produced in the bone marrow. They are formed with a nucleus, which they lose as they mature and enter the blood stream. Immature RBCs in the blood stream that contain nuclear remnants are called **reticulocytes** (re-tik'u-lo-sits) or **retics.** Mature RBCs have a life span of approximately 120 days, after which they begin to disintegrate and are removed from the blood stream by the spleen and liver. RBCs are described as anuclear (no nucleus), biconcave (indented from both sides) disks approximately 7 to 8 microns in diameter. RBCs have **intravascular** function, which means that they do their job within the blood vessels. An old term for RBCs is red corpuscles.

Key Point ➤ The main component of RBCs is **hemoglobin (Hgb or Hb),** which enables them to transport oxygen and carbon dioxide and also gives them their red color.

LEUKOCYTES

Leukocytes, or white blood cells (WBCs), are cells containing a nucleus. The average adult has from 5,000 to 10,000 WBCs per cubic millimeter of blood. WBCs are formed in the bone marrow and lymphatic tissue. They are said to have **extravascular** function because they are able to leave the blood stream and do their job in the tissues. WBCs may appear in the blood stream for only 6 to 8 hours but reside in the tissues for days, months, or even years. The life span of WBCs varies with the type.

Key Point ➤ The process by which WBCs are able to pass through the walls of the capillaries to enter the tissues is called **diapedesis** (di'a-ped-e'sis). "Dia" (Greek for through), ped from "pedan" (leap), esis (condition or state)

The main function of WBCs is to destroy pathogens. Some accomplish this by a method called **phagocytosis** (fag'o-si-to'sis), in which the pathogen is surrounded and engulfed by the WBC. Other WBCs produce antibodies that destroy pathogens indirectly or release substances that attack foreign matter. An old term for WBCs is white corpuscles.

There are different types of WBCs, each identified by their size, shape of the nucleus, and whether or not there are granules present in the cytoplasm when the cells are stained with a special blood stain called **Wright's stain.** WBCs containing easily visible granules are called **granulocytes** (gran'u-lo-sites'). WBCs lacking easily visible granules are called **agranulocytes.**

Granulocytes

Granulocytes can be differentiated by the color of their granules when stained with Wright's stain. There are three types of granulocytes: neutrophils, eosinophils, and basophils.

- **Neutrophils** (nu'tro-fils): Neutrophils are normally the most numerous of the WBCs, averaging 65% of the WBC total. The granules of neutrophils are fine in texture and stain lavender. Because a typical neutrophil is **polymorphonuclear (PMN),** meaning its nucleus has several lobes or segments, neutrophils are sometimes referred to as **PMNs, polys,** or **segs.** Neutrophils are one of the main phagocytic cells. The life span of a neutrophil is from about 6 hours to a few days.

 Key Point ➤ The presence of increased numbers of neutrophils is associated with bacterial infections.

- **Eosinophils** (e'o-sin'o-fils): The granules of **Eos** are bead-like and stain bright orange-red. The nucleus of an eosinophil has two lobes. Up to 3% of the WBCs of a normal adult are Eos. Eos ingest and detoxify foreign protein and help turn off immune reactions. Eos increase with allergies and parasitic infestations such as pinworms. The life span of an eosinophil is from 8 to 12 days.
- **Basophils** (ba'so-fils): Basophils **(basos)** are the least numerous of the WBCs, comprising less than 1% of the WBC population. The granules of basophils are large, stain dark blue, and often obscure the nucleus. Nuclei of basos are often in the shape of an "S." Basos release histamine and heparin, which enhance the inflammatory response. Basos are thought to live several days.

Agranulocytes

There are two types of agranulocytes: monocytes and lymphocytes.

- **Monocytes:** Monocytes **(monos)** are the largest of the WBCs. They comprise from 1% to 7% of the WBC population. Monos have fine, gray-blue cytoplasm and a large, dark-staining nucleus. Monos destroy pathogens by phagocytosis. They are sometimes referred to as macrophages after they leave the blood stream. The life span of a mono is several months.
- **Lymphocytes:** Lymphocytes are the second most numerous of the WBCs. They comprise approximately 15% to 30% of the WBC population. A typical lympho-

cyte has a large, round, dark purple nucleus that occupies the majority of the cell. The nucleus is surrounded by a thin rim of pale blue cytoplasm. The majority of lymphocytes stay in the lymph tissue, where they play an important role in immunity. Two main types of lymphocytes are **T-lymphocytes,** which directly attack infected cells, and **B-lymphocytes,** which give rise to plasma cells that produce immunoglobulins (antibodies) that are released into the blood stream, where they circulate and attack foreign cells. The life span of lymphocytes varies from only a few hours to a number of years.

THROMBOCYTES

Thrombocytes (throm′bo-sits), better known as **platelets,** are the smallest of the formed elements. Platelets are actually parts of a large cell called a **megakaryocyte** (meg′a-kar′e-o-sit′), which is found in the bone marrow. The number of platelets in the blood (platelet count) of the average adult is from 150,000 to 400,000 per cubic millimeter. Platelets are essential to **coagulation** (the blood clotting process) and are the first cell on the scene when an injury occurs (see Hemostasis section in this chapter). The life span of a platelet is around 10 days.

Blood Type

An individual's blood type (also called blood group) is inherited and is determined by the type of antigen present on his or her red blood cells. Some blood type antigens cause formation of antibodies to the opposite blood type. If a person receives a blood transfusion of the wrong type, the person's antibodies may react with the donor RBCs and cause them to **agglutinate** (a-gloo′ti-nat) (clump together) and **lyse** (līs) (be destroyed). Such a reaction, which can be fatal, is called a **transfusion reaction.** A person will not normally produce antibodies against his or her own RBC antigens. The most commonly used method of blood typing recognizes two blood group systems: the ABO system and the Rh factor system.

ABO Blood Group System

The **ABO blood group system** recognizes four blood types, A, B, AB, and O, based on the presence or absence of two antigens identified as A and B. An individual who is type A has the A antigen; type B has the B antigen; type AB has both antigens; and type O has neither A nor B. Type O is the most common type and type AB is the least common.

Unique to the ABO system are preformed antibodies (also called agglutinins) present in a person's blood that are directed against the opposite blood type. Type A blood will have an antibody (agglutinin) directed against type B called anti-B. A person with type B has anti-A; type O has both anti-A and anti-B; and type AB has neither. Table 6-1 shows the antigens and antibodies present in the four ABO group blood types.

Individuals with type AB blood were once referred to as **universal recipients** because they have neither A nor B antibody to the RBC antigens and can theoretically receive any ABO type blood. In the same manner, type O individuals were once called

Table 6-1

ABO Blood Group System

Blood Type	RBC Antigen	Plasma Antibodies (Agglutinins)
A	A	Anti-B
B	B	Anti-A
AB	A and B	Neither anti-A nor anti-B
O	Neither	Anti-A and anti-B

universal donors because they have neither A nor B antigen on their RBCs and in an emergency their type can theoretically be given to anyone. However, type O blood *does* contain plasma antibodies to both A and B antigens, and when given to an A or B type recipient, it can cause a mild transfusion reaction. To avoid reactions, patients are now given type-specific blood, even in emergencies.

Rh Blood Group System

The **Rh blood group system** is based upon the presence or absence of an RBC antigen called the D antigen, also known as Rh factor. An individual whose RBCs have the D antigen is said to be positive for the Rh factor, or **Rh positive (Rh+).** An individual whose RBCs lack the D antigen is said to be **Rh negative (Rh−).** It is important that a patient receive the correct Rh type blood and the correct ABO type. Approximately 85% of the population is Rh+.

Unlike the ABO system, antibodies to the Rh factor (anti-Rh antibodies) are not preformed in the blood of Rh− individuals. However, an Rh− individual who receives Rh+ blood can become **sensitized.** This means that the individual may produce antibodies against the Rh factor. In addition, an Rh− woman who is carrying an Rh+ fetus may become sensitized by the RBCs of the fetus, most commonly by leakage of the fetal cells into the mother's circulation during childbirth. This may lead to the destruction of the RBCs of a subsequent Rh+ fetus because Rh antibodies produced by the mother can cross the placenta into the fetal circulation. When this occurs, it is called **hemolytic disease of the newborn (HDN).**

 Key Point ➤ A previously unsensitized Rh− mother can be given **Rh immune globulin (RhIg),** such as RhoGam, at certain times during her pregnancy and immediately after the baby's birth if the baby is Rh+. RhIg will destroy any Rh+ fetal cells that may have entered her blood stream and prevent sensitization.

Compatibility Testing/Crossmatch

Other factors in an individual's blood can cause adverse reactions during a blood transfusion, even with the correct ABO and Rh type blood. For this reason, a compatibility test or **crossmatch** is performed using the patient's serum and cells and the donor's serum and cells before a unit of blood is determined **compatible** for transfusion. Recently invented artificial blood, made by chemically altering donor blood, is being tested on humans. This blood is designed to be given to any blood type and poses no risk of transmitting disease.

Types of Blood Specimens

Serum

Blood that has been removed from the body will coagulate or clot within 30 to 60 minutes. The clot consists of the blood cells enmeshed in a fibrin network (see Hemostasis section in this chapter). The remaining fluid portion is called **serum** and can be separated from the clot by centrifugation (spinning the clotted blood at high rpms in a machine called a centrifuge). Normal fasting serum is a clear, pale yellow fluid. Serum has the same composition as plasma except it does not contain fibrinogen, because the fibrinogen was used in the formation of the clot. Many laboratory tests, especially chemistry and immunology tests, are performed on serum.

Plasma

Most coagulation tests cannot be performed on serum because the coagulation factors, particularly fibrinogen, have been used up in the process of clot formation. In addition, some chemistry test results are needed immediately (STAT) to respond to emergency situations; having to wait a minimum of 30 minutes for a specimen to clot would be unacceptable. If the blood is prevented from clotting, the coagulation factors are preserved and the specimen can be centrifuged immediately. Blood can be prevented from clotting by adding a substance called an **anticoagulant.** Most anticoagulants work by either binding calcium, which is critical to the coagulation process, or inhibiting the clotting component thrombin (see Anticoagulants, Chapter 7). When a blood specimen containing an anticoagulant is centrifuged, it will separate into three distinct layers (Fig. 6-13): a bottom layer of red blood cells; a thin, fluffy-looking, white-colored middle layer of WBCs and platelets referred to as the **buffy coat;** and a top layer of clear liquid called **plasma** that can be separated from the cells and used for testing. Normal fasting plasma is a clear to slightly hazy pale yellow fluid visually indistinguishable from serum. The major difference between plasma and serum is that plasma contains fibrinogen. Many laboratory tests can now be performed on either serum or plasma.

Whole Blood

Some tests, including most hematology tests and some chemistry tests such as ammonia and glycohemoglobin, cannot be performed on clotted blood. These tests need to be performed on **whole blood** or blood that is in the same form as when it circulated in the blood stream. This means the blood specimen must *not* be allowed to clot or separate. To obtain a whole blood specimen, it is necessary to add an anticoagulant. In addition, because the components will separate if the specimen is allowed to stand undisturbed, the specimen must be mixed for a minimum of 2 minutes before performing the test.

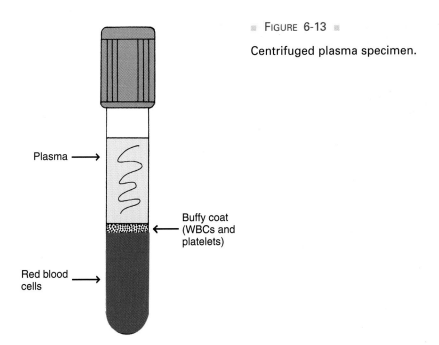

■ FIGURE 6-13 ■

Centrifuged plasma specimen.

Blood Disorders

- Anemia: an abnormal reduction in the number of RBCs in the circulating blood.
- Leukemia: an increase in WBCs characterized by the presence of a large number of abnormal forms.
- Leukocytosis: an abnormal increase in WBCs in the circulating blood.
- Leukopenia: an abnormal decrease in WBCs.
- Polycythemia: an abnormal increase in RBCs.
- Thrombocytosis: increased platelets.
- Thrombocytopenia: decreased platelets.

Diagnostic Tests

- ABO and Rh type
- Bone marrow examination
- Complete blood count (CBC)
- Crossmatch
- Differential (diff)
- Eosinophil (Eos) count
- Erythrocyte sedimentation rate (ESR)
- Ferritin
- Hematocrit (HCT)
- Hb or Hgb
- Hemogram

- Indices (MCH, mean corpuscular hemoglobin; MCV, corpuscular volume; MCHC, mean corpuscular hemoglobin concentration)
- Iron
- Reticulocyte (retic) count
- Total iron binding capacity (TIBC)

HEMOSTASIS

Hemostasis (he'mo-sta'sis) (Fig. 6-14) is the process by which the body stops the leakage of blood from the vascular system after injury. If an injury occurs to a blood vessel, the hemostatic process is set in motion to repair the injury. Hemostasis, also called the **coagulation** process, proceeds in four stages. Stages 1 and 2 are referred to as **primary hemostasis,** and stages 3 and 4 are referred to as **secondary hemostasis.**

Primary Hemostasis

Stage 1: **Vasoconstriction.** The damaged vessel constricts (narrows) to decrease the flow of blood to the injured area.

Stage 2: **Platelet plug formation.** Injury to the blood vessel exposes protein material in the basement membrane. Contact with this material causes the platelets to degranulate and stick to one another **(platelet aggregation)** and adhere to the injured area **(platelet adhesion),** forming a "platelet plug." Normal platelet plug formation depends on an adequate concentration of platelets in the blood (determined by a platelet count), normal functioning of platelets, and blood vessel integrity.

 Key Point ➤ A bleeding time (BT) test assesses platelet plug formation.

For some injuries, such as a needle puncture of a vein, platelet plug formation is sufficient to seal the site and the hemostatic process goes no further. For larger injuries, the process continues to what is called **secondary hemostasis** involving formation of a tougher "fibrin" clot formed of RBCs, platelets, and fibrin.

Secondary Hemostasis

- **Fibrin clot formation.** Fibrin clot formation involves the interaction of a series of coagulation **factors** designated by Roman numerals in the order of discovery. Once activated, each factor activates the next factor in sequence, somewhat like a waterfall or cascade. This **coagulation cascade** can be initiated by two separate pathways, the intrinsic and the extrinsic, both of which eventually join to form a common pathway that ends in the formation of a fibrin clot. Both pathways require the presence of calcium for proper function.
- **Intrinsic pathway.** The intrinsic pathway involves coagulation factors circulating within the blood stream. Functioning of the intrinsic pathway is measured by the **activated partial thromboplastin test (APTT or PTT),** which is also useful in monitoring heparin therapy.

PRIMARY HEMOSTASIS

Stage 1: Vasoconstriction

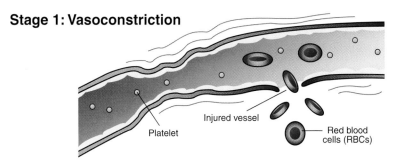

Injured vessel

Platelet

Red blood
cells (RBCs)

Stage 2: Platelet Plug Formation

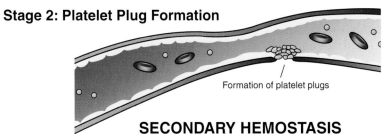

Formation of platelet plugs

SECONDARY HEMOSTASIS

Coagulation Cascade

Stage 3: Fibrin Clot Formation

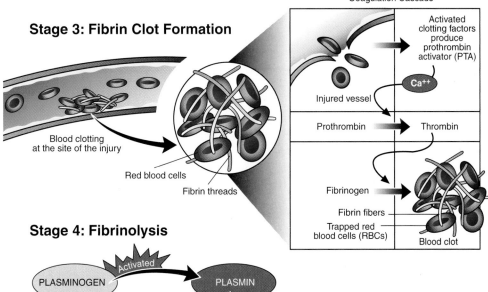

Blood clotting
at the site of the injury

Red blood cells

Fibrin threads

Activated
clotting factors
produce
prothrombin
activator (PTA)

Ca++

Injured vessel

Prothrombin → Thrombin

Fibrinogen

Fibrin fibers

Trapped red
blood cells (RBCs)

Blood clot

Stage 4: Fibrinolysis

PLASMINOGEN → Activated → PLASMIN

Blood clot

Fibrin
degradation products

FIGURE 6-14

Hemostasis.

- **Extrinsic pathway.** The extrinsic pathway is initiated by the release of thromboplastin from injured tissue. The PT measures the functioning of the extrinsic pathway and is used to monitor coumarin therapy.
- **Common pathway.** This pathway involves the conversion of prothrombin (factor II) to thrombin by the action of **prothrombin activator** generated earlier in the coagulation process as a consequence of vessel injury. Calcium ions are necessary for this reaction to occur. Thrombin splits fibrinogen (factor I) into strands of protein called fibrin. The fibrin creates a netlike structure that traps blood cells and platelets forming a **hemostatic plug** (blood clot), which seals the opening in the injured blood vessel and stops the bleeding.

Stage 4: **Fibrinolysis** (fi'brin-ol'i-sis). Fibrinolysis involves the ultimate removal or dissolution of the blood clot once healing has occurred. This process is possible because activation of the clotting process also releases substances that lead to the conversion of plasminogen to plasmin. Plasmin is an enzyme that breaks the fibrin into small fragments called **fibrin degradation products (fibrin split products),** which are then removed by reticuloendothelial cells (phagocytic cells).

Key Point ➤ The coagulation process is kept in check and limited to local sites by the action of natural inhibitors circulating in the plasma along with the coagulation factors. The inhibitors bind with coagulation factors that escape the clotting site and those remaining after clotting is complete.

The Role of the Liver in Hemostasis

The liver plays an important role in the hemostatic process. It is responsible for the synthesis (manufacture) of coagulation factors, such as fibrinogen and prothrombin. It produces the bile salts necessary for the absorption of vitamin K, which is also necessary to the synthesis of the coagulation factors. In addition, mast cells (tissue basophils) in the liver produce heparin. When the liver is diseased, synthesis of coagulation factors is impaired and bleeding may result.

Hemostatic Disorders

- DIC: a pathologic form of diffuse coagulation in which coagulation factors are consumed to such an extent that bleeding occurs.
- Hemophilia (he'mo-fil'e-a): a hereditary condition characterized by bleeding resulting from increased coagulation time. The most common type of hemophilia is the result of factor VIII deficiency.
- Thrombocytopenia (throm'bo-si'to-pe'ne-a): an abnormal decrease in platelets.

Diagnostic Tests

- BT
- D-dimer
- Factor assays

- Fibrin degradation products (FDP)
- Prothrombin time (PT)
- Partial thromboplastin time/activated partial thromboplastin time (PTT/APTT)

THE LYMPHATIC SYSTEM

Functions

The lymphatic system (Fig. 6-15) returns tissue fluid to the blood stream, protects the body by removing microorganisms and impurities, processes lymphocytes, and delivers fats absorbed from the small intestine to the blood stream. Lymph vessels spread throughout the entire body much like blood vessels.

Structures

The lymphatic system is made up of fluid called **lymph** and **lymphatic vessels, ducts,** and **nodes** (masses of lymph tissue) through which the lymph flows.

Lymph Flow

Body cells are bathed in tissue fluid acquired from the blood stream. Water, oxygen, and nutrients continually diffuse through the capillary walls into the tissue spaces. Much of the fluid diffuses back into the capillaries along with waste products of metabolism. Excess tissue fluid filters into lymphatic capillaries, where it is called **lymph.** Lymph fluid is similar to plasma, but is 95% water.

Lymphatic capillaries join with larger and larger lymphatic vessels until they empty into one of two terminal vessels, either the **right lymphatic duct** or the **thoracic duct.** These ducts then empty into large veins in the upper body. Lymph moves through the vessels primarily owing to skeletal muscle contraction, much as blood moves through the veins. As with veins, lymphatic vessels have valves to keep the lymph flowing in the right direction.

Before reaching the ducts, the lymph passes through a series of structures called **lymph nodes,** which trap and destroy bacteria and foreign matter. The nodes also function in the production of lymphocytes. Lymph nodes are made of a special kind of tissue called **lymphoid tissue.** Lymphoid tissue has the ability to remove impurities and process lymphocytes. The tonsils, thymus, gastrointestinal tract, and spleen also contain lymphoid tissue.

Key Point ➤ Axillary lymph nodes are often removed as part of breast cancer surgery. Removal of the nodes can impair lymph drainage and interfere with removal of bacteria and foreign matter.

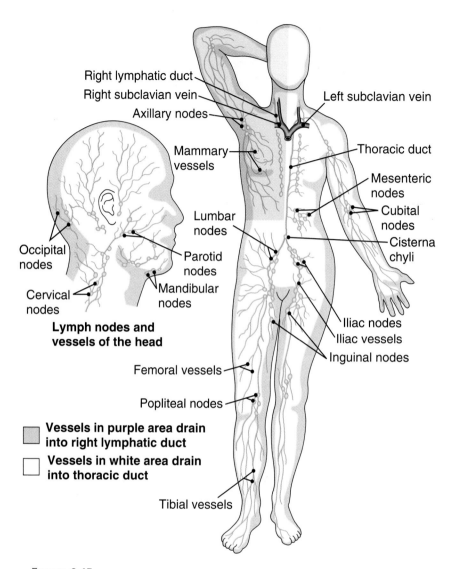

Right lymphatic duct

Right subclavian vein

Axillary nodes

Left subclavian vein

Mammary vessels

Thoracic duct

Mesenteric nodes

Lumbar nodes

Cubital nodes

Cisterna chyli

Occipital nodes

Parotid nodes

Cervical nodes

Mandibular nodes

Lymph nodes and vessels of the head

Iliac nodes

Iliac vessels

Inguinal nodes

Femoral vessels

Popliteal nodes

Vessels in purple area drain into right lymphatic duct

Vessels in white area drain into thoracic duct

Tibial vessels

▓ FIGURE 6-15 ▓

Lymphatic system. (Used with permission from Cohen, B. J. & Wood, D. L. (2000). *Memmler's structure and function of the human body* (7th ed.). Philadelphia: Lippincott Williams & Wilkins, p. 232.)

Lymphatic System Disorders

- Lymphangitis (lim-fan-ji'tis): inflammation of the lymph vessels.
- Lymphadenitis (lim-fad'e-ni-tis): inflammation of lymph nodes. Inflamed lymph nodes may not be able to filter pathogens from the lymph before it returns to the blood stream. This could lead to **septicemia** (sep-ti-se'me-ah).
- Lymphadenopathy (lim-fad'e-nop'ah-the): disease of the lymph nodes, often associated with enlargement such as seen in mononucleosis.
- Splenomegaly (splen'no-meg'ah-le): spleen enlargement.
- Hodgkin's disease: a chronic, malignant disorder, common in males, characterized by lymph node enlargement.
- Lymphosarcoma (lim-fo-sar-ko'mah): a malignant lymphoid tumor.
- Lymphoma: the term for any lymphoid tumor, benign or malignant.

Diagnostic Tests

- Biopsy
- Complete blood count (CBC)
- Mononucleosis test (Monospot)
- Culture and sensitivity (C & S)
- Bone marrow biopsy

STUDY & REVIEW QUESTIONS

1. The thin membrane lining the heart that is continuous with the lining of the blood vessels is the

   a. endocardium.   c. myocardium.
   b. epicardium.   d. pericardium.

2. The chamber of the heart that receives blood from the systemic system is the

   a. left atrium.   c. right atrium.
   b. left ventricle.   d. right ventricle.

3. The mitral valve in the heart is also called the

   a. aortic valve.   c. pulmonary semilunar valve.
   b. bicuspid valve.   d. tricuspid valve.

4. The ECG shows P waves resulting from

   a. atrial contractions.   c. recovery of the electrical charge.
   b. delayed contractions.   d. ventricular contraction.

5. When taking a blood pressure, the systolic pressure is the pressure reading when the

   a. artery is compressed and blood flow is cut off.
   b. cuff is completely deflated.
   c. first heart sounds are heard as the cuff is deflated.
   d. muffled sound is heard as the cuff is deflated.

6. The purpose of the pulmonary system is to

   a. carry blood to and from the lungs.
   b. carry nutrients to the cells.
   c. deliver blood to the systemic system.
   d. remove impurities from the blood.

7. Which of the following blood vessels are listed in the proper order of blood flow?

   a. aorta, superior vena cava, vein   c. capillary, venule, vein
   b. arteriole, venule, capillary   d. vein, venule, capillary

Continued

STUDY & REVIEW QUESTIONS *(CONTINUED)*

8. A vein is defined as a blood vessel that carries

   a. blood away from the heart.   c. deoxygenated blood.

   b. blood to the heart.   d. oxygen rich blood.

9. While selecting a vein for venipuncture you feel a distinct pulse. What you are feeling is a/an

   a. artery.   c. valve.

   b. nerve.   d. vein.

10. The internal space of a blood vessel is called the

   a. atrium.   c. septum.

   b. lumen.   d. valve.

11. The longest vein and the largest artery in the body in that order are

   a. cephalic and femoral.   c. inferior vena cava and brachial.

   b. great saphenous and aorta.   d. pulmonary and femoral.

12. The first choice vein to select for venipuncture is the

   a. accessory cephalic.   c. cephalic.

   b. basilic.   d. median cubital.

13. Which of the following is described as an anuclear, biconcave disk?

   a. erythrocyte   c. leukocyte

   b. granulocyte   d. thrombocyte

14. An individual's blood type—A, B, AB, or O—is determined by the presence or absence of which of the following on the red blood cells?

   a. antigens   c. chemicals

   b. antibodies   d. hormones

15. The main difference between plasma and serum is that plasma

   a. contains fibrinogen, serum does not.

   b. contains nutrients, plasma does not.

   c. looks clear, serum looks cloudy.

   d. looks dark yellow, serum looks pale yellow.

Continued

STUDY & REVIEW QUESTIONS *(CONTINUED)*

16. Which is the correct sequence of events after vessel injury?
    a. platelet aggregation, vasoconstriction, fibrin clot formation
    b. vasoconstriction, platelet aggregation, fibrin clot formation
    c. vasodilation, platelet adhesion, fibrin clot formation
    d. fibrinolysis, platelet adhesion, vasoconstriction

17. Lymph originates from
    a. joint fluid.
    b. plasma.
    c. serum.
    d. tissue fluid.

18. A heart disorder that is characterized by fluid buildup in the lungs is called
    a. aortic stenosis.
    b. bacterial endocarditis.
    c. congestive heart failure.
    d. MI.

Bibliography and Suggested Readings

Cohen, B. J., & Wood, D. L. (2000). Memmler's *Structure and function of the human body* (7th ed.). Philadelphia: Lippincott-Williams & Wilkins.

Cohen, B. J., & Wood, D. L. (2000). Memmler's *The human body in health and disease* (9th ed.). Philadelphia: Lippincott Williams & Wilkins.

Fischbach, F. (2000). *Laboratory diagnostic tests* (6th ed.). Philadelphia: Lippincott-Williams & Wilkins.

Herlihy, B., & Maebius, N. K. (2000). *The human body in health and illness*. Philadelphia: W.B. Saunders.

Quinley, E. (1993). *Immunohematology: Principles and practice*. Philadelphia: J. B. Lippincott.

Stevens, M.L. (1997). *Fundamentals of clinical hematology*. Philadelphia: W.B. Saunders.

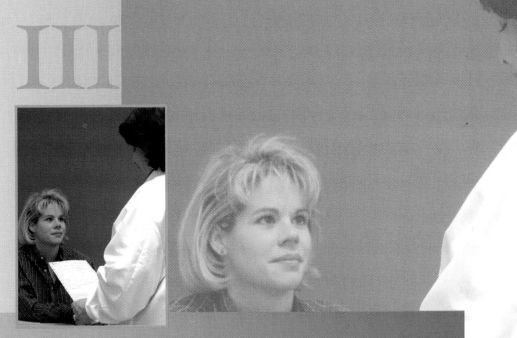

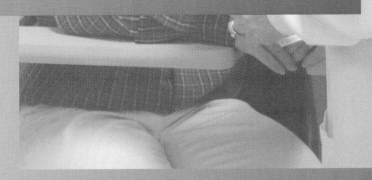

Blood Collection Procedures

7

BLOOD COLLECTION EQUIPMENT, ADDITIVES, AND ORDER OF DRAW

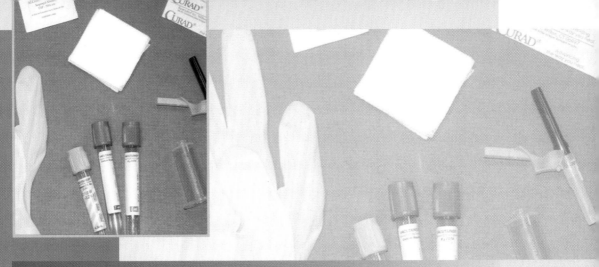

OBJECTIVES

Upon successful completion of this chapter, the reader will be able to:

1 Define the key terms and abbreviations listed at the beginning of this chapter.

2 List and describe the equipment and supplies needed to collect blood by venipuncture.

3 Compare and contrast antiseptics and disinfectants and give examples of each.

4 Identify and describe the various types of tourniquets, and explain the purpose and effects of using a tourniquet for venipuncture.

5 List and describe evacuated tube system and syringe system components and explain how each system works.

6 Identify the general categories of additives used in blood collection, list the various additives within each category, and describe how each additive works.

7 Describe the color coding used to identify the presence or absence of additives in blood collection tubes, and name the additive, laboratory departments and individual tests associated with the various color-coded tubes.

8 List the "order of draw" for collecting multiple tubes and explain why it is important.

INTRODUCTION

The primary duty of the phlebotomist is to collect blood specimens for laboratory testing. Blood is collected by several methods, including arterial puncture, skin puncture, and venipuncture. This chapter describes general blood collection equipment and supplies commonly needed regardless of the method of collection, as well as blood collection equipment specific to venipuncture. Arterial puncture equipment and skin puncture equipment are described in their respective chapters.

GENERAL BLOOD COLLECTION EQUIPMENT

The following are equipment and supplies commonly needed for all methods of collecting blood specimens.

Blood-Drawing Station

A blood-drawing station is a special area of a medical laboratory or clinic equipped for performing phlebotomy procedures on patients, primarily outpatients sent by their physicians for laboratory testing. As a minimum, a blood-drawing station includes a table for supplies, a special chair where the patient sits during the blood collection procedure, and a bed or reclining chair for patients with a history of fainting, people donating blood, and other special situations. A bed or padded table is also needed for performing heel sticks or other procedures on infants and small children.

Phlebotomy Chairs

Special **phlebotomy chairs** (Fig. 7-1) are available from a number of manufacturers. A phlebotomy chair should be comfortable for the patient and have adjustable armrests to achieve proper positioning of either arm. There should be a safety device to lock the armrest in place to prevent the patient from falling out should he or she become faint.

Carts and Trays

Carts and trays make blood-drawing equipment portable. This is especially important in a hospital setting and other instances where the patient cannot come to the laboratory.

Carts

Phlebotomy carts (Fig. 7-2) are generally made of stainless steel or strong synthetic material. They have swivel wheels, which glide the carts smoothly and quietly down hospital hallways and in and out of elevators. They normally have several shelves to carry adequate supplies for obtaining blood specimens from many patients. Carts are commonly used for early morning hospital phlebotomy rounds when many patients need lab work and for scheduled "sweeps" (rounds that occur at regular intervals throughout the day). Carts are bulky and a potential source of nosocomial infections and are not normally brought into patient rooms. Instead, they are parked outside in the hallway. A tray of supplies to be taken into the room is often carried on the cart.

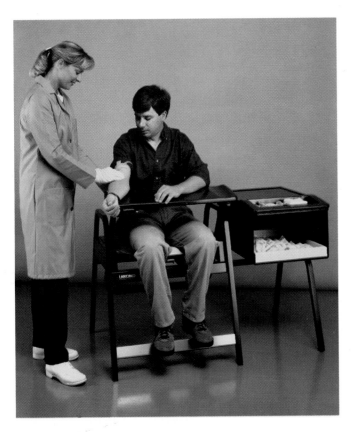

■ FIGURE 7-1 ■

Phlebotomy chair with attached storage unit. (Courtesy Labconco, Kansas City, MO.)

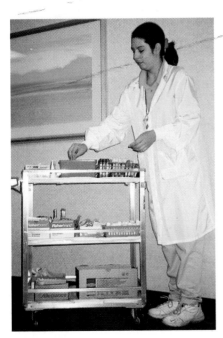

■ FIGURE 7-2 ■

Phlebotomy cart.

Trays

Phlebotomy trays (Fig. 7-3) come in a variety of styles and sizes designed to be easily carried by the phlebotomist and to contain enough equipment for numerous blood draws. They are convenient for "stat" or emergency situations or when relatively few patients need blood work.

 Key Point ➤ Keeping carts and trays adequately stocked with supplies is an important duty of the phlebotomist.

Gloves and Glove Liners

CDC/HICPAC Standard Precautions guidelines and the Occupational Safety and Health Administration (OSHA) Bloodborne Pathogen Standard, require the wearing of gloves when performing phlebotomy procedures. A new pair of gloves must be used for each patient and removed when the procedure is completed. Nonsterile, disposable latex, nitrile, neoprene, thermoplastic elastomer, polyethylene, and vinyl examination gloves are acceptable for most phlebotomy procedures. Glove quality is regulated by The Food and Drug Administration (FDA).

 Key Point ➤ Hand washing after glove removal is essential. Any type of glove may contain defects and some studies suggest that vinyl gloves may not provide an adequate barrier to viruses.

A good fit is essential. Some gloves come lightly dusted with powder to make them more comfortable to wear and easier to slip on and off. However, the phlebotomist

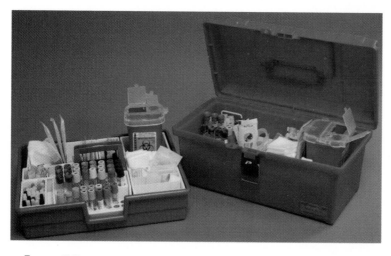

■ FIGURE 7-3 ■

Two types of phlebotomy trays: covered phlebotomy tray and phlebotomy tray with drawer.
(Post Medical Inc., Atlanta, GA.)

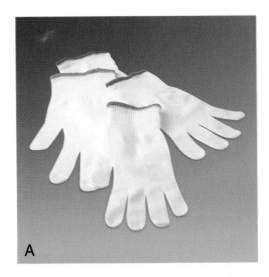
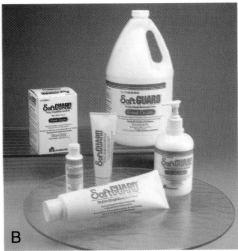

■ FIGURE 7-4 ■

(A) UltraFIT glove liners. (B) SoftGUARD Barrier hand cream.   (Courtesy Eric Scientific Company, Portsmouth, NH.)

should be aware that glove powder can be a source of contamination for some tests, especially those collected by skin puncture. In addition, powder has been known to cause allergies in some users. Powder in latex gloves can help suspend latex particles in the air and pose a danger to those with latex allergy. Special glove liners (Fig. 7-4, A) designed to be worn under latex or plastic gloves are available for people who develop allergies or dermatitis from wearing gloves. Barrier hand creams (Fig. 7-4, B) that help prevent skin irritation and are compatible with latex gloves are also available.

Antiseptics

Antiseptics are substances or solutions used to prevent sepsis, a disease state resulting from the presence of microorganisms or their toxic products in the blood stream. Antiseptics are bacteriostatic, that is, they prevent or inhibit the growth of bacteria, but do not necessarily kill them. They are considered safe to use on human skin and are used to clean the skin before blood collection. Antiseptics used for blood collection include the following.

- 70% isopropyl alcohol (isopropanol): the most common antiseptic used for routine blood collection, usually in the form of individually wrapped prep pads.
- Povidone-iodine: in several forms, including swab sticks and sponge pads for blood culture collection and prep pads for blood gas collection.
- 0.5% chlorhexidine gluconate: often used for those allergic to iodine.
- Benzalkonium chloride (e.g., zephiran chloride): alternate antiseptic.

Key Point ➤ Cleaning with an antiseptic reduces the number of microorganisms but does not sterilize the site.

Disinfectants

Disinfectants are chemical substances that are bacteriocidal (kill bacteria). They are used to remove or kill bacteria and other microorganisms on surfaces and instruments, but do not necessarily kill bacterial spores. They are not safe for use on human skin. Disinfectants are regulated by the Environmental Protection Agency (EPA).

 Key Point ➤ Household bleach (5.25% sodium hypochlorite) in a 1:10 dilution will kill human immunodeficiency virus and hepatitis viruses and is commonly used to wipe surfaces and clean up blood spills. Fresh bleach solutions should be made daily.

Gauze Pads/Cotton Balls

Clean 2 × 2 inch gauze pads folded in fourths are used to hold pressure over the site after venipuncture or skin puncture. Special gauze pads with plastic backing are available to help prevent contamination of gloves from blood at the venipuncture site. The use of cotton balls is not recommended because they have a tendency to stick to the site and reinitiate bleeding when removed.

Bandages

Adhesive bandages are used to cover a venipuncture or skin puncture site after the bleeding has ceased. Paper, cloth, or knitted tape placed over a folded gauze square can also be used, especially for patients who are allergic to adhesive bandages. Two-inch-wide roll gauze or self-adhesive gauze such as Coban (a special type of gauze that sticks to itself but not the skin) is occasionally used over a gauze pad or cotton ball to form a pressure bandage after arterial puncture or after venipuncture if patients have bleeding problems. Bandages are not to be used on babies younger than 2 years of age because of the danger of aspiration and suffocation. Latex-free bandages are available for those with latex allergies.

Needle and Sharps Disposal Containers

Regardless of whether or not they contain safety features, used needles, lancets, and other sharp objects must be disposed of immediately in special containers usually referred to as **"sharps" containers** (Fig. 7-5). A variety of styles and sizes are available from a number of different manufacturers. Some are red, orange, or other bright colors for easy identification; others are clear or opaque, which makes it easier to tell when they are full. All must be clearly marked with a biohazard symbol. Sharps containers must be rigid, puncture-resistant, leak-proof, disposable, and have locking lids that seal in the contents when full, after which they must be properly disposed of as biohazardous waste.

Slides

Precleaned 25 × 75 mm (1 × 3 inch) glass microscope slides are used to make blood films for hematology determinations. Slides are available either plain or with a frosted area at one end where the patient's name or other information can be written in pencil.

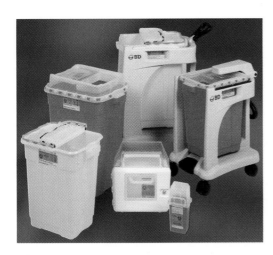

◈ FIGURE 7-5 ◈

Several styles of sharps containers.   (Courtesy Becton-Dickinson, Franklin Lakes, NJ)

Pen

A phlebotomist should always carry a pen with indelible or non–smear ink to label tubes and record other patient information.

Watch

A watch, preferably one with a sweep second hand or timer, is needed by the phlebotomist to determine specimen collection times accurately and to time special tests.

ARTERIAL PUNCTURE EQUIPMENT

See Chapter 12.

SKIN PUNCTURE EQUIPMENT

See Chapter 10.

VENIPUNCTURE EQUIPMENT

The following equipment is used for venipuncture procedures in addition to the general blood collection supplies and equipment.

Vein Locating Device

Transillumination means to inspect an organ by passing light through its walls. A transilluminator device such as the Venoscope II (Fig. 7-6) is an optional but useful tool for locating veins that are difficult to see or feel on all populations from neonates through adults. The Venoscope II uses an array of high-intensity light-emitting diode (LED) lights to transilluminate the patient's subcutaneous tissue and highlight the veins, which absorb the light rather than reflecting it and stand out as dark lines. When us-

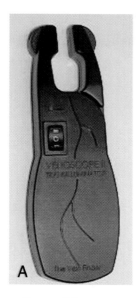
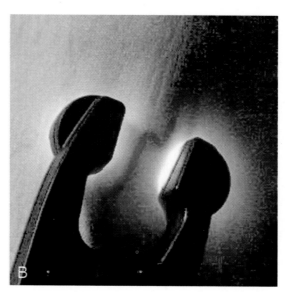

■ FIGURE 7-6 ■

(*A*) Venoscope II transilluminator device. (*B*) A vein appears as a dark line between the arms of the Venoscope II.   (Venoscope, L.L.C.)

ing the device, ambient lighting is dimmed to provide the contrast needed to see the vein. The device is then placed on the skin with the light directed into the subcutaneous tissues and moved longitudinally until a dark line is detected. If the vein is patent (unobstructed), pressing down on the arms of the device will cause it to blanch and releasing pressure will allow blood to flow again.

Tourniquet

A **tourniquet** (Fig. 7-7) is applied to a patient's arm before venipuncture. Proper tourniquet application allows arterial blood flow into the area below the tourniquet, but obstructs venous flow away from the area. This causes the veins to enlarge and makes them easier to find and pierce with a needle. Obstruction of blood flow can change blood components if the tourniquet is left in place for more than 1 minute, so a tourniquet must fasten in a way that is easy to release with one hand during blood collection procedures or in emergency situations such as when a patient starts to faint or the needle accidentally backs out of the arm during venipuncture.

There are a number of different types of tourniquets and most are available in both adult and pediatric sizes. The most commonly used tourniquet is a flat strip of stretchable latex, 15 to 18 inches long. A length of latex Penrose drain tubing can also be used. Latex does not readily support bacterial growth and if soiled can easily be wiped clean with disinfectant. Inexpensive disposable latex tourniquets are available. These can be used more than once, but are normally thrown away if they become contaminated with blood. Stretchable vinyl tourniquets are now available for general use or when employees or patients are allergic to latex.

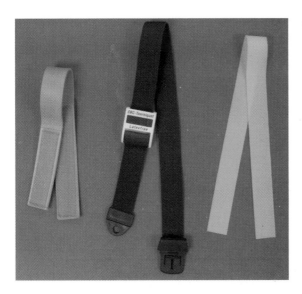

■ FIGURE 7-7 ■

Several types of tourniquets (left to right): Velcro closure, Buckle closure, and latex strap.

Velcro-closure tourniquets are also available. They usually are made of elastic material with a long band of Velcro or similar interlocking material that allows a wide range of adjustment capability. Two disadvantages of these tourniquets are that they may not fit around the arms of extremely obese patients, and they cannot be easily cleaned when soiled with blood or otherwise contaminated.

Several manufacturers make a type of tourniquet with stretchable webbing and a buckle closure. This type stays on the patient's arm when released and can be tightened again if necessary. Although older tourniquets of this type could not be easily cleaned, most new ones can be cleaned with disinfectant and some can even be put in the autoclave.

 Key Point ➤ A blood pressure cuff may be used in place of a tourniquet by those familiar with its operation. The patient's blood pressure is taken and the pressure is then maintained below the patient's diastolic pressure.

Needles

Needles used for phlebotomy include **multisample needles** (see Evacuated Tube System in this chapter), **hypodermic needles** (see Syringe System in this chapter), and **winged infusion (butterfly) needles** used with both the evacuated tube system and the syringe system. Needles are available with and without safety features.

 Key Point ➤ According to OSHA regulations, needles must have safety features to minimize the chance of accidental needlesticks or they must be used with equipment that contains safety features that shield the needle after use.

Safety features must provide a barrier between the hands of the user and the needle after use, and allow the user's hand to remain behind the needle at all times. Safety features include shields that cover the needle after use, blunting devices, and equipment with devices that retract the needle after use. Safety features must provide immediate permanent containment and be activated using a one-handed behind-the-needle technique. The FDA is responsible for clearing medical devices for marketing. Box 7-1 lists desirable characteristics of safety features that the FDA agrees are important in preventing percutaneous injury.

Box 7-1

DESIRABLE CHARACTERISTICS OF SAFETY FEATURES

1. The safety feature is a fixed safety feature that provides a barrier between the hands and the needle after use; the safety feature should allow or require the worker's hands to remain behind the needle at all times.
2. The safety feature is an integral part of the device and not an accessory.
3. The safety feature is in effect before disassembly and remains in effect after the disposal to protect users and trash handlers and for environmental safety.
4. The safety feature is as simple as possible, requiring little or no training to use effectively.

All blood collection needles are sterile, disposable, and designed for single use only. They are silicon coated to help them penetrate the skin smoothly. Hypodermic needles and butterfly needles normally come sealed in sterile pull-apart packages. Multisample needles are commonly enclosed in sealed twist-off shields or caps that cover both ends.

Key Point ➤ It is important to examine the packaging or seal of a needle before use. If the packaging is open or the seal is broken, the needle is no longer sterile and should not be used.

Specific terminology is used to refer to the parts of a needle. The end that pierces the vein is called the **bevel** because it is "beveled" or cut on a slant. A bevel allows the needle to easily slip into the skin and vein without coring (removal of a portion of the skin or vein). The cylindrical portion is called the **shaft.** The end that attaches to the blood collection device is called the **hub.**

Key Point ➤ It important to visually inspect a needle before venipuncture. Needles are mass manufactured and on rare occasions contain defects such as blocked, blunt, or bent tips or rough bevels or shafts that could injure a patient's vein, cause unnecessary pain, or result in failure to collect blood.

Needles come in various sizes, as indicated by gauge and length.

Gauge

Needle **gauge** is a number that relates to the diameter of the lumen (internal space) or "bore" of the needle. The needle diameter and the gauge number have an inverse (opposite) relationship, that is, the larger the gauge number, the smaller the actual diameter of the needle.

Manufacturers **color code** needles according to gauge for easy identification. Generally, multisample needles have color-coded caps and hubs (Fig. 7-8), syringe needles have color-coded hubs. Butterfly needles often have color-coded "wings." Syringe and butterfly needle packaging may also contain color coding. Needle color codes vary among manufacturers.

Although blood typically flows more quickly through large diameter needles, needle gauge is selected according to the size and condition of the patient's vein, the type of procedure, and the equipment being used. Appropriate needles for the collection of most blood specimens for laboratory testing include gauges 20 through 23; however, a 21-gauge needle is considered the standard for most routine phlebotomy situations. Common venipuncture needle gauges with needle type and typical use are shown in Table 7-1.

Multisample needles are generally available in gauges required for routine venipuncture, normally gauges 20 through 22. Syringe needles and butterflies are available in many gauges but it is important to use only those gauges appropriate for blood collection.

Key Point ➤ It is important to select the appropriate needle for the situation. A needle that is too large may damage a vein needlessly and a needle that is too small may hemolyze (damage red blood cells [RBCs], causing the release of hemoglobin into the serum or plasma) the specimen.

Length

Needles are available in various lengths. Most multisample needles come in 1 inch or 1-½ inch lengths. Syringe needles come in many lengths; however, 1 inch and 1-½ inch needles are most commonly used for venipuncture. Butterfly needles are commonly ½ to ¾ of an inch long. Some of the new self-sheathing needles come in slightly longer lengths to accommodate resheathing features. Length selection depends primarily upon

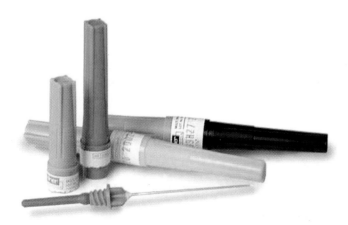

※ FIGURE 7-8 ※

Multisample needles with color-coded caps; yellow 20g, green 21g, and black 22g. (Greiner Bio-One, Kremsmünster, Austria.)

Table 7-1

Gauge	Needle Type	Typical use
15–17	Special needle attached to collection bag	Collection of donor units, autologous blood donation, and therapeutic phlebotomy
18	Hypodermic	Used primarily as a transfer needle rather than for blood collection Safety issues have diminished their use
20	Multisample, hypodermic	Sometimes used when large-volume tubes are collected or large-volume syringes are used on patients with normal-size veins
21	Multisample, hypodermic	Considered the standard venipuncture needle for routine venipuncture on patients with normal veins or syringe blood culture collection
22	Multisample, hypodermic	Used on older children and adult patients with small veins or syringe draws on difficult veins
23	Butterfly	Used on veins of infants and children and difficult or hand veins of adults
25	Butterfly	Venipuncture on premature infants and other neonates

Common Venipuncture Needle Gauges with Needle Type and Typical Use

user preference and also the depth of the vein. Many phlebotomists prefer to use the 1-inch needle in routine situations because it is less intimidating to the patient. It is also less intimidating to a phlebotomy student. However, some phlebotomists feel that the 1-$\frac{1}{2}$ inch needle allows for easier placement of the anchoring thumb.

Evacuated Tube System

The most common and preferred system for collecting blood samples is the **evacuated tube system (ETS)** (Fig. 7-9). It is a closed system in which the patient's blood flows through a needle inserted into a vein, directly into a collection tube without being exposed to the air. The system allows numerous tubes to be collected using a single venipuncture. Evacuated tube systems are available from several manufacturers. Although the design of individual elements may vary slightly by manufacturer, all ETS systems have three basic components, a special blood-drawing needle, a plastic holder that secures the needle and holds the evacuated tubes, and the various types of evacuated tubes.

Key Point ➤ Unless a component is specifically designed for use with multiple systems, it is recommended that all ETS components come from the same manufacturer. Mixing components from different manufacturers can lead to problems, such as needles coming unscrewed and tubes popping off during venipuncture procedures.

Multisample Needles

ETS needles are called multisample needles because they allow multiple tubes of blood to be collected during a single venipuncture. They are threaded in the middle and have a beveled point on each end. One end of the needle is longer and has a

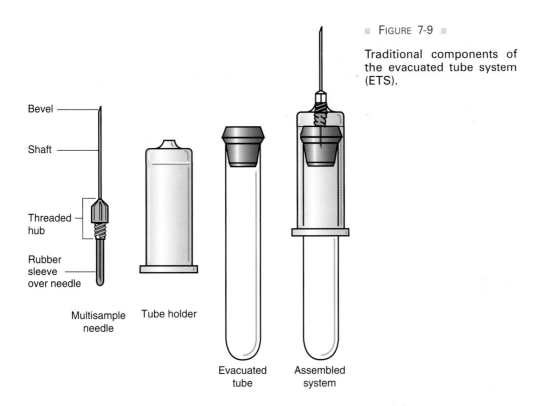

FIGURE 7-9

Traditional components of the evacuated tube system (ETS).

Bevel

Shaft

Threaded hub

Rubber sleeve over needle

Multisample needle

Tube holder

Evacuated tube

Assembled system

longer bevel and is used to pierce the patient's skin and enter the vein. The threaded portion of the needle screws into a tube holder, leaving the longer end exposed and the shorter end inside the tube holder. The shorter end is what penetrates the rubber stopper of a collection tube. It has a retractable rubber sleeve or sheath that pushes back when it goes into a tube stopper allowing blood to flow into the tube, but recovers the end of the needle when the tube is removed. This prevents leakage of blood when changing tubes during a multiple-tube draw, and when the tube is removed before withdrawing the needle from a vein. ETS multisample needles are available with or without safety features. An example of an ETS needle with safety features is shown in Figure 7-10.

Key Point ➤ ETS needles without safety features must be used with holders that contain safety features.

Needle and Tube Holders

A traditional needle and tube **holder** (Fig. 7-11), sometimes referred to as a tube hub or adapter, is a clear, plastic cylinder with a small opening at one end where the threaded needle is screwed in and a large opening at the other end to accept the evacuated tube. There are flanges or extensions on the sides of the tube end that aid in tube placement and removal.

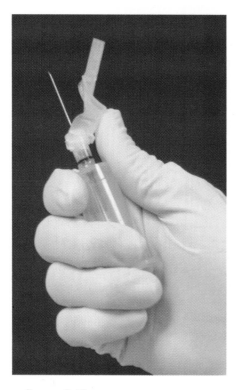

■ FIGURE 7-10 ■

BD Eclipse multisample safety needle attached to traditional tube holder.
(Courtesy Becton-Dickinson, Franklin Lakes, NJ.)

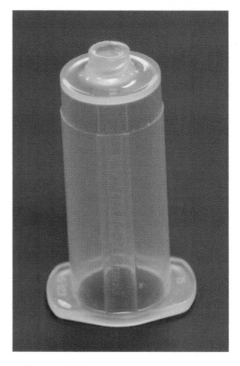

■ FIGURE 7-11 ■

Traditional needle and tube holders.

Holders come in several sizes; ones that fit regular diameter tubes, smaller ones that fit small diameter tubes used for pediatric patients or difficult draws, and special large ones for large diameter blood culture bottles. Some blood culture bottle holders have adapter inserts that narrow the diameter of the holder to allow collection of evacuated tubes after collecting blood culture specimens. Adapter inserts are also available so that small diameter tubes can be collected in regular-size tube holders. Holders are available with or without safety features. Safety features include shields that cover the needle and devices that manually or automatically retract the needle into the holder after it is withdrawn from the vein. Two types of holders with safety features are shown in (Fig. 7-12).

Key Point ➤ According to OSHA regulations, tube holders must be used with needles that have safety devices or a safety device to shield the needle must be incorporated into the tube holder.

Evacuated Tubes

Evacuated tubes (Fig. 7-13) are used with both the evacuated tube system and the syringe method of obtaining blood specimens. With the evacuated tube system, blood is collected directly into the tube during venipuncture. With the syringe method, blood is collected in a syringe and must be transferred into the tubes.

Evacuated tubes are made of glass or plastic and come in different sizes and volumes ranging from 2 to 15 mL. The size of tube is selected according to the age of the patient, the amount of blood needed for the test, and the size and condition of the patient's vein. Most laboratories stock several sizes of each type of tube in order to accommodate various needs.

Glass evacuated tubes are often coated on the inside with silicon to fill tiny cracks and other imperfections and create a smooth surface. The smooth surface prevents destruction of RBCs and helps keep blood from sticking to the sides of the tube. The silicon coating also prevents activation of the clotting factors in tubes used for coagulation studies.

Evacuated tubes fill with blood automatically because a **vacuum** (artificially created absence of air or negative pressure) exists in the tube. The vacuum is premeasured by the manufacturer so that the tube will draw the precise volume of blood indicated. To reach its stated volume, a tube with normal vacuum will fill with blood until the vacuum is exhausted. A tube that has lost all or part of its vacuum will, respectively, fail to fill with blood or will fill incompletely.

 Key Point ➤ A tube that is not filled to its stated capacity is called a partial or **"short draw."** Partially filled tubes can lead to inaccurate results for some tests.

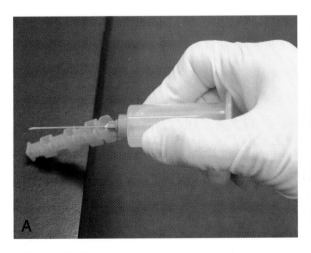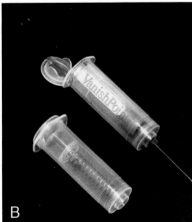

■ FIGURE 7-12 ■

Safety tube holders. (*A*) Venipuncture Needle-Pro with needle resheathing device. (*B*) Vanishpoint tube holder with needle retracting device.   (Retractable Technologies, Little Elm, Tx.)

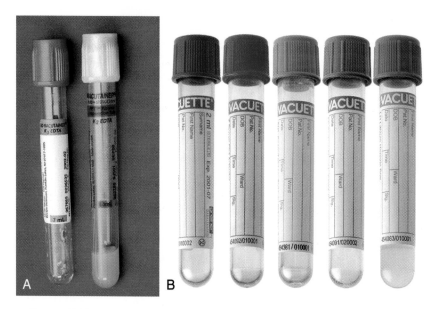

■ FIGURE 7-13 ■

Evacuated tubes. (*A*) BD Vacutainer Plus Plastic brand evacuated tubes. (Courtesy Becton-Dickinson, Franklin Lakes, NJ.). (*B*) Vacuette evacuated tubes. (Courtesy Greiner Bio-One Kremsmünster, Austria.)

Some manufacturers offer special **"short draw" tubes** designed to partially fill without compromising test results. These tubes are used in situations where it is difficult or inadvisable to draw larger quantities of blood.

Key Point ➤ Tubes do not fill all the way to the stopper. When filled properly, there is always a consistent amount of space between the level of blood in the tube and the tube stopper.

Evacuated tubes sometimes contain **additives.** A tube additive is any substance placed within a tube other than the tube stopper or the coating of the tube. Manufacturers guarantee additive integrity and tube vacuum until an expiration date printed on the label provided the tubes are stored between 4 and 25°C. Additive integrity and tube vacuum can be compromised if tubes are not stored properly. Premature loss of vacuum can occur from opening the tube, dropping the tube, advancing the tube too far onto the needle before venipuncture, or pulling the needle bevel partially out of the skin during venipuncture.

Key Point ➤ Always check the expiration date on a tube before using it. Never use a tube that has expired or has been dropped. Discard it instead.

TUBE STOPPERS

Tube stoppers (tops or closures) are commonly made of rubber or plastic. Some tubes have a rubber stopper covered by a plastic shield. The plastic shield is designed to protect lab personnel from blood remaining on the stopper after the tube is removed from the needle and when the stopper is removed from the tube. The rigidity of the plastic also prevents a "thumb roll" technique and subsequent aerosol (misting) of contents when removing the stopper from the tube.

COLOR CODING

Tube stoppers are color coded to indicate the presence and type of additive or the absence of additive in the tube. Color coding of plastic stoppers varies slightly from that of regular stoppers. In addition, although color coding is generally universal, some stopper colors may vary slightly by manufacturer. Common stopper colors, what they indicate, and what department uses them are shown in Table 7-2. Laboratory personnel normally identify tubes by color, referring to them as red tops, green tops, and so forth. For reference, two manufacturers' tube guides are shown on the last two pages of this book.

NONADDITIVE TUBES

Blood collected in tubes without additives will clot within 60 minutes. Fluid eventually separates from the clotted blood and is used for testing. The fluid is called serum because it does not contain fibrinogen. A clotted specimen must be centrifuged to separate the serum from the clot and remove any loose cells before the serum can be used for testing. Nonadditive tubes are used to obtain serum for chemistry and serology tests and for blood bank determinations. They are usually made of glass and have plain red rubber or plastic stoppers or royal blue stoppers with red on the label.

 Key Point ➤ Check tube labels carefully because some plastic tubes with plain red stoppers contain an additive that activates clotting and cannot be used for blood bank tests.

ADDITIVE TUBES

ETS tubes often contain additives. Blood collected in tubes that contain additives may or may not clot, depending on the type of additive(s) they contain. Color coding of the tube stopper (Table 7-2) identifies the type of additive in the tube. The amount of additive in a tube is designed to function optimally with the amount of blood required to fill the tube to the capacity or volume indicated by the manufacturer. An additive tube that has been under or overfilled will have an incorrect additive to blood ratio, which can cause inaccurate test results.

 Key Point ➤ To ensure delivery of a quality specimen, it is important to allow additive tubes to fill with blood until the vacuum is exhausted and the tube appears to contain a normal volume of specimen.

Table 7-2

Stopper Colors, Additives, and Departments

Stopper Color	Additives	Department(s)
Red (glass tube)	None	Chemistry, blood bank, serology/immunology
Light blue	Sodium citrate	Coagulation
Red (plastic tube)	Silica particles	Chemistry
Red and gray mottled Gold Hemogard	Gel separator/silica particles	Chemistry
Green and gray mottled Light green Hemogard	Gel separator/lithium heparin	Chemistry
Green	Lithium heparin Sodium heparin	Chemistry
Lavender	Ethylenediaminetetraacetate acid (EDTA)	Hematology, blood bank, chemistry
Gray	Sodium fluoride	Chemistry
Royal blue	None (red label) EDTA (lavender label) Sodium heparin (green label)	Chemistry
Yellow	Acid citrate dextrose (ACD)	Blood bank
Yellow	Sodium polyanetholesulfonate (SPS)	Microbiology

TRACE ELEMENT–FREE TUBES

Although stopper colors normally indicate the presence or absence of additive in a tube, royal blue stoppers are used to identify **trace element–free tubes.** These tubes are used for trace element tests, toxicology studies, and nutrient determinations. These substances are measured in such small quantities that trace elements commonly found in the glass or stopper material of evacuated tubes may leach into the specimen and falsely elevate test results. Trace element–free tubes are made of materials that have been specially manufactured to be as free of trace elements as possible. Inserts that come inside cartons of these tubes give a detailed analysis of residual amounts of trace elements contained in the tubes. Royal blue stopper tubes contain ethylenediaminetetraacetic acid (EDTA), heparin, or no additive to meet various test requirements. Color coding on the label indicates the type of additive or the absence of additive in the tube, lavender for EDTA, green for heparin, and red for no additive.

Syringe System

Although the evacuated tube system is the preferred method of blood collection, a **syringe system** (Fig. 7-14) is sometimes used for patients with difficult veins. The syringe system consists of a sterile Luer-Lok **(hypodermic)** needle attached to a disposable plastic **syringe.** Blood specimens collected using a syringe system must be transferred to evacuated tubes. This was formerly accomplished by inserting the syringe needle into the tube stopper, a practice now considered unsafe. **Syringe transfer devices** (Fig. 7-15) are available to allow safe transfer of blood to collection tubes without using the collection needle.

Needles

Syringe needles (Fig. 7-14) come in a wide range of gauges for many different uses. Only those gauges appropriate for phlebotomy procedures should be used, generally 21 to 23 gauge. Syringe needles also come in different lengths, with 1 inch and 1-½ inch lengths most commonly used for blood drawing. Syringe needles are available with or without safety features. Syringe needles with safety devices are shown in Figure 7-16.

 Key Point ➤ Syringe needles used for phlebotomy procedures must have resheathing devices to minimize the chance of accidental needlesticks. Needles used for intradermal skin tests must have resheathing devices or be used with syringes that have devices that cover or retract the needle after use.

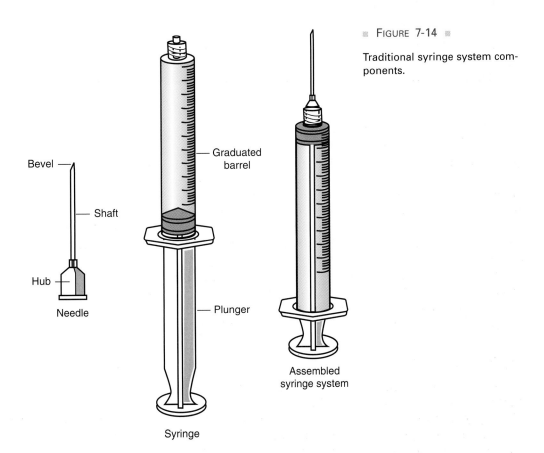

▓ FIGURE 7-14 ▓

Traditional syringe system components.

Bevel

Shaft

Hub

Needle

Graduated barrel

Plunger

Syringe

Assembled syringe system

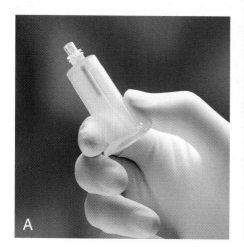
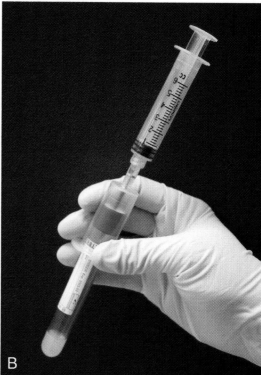

■ FIGURE 7-15 ■

Syringe transfer devices. (*A*) BD Transfer device. (Courtesy Becton-Dickinson, Franklin Lakes, NJ)
(*B*) Greiner Transfer device attached to syringe.

Syringes

Syringes (Fig. 7-14) come in various sizes, however 2 to 10 mL syringes are most commonly used for phlebotomy procedures. Syringe size is selected according to the size and condition of the patient's vein and the amount of blood to be collected.

Syringes have two parts, a **barrel** with graduated markings in either milliliters (mL) or cubic centimeters (cc), and a **plunger** that fits tightly into the barrel of the syringe. Most syringes come in sterile pull-apart packages. When drawing venous blood with a syringe, the phlebotomist must slowly retract (pull back on) the plunger creating a vacuum that causes the barrel of the syringe to fill with blood. Needles used with syringes must have resheathing devices or the syringe must have a device to cover the needle after use. Safety syringes (Fig. 7-17) with shields that slide over the needle after use are available. Needle resheathing devices that attach to the syringe before needle attachment (Fig. 7-18) are also available. They allow the needle to be safely covered, removed, and a transfer device attached to fill the evacuated tubes.

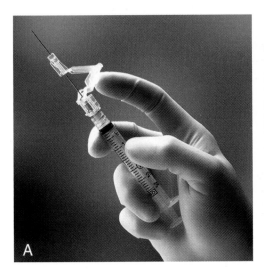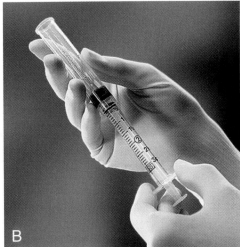

A B

■ FIGURE 7-16 ■

(*A*) Syringe with BD SAFETYGLIDE hypodermic needle attached. (*B*) BD SAFETY-LOK Syringe SIMS Portex.   (Courtesy Becton-Dickinson, Franklin Lakes, NJ.)

Winged Infusion Set

A **winged infusion set** or **butterfly,** as it is commonly called, is an indispensable tool for collecting blood from small or difficult veins such as hand veins or veins of elderly and pediatric patients. It allows much more flexibility and precision than a needle and syringe. A winged infusion set consists of a ½- to ¾-inch stainless steel needle permanently connected to a 5- to 12-inch length of tubing with either a luer attachment on the end for syringe use or a luer connected to a multisample Luer adapter for use with the evacuated tube system. Multiple sample Luer adapters are also available separately to convert a luer attachment butterfly so that it can be used with the evacuated tube system (Fig. 7-17).

Key Point ➤ The first tube collected with a butterfly will underfill because of the air in the tubing. If the tube contains an additive, the blood to additive ratio will be affected. If an additive tube is the first tube to be collected, draw a few milliliters of blood into a nonadditive red top and discard it before collecting the first tube. This is referred to as collecting a "clear" or discard tube.

Plastic extensions that resemble butterfly wings (thus the name butterfly) are attached to the needle where it is joined to the tubing. During use the needle is held from above by gripping the "wings" together between the thumb and index finger, allowing the user to achieve the shallow angle of needle insertion required to access small veins.

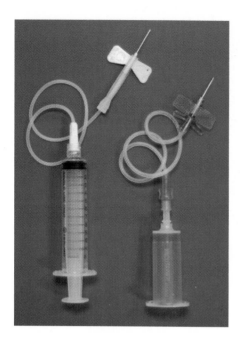

■ FIGURE 7-17 ■

Winged infusion sets attached to a syringe (left) and an evacuated tube holder by means of a Luer adapter.

Butterfly needles come in various gauges, with a 23 gauge being the one most commonly used in difficult phlebotomy situations. In rare situations a 25-gauge butterfly is used to collect blood from scalp or other tiny veins of premature infants and other neonates.

 Key Point ➤ Using a needle smaller than 23 gauge increases the chance of hemolyzing the specimen.

As with other types of blood collection needles, butterfly needles are required to contain safety devices to reduce the possibility of accidental needle sticks. Butterfly safety devices that are manually or sometimes automatically activated either before, during, or after needle removal include locking shields that slide over the needle, blunting devices, and needle retracting devices. See Figure 7-18 for examples of safety butterflies.

Combination Systems

The S-Monovette Blood Collection System (Sarstedt, Inc., Newton, NC) shown in Figure 7-19 is a complete system for blood collection in which the blood collection tube and collection apparatus are combined in a single unit. The unit allows the specimen to be collected by either an evacuated tube or syringe system technique. The units are available with regular or butterfly-style needles. Safety devices are available to contain the needle immediately after use.

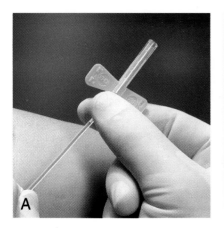
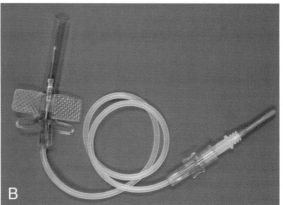
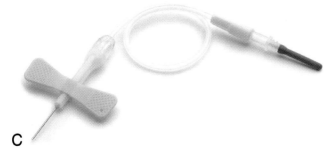

■ FIGURE 7-18 ■

Examples of safety winged infusion sets. (*A*) SAFETY-LOK Blood Collection Set for use with the evacuated tube system.   (Becton Dickinson Vacutainer Systems, Franklin Lakes, NJ.) (*B*) Monoject Angel Wing blood collection set.   (Kendall CO, LP, Mansfield, MA.) (*C*) Vacuette safety blood collection systems.   (Greiner Bio-One, Kremsmunster, Austria.)

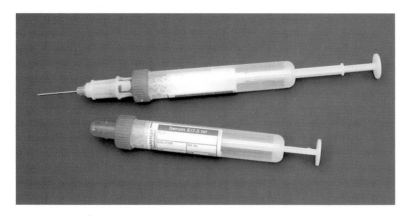

■ FIGURE 7-19 ■

S-Monovette Blood Collection System.   (Sarstedt, Inc., Newton, NC.)

BLOOD COLLECTION ADDITIVES

Blood collection tubes and other collection devices often contain additives to aid in blood specimen collection. There are a number of different types of additives used and each type has a specific function. Whether or not an additive is required during specimen collection generally depends upon the type of test and the method used to perform it. Consequently, additives should not be used arbitrarily or mixed together.

Key Point ➤ *Never* transfer blood collected in an additive tube into another additive tube because different additives may interfere with each other or the testing process. Even if the additives are the same, mixing them will create an excess of additive and possible interference in testing.

Additives are available in both liquid and dry forms. Tubes containing freeze-dried or powdered additive should be lightly tapped before use to settle the additive to the bottom of the tube. Additive tubes must be gently inverted anywhere from 3 to 10 times (number of inversions depends upon the type of additive) immediately after collection to ensure adequate mixing of the additive with the specimen.

Key Point ➤ *Never* shake or otherwise vigorously mix a specimen because it can cause hemolysis, which makes most specimens unsuitable for testing.

The most common additives are categorized by function as follows.

Anticoagulants

Anticoagulants are substances that prevent blood from coagulating or clotting. Clotting is prevented by either of two methods: chelating (binding) or precipitating calcium so it is not available for the coagulation process or inhibiting the formation of thrombin needed to convert fibrinogen to fibrin in the coagulation process. When a test requires either whole blood or a plasma specimen, it must be collected in a tube that contains an anticoagulant.

A blood specimen that has been collected in a tube containing an anticoagulant is called a whole blood specimen. The cells in a whole blood specimen will separate from the fluid and settle to the bottom of the tube on standing or when centrifuged. The red blood cells are heaviest and settle first. The lighter white blood cells and platelets settle on top of the red cell layer producing a thin white layer called the buffy coat. The clear to slightly hazy fluid on top is called plasma because clotting has been prevented and the fluid still contains fibrinogen.

Key Point ➤ Because the cells are free-flowing and not clotted, they can be resuspended by intentional or inadvertent mixing of the specimen.

There are different types of anticoagulants, each designed for use in certain types of testing. It is important to use the correct anticoagulant for the type of test performed. The most common anticoagulants are EDTA, citrates, heparin, and oxalates.

> *Memory Jogger* ➤ Remember the most common anticoagulants by the acronym "ECHO" created using the first letter of each one. "E" for EDTA, "C" for citrates, "H" for heparin, and "O" for oxalates.

EDTA

EDTA prevents coagulation by binding or chelating calcium. It is commonly available in several forms: spray-dried dipotassium (K_2)EDTA, disodium (Na_2)EDTA freeze-dried powder, or tripotassium (K_3)EDTA liquid. EDTA is increasingly being used for blood bank studies; however, it is primarily used to provide whole blood specimens for hematology studies because it preserves cell morphology and inhibits platelet aggregation or clumping which can negatively affect test results. EDTA specimens must be mixed immediately after collection to prevent platelet clumping and microclot formation. Eight to ten inversions are required for proper mixing.

Key Point ➤ If microclots are detected in a hematology specimen it cannot be used for testing and must be recollected.

The National Committee for Clinical Laboratory Standards (NCCLS) and The International Council for Standardization in Haematology recommend spray-dried (K_2)EDTA for blood cell counting and sizing because liquid (K_3)EDTA dilutes the specimen and results in lower hemoglobin values, RBC and white blood cell (WBC) counts, platelet counts, and packed cell volume. The dilution effect is even more pronounced if the tubes are incompletely filled, so it is important that the tubes be filled until their normal vacuum is exhausted. (Some manufacturers such as Becton Dickinson Vacutainer Systems are discontinuing liquid (K_3)EDTA tubes for these reasons.) Proper filling of tubes is important for all types of EDTA because the excess of EDTA that results when tubes are underfilled causes RBCs to shrink and changes the staining characteristics of WBCs.

Key Point ➤ Prolonged contact with EDTA can also change the staining characteristics of WBCs. Consequently, blood smears made from EDTA specimens should be made within 1 hour of specimen collection.

EDTA is contained in lavender (purple) stopper tubes, royal blue stopper tubes with lavender on the label, and microcollection containers with lavender stoppers. New EDTA tubes especially designed for blood bank use have pink plastic stoppers and a special cross match label for patient information required by the American Association of Blood Banks (AABB).

Memory Jogger ➤ An easy way to remember that lavender (purple) stopper tubes contain EDTA and are used for hematology studies is to think of the nonsense word phedta (fa he' ta), pronounced like the popular Mexican food, *fajita;* where "p" stands for purple, "h" stands for hematology, and EDTA is the anticoagulant in the tube.

Citrates

Citrates prevent coagulation by binding or chelating calcium. The most common citrate is **sodium citrate** contained in light blue stopper tubes. It is used for coagulation specimens because it does the best job of preserving the coagulation factors, and adding calcium back to the specimen during testing can easily reverse its binding effects. Coagulation tests are performed on plasma, so specimens must be centrifuged to separate the plasma from the cells. Coagulation specimens require immediate mixing to prevent activation of the coagulation process and microclot formation, which invalidate test results. Light blue top tubes require three to four inversions for proper mixing.

 Key Point ➤ There is a critical 9:1 ratio of blood to anticoagulant in light blue sodium citrate tubes, so it is important to fill them to the stated capacity. Underfilled light blue tubes do not contain the proper ratio and will not be accepted for testing by most laboratories.

Memory Jogger ➤ Use the jingle, "Spring creates colorful light blue pansies" to remember that sodium citrate tubes go to the coagulation department and have light blue stoppers. The "S" in spring is for sodium, "C" in creates is for citrate, "C" in colorful is for the coagulation department, light blue is the color of the tube, and "P" in pansies is for the plasma used in testing.

Heparin

Heparin prevents clotting primarily by inhibiting thrombin. It inhibits thrombin by accelerating the action of a naturally occurring coagulation inhibitor called antithrombin III (ATIII), increasing its activity by up to 1,000 times. ATIII neutralizes or inhibits thrombin and further conversion of prothrombin to thrombin. Clotting is prevented because thrombin is needed to convert fibrinogen into the fibrin necessary for clot formation.

Memory Jogger ➤ A way to remember that heparin inhibits thrombin formation is: there is an "h" in heparin, and an "h" in inhibits. In addition, heparin and thrombin both end in "in," and inhibits begins in "in."

There are three heparin formulations: ammonium, lithium, and sodium heparin. Lithium heparin causes the least interference in chemistry testing and is the most widely used anticoagulant for plasma and whole blood chemistry determinations. Although serum specimens are sometimes preferred for routine chemistry tests, heparinized plasma is often used for immediate chemistry determinations to save the time required for a specimen to clot before serum can be obtained.

Key Point ➤ Heparinized whole blood or plasma is preferred over serum for potassium tests because potassium is released from platelets into the serum when blood clots and can falsely elevate results.

Heparinized specimens must be mixed immediately upon collection to prevent clot formation and fibrin generation. Eight to ten inversions are required for proper mixing. Gentle mixing is essential to prevent hemolysis. Hemolyzed specimens are unsuitable for many chemistry tests. Heparin is contained in tubes and microcollection containers that have green stoppers, and royal blue stopper tubes with green on the label.

Key Point ➤ It is important to choose the right heparin formulation for the type of test. Lithium heparin must not be used to collect lithium levels. Sodium heparin must not be used to collect sodium specimens or electrolyte panels because sodium is part of the panel. In addition, heparinized blood should not be used to make blood smear slides for hematology because heparin interferes in the staining process.

Memory Jogger ➤ Use the jingle, "Greenhouses have colorful plants" to remember that green tubes contain heparin used to collect chemistry tests that require plasma samples for testing. "Green" in greenhouses is the color of the tube. The "H" in have stands for the heparin in the tube. The "C" in colorful stands for chemistry. The "P" in plants stands for the plasma used for testing.

Oxalates

Ammonium, lithium, potassium, and **sodium oxalate** all prevent coagulation by precipitating calcium. However, potassium oxalate is the most widely used. Oxalates are commonly added to tubes containing glucose preservatives (see antiglycolytic agents) to provide plasma for glucose testing. Oxalates are most commonly found in tubes and microcollection containers with gray stoppers. Oxalate specimens must be mixed immediately upon collection to prevent clot formation and fibrin generation. Eight to ten inversions are required for proper mixing.

Key Point ➤ It is important to fill oxalate tubes to the stated capacity because excess oxalate causes hemolysis, the destruction of red blood cells and release of hemoglobin into the plasma.

> *Memory Jogger* ➤ Think of the word "GO" to remember that gray tubes contain oxalate. "G" stands for "gray" and "O" stands for "oxalate," or picture a "gray ox" where "gray" stands for the tube and "ox" stands for "oxalate."

Special Use Anticoagulants

The following anticoagulants are combined with other additives and have additional properties for special use situations.

Acid Citrate Dextrose

Acid citrate dextrose (ACD) solution is available in two formulations, solution A and solution B, and is used for certain immunohematology tests such as DNA testing and human leukocyte antigen phenotyping used in paternity evaluation and to determine transplant compatibility. The acid citrate in ACD solution prevents coagulation by binding calcium with little effect on cells and platelets. The dextrose acts as both a red blood cell nutrient and a preservative because it maintains red cell viability. ACD tubes require 8 to 10 inversions immediately after collection to prevent clotting. ACD tubes have yellow stoppers.

Citrate-Phosphate-Dextrose

Citrate-phosphate-dextrose (CPD) and CPD with adenine (CPDA-1) are used in collecting units of blood for transfusion purposes. The citrate prevents clotting by chelating calcium. Sodium biophosphate stabilizes the pH, and dextrose provides energy to the cells and helps keep them alive.

Sodium Polyanethol Sulfonate

Sodium polyanethol sulfonate (SPS) also prevents coagulation by binding calcium. It is used for blood culture collection because, in addition to being an anticoagulant, it inhibits complement (proteins in serum that destroy bacteria) and phagocytosis (ingestion of bacteria by leukocytes) and reduces the activity of certain antibiotics. SPS tubes also have yellow stoppers.

Antiglycolytic Agents

An **antiglycolytic agent** is a substance that inhibits **glycolysis,** or metabolism of glucose (blood sugar) by the cells of the blood. If glycolysis is not prevented, the glucose concentration in a blood specimen decreases at a rate of 10 mg/dL per hour.

Key Point ➤ Glycolysis occurs faster in newborns because their metabolism is increased and in patients with leukemia because of high metabolic activity of WBCs.

The most common antiglycolytic agents are **sodium fluoride** and **lithium iodo-acetate.** Glucose stability is preserved for 24 hours in iodoacetate and for up to 3 days in sodium fluoride. Sodium fluoride also inhibits the growth of bacteria. Antiglycolytic agents are commonly used in combination with ammonium or potassium oxalate, or lithium heparin to provide plasma specimens. Sodium fluoride and lithium iodoacetate tubes have gray stoppers.

Key Point ➤ Sodium fluoride tubes are used to collect ethanol specimens to prevent either a decrease in alcohol concentration because of glycolysis since ethanol is mostly sugar, or an increase because of fermentation by bacteria.

Clot Activators

A **clot activator** is a substance that initiates or enhances coagulation. Clot activators include substances that provide increased surface for platelet activation, such as glass or **silica** particles and inert clays such as **Celite, kaolin,** or **siliceous earth,** and clotting factors such as thromboplastin and thrombin. Silica particles are the clot activators in serum separator tubes. Silica particles cause the blood to clot within 15 to 30 minutes. Thrombin is an additive in a special type of light blue tube, Becton Dickinson orange Hemogard stopper tubes, and mottled yellow and black rubber stopper tubes used for a few coagulation studies. Blood collected in thrombin tubes generally clots within 5 minutes. Celite tubes and kaolin tubes are available for use with the Hemochron Response Whole Blood Coagulation System used for point-of-care coagulation testing. Tubes containing clot activators require a minimum of five gentle inversions for complete and rapid clotting to occur.

Thixotropic Gel Separator

A **thixotropic gel separator** is an inert (nonreacting) synthetic substance that forms a physical barrier between the cells of a specimen and the serum or plasma when the specimen is centrifuged. The physical separation prevents the cells from continuing to metabolize substances, particularly glucose, in the serum or plasma. The gel, which is initially contained in or near the bottom of the collection tube, has a density between that of the cells and the serum or plasma. When the specimen is centrifuged, the gel undergoes a change in viscosity (thickness) and moves to a position between the cells and the serum or plasma portions of the specimen, forming the physical barrier. Serum specimen tubes that contain the gel have gold plastic stoppers or mottled red/gray rubber stoppers and are called **serum separator tubes (SSTs).** Heparinized tubes that contain the gel have light green plastic or mottled gray/green rubber stoppers and are called **plasma separator tubes (PSTs).** EDTA tubes that contain the gel have special lavender stoppers and are called **plasma preparation tubes (PPTs).**

ORDER OF DRAW

The order in which tubes are collected during a multiple tube draw, filled from a syringe after a draw, or obtained by skin puncture can lead to interference in testing caused by contamination of the specimen by additive carryover, tissue thromboplastin, or microorganisms. The order of draw is a special sequence of tube collection that was developed to minimize these problems.

Key Point ➤ Order of draw may vary among institutions. Consult institution protocol before using a specific order of draw.

Carryover/Cross-Contamination

Carryover or cross-contamination is the transfer of additive from one tube to the next. It can occur when blood in a tube that contains an additive is allowed to come in contact with the stopper puncturing needle during ETS blood collection or when transferring blood from a syringe into multiple tubes. Blood remaining on or within the needle may then be transferred to the next tube drawn or filled, contaminating that tube and possibly affecting test results on that specimen.

EDTA has been the source of more carryover problems than any other additive. Heparin causes the least interference in tests other than coagulation tests because it also occurs in blood naturally.

Box 7-2 lists some of the most common tests affected by additive contamination. However, remembering which tests the various additives affect can be difficult. The order of draw eliminates confusion by presenting a sequence of collection that results in the least amount of interference should carryover occur. Carryover can also be minimized by making certain that specimen tubes fill from the bottom up during collection and that the contents of the tube do not come in contact with the stopper puncturing needle during the draw or when transferring blood into tubes from a syringe.

Box 7-2

COMMON TESTS AFFECTED BY ADDITIVE CONTAMINATION

Tests Affected by Ethylenediaminetetraacetic Acid Contamination

Calcium	Protime
Partial thromboplastin	Serum iron
Potassium	Sodium

Tests Affected by Heparin Contamination

Activated clotting time
Partial thromboplastin
Protime

Tests Affected by Potassium Oxalate Contamination

Partial thromboplastin	Protime
Potassium	Red cell morphology

Tissue Thromboplastin Contamination

Tissue thromboplastin is a clotting factor that activates the coagulation process. It is released when skin is pierced and is present in skin puncture blood. It is picked up by the needle during venipuncture and flushed into the first tube as it fills during ETS collection or mixed with blood collected in a syringe. Because it activates the coagulation process, it can interfere with coagulation tests. Although it is no longer considered a significant problem for prothrombin time (PT) and partial thromboplastin time (PTT) tests unless the draw is difficult and involves extra manipulation of the needle, it can be a significant problem for special coagulation tests such as factor VIII tests. Therefore if coagulation tests other than PT or PTT are the only tests ordered or they are first in the sequence of other tests ordered, a "clear" or "discard" tube should be drawn first. This involves collecting a few milliliters of blood into a nonadditive red top tube and discarding it before collecting a coagulation tube. In addition, a coagulation tube should not be the first tube collected when a butterfly is used because the air in the tubing displaces blood in the tube and changes the critical 9:1 blood to additive ratio. Drawing a discard tube first eliminates this problem also.

 Key Point ➤ A discard tube should be drawn first to protect the blood to additive ratio of any additive tube that is first in a sequence of tubes collected using a butterfly.

Microbial Contamination

Microbial contamination can lead to false-positive blood cultures. Blood cultures detect microorganisms in the blood and require special site cleaning measures before collection to prevent contamination of the specimen by microorganisms normally found on the skin. Blood cultures are collected first in the order of draw to ensure that they are collected when sterility of the site is optimal and to prevent microbial contamination of the needle from the unsterile tops of tubes used to collect other tests. Blood cultures, however, are typically drawn separately and do not often factor into the sequence of collection.

NCCLS Order of Draw

The NCCLS recommends the same order of draw for the collection of evacuated tubes or filling evacuated tubes from a syringe. The NCCLS order of draw and the rationale behind it are summarized in Table 7-3.

Memory Jogger ➤ Remember the most common tubes in the order of draw by the phrase "stop, red light, stay put, green light, go." The first letter of each word in the phrase stands for a tube in the order of draw: S (sterile), R (red), L (light blue), S (serum separator tube or SST), P (plasma separator tube or PST), G (green), L (lavender), and G (gray).

Table 7-3

NCCLS Order of Draw, Stopper Color, and Rationale for Collection Order

Order of Draw	Tube Stopper Color	Rationale for Collection Order
Blood cultures (sterile collections)	Yellow sodium polyanetholesulfonate (SPS) (or sterile media containers)	Minimizes chance of microbial contamination.
Plain (nonadditive) tubes	Red	Prevents contamination by additives in other tubes.
Coagulation tubes	Light blue	Second or third position in order of draw prevents tissue thromboplastin contamination. Must be the first additive tube in the order because all other additive tubes affect coagulation tests.
Serum separator gel tubes (SSTs)	Red and gray rubber Gold plastic	Prevents contamination by additives in other tubes. Comes after coagulation tests because silica particles activate clotting and affect coagulation tests. Carryover of silica into subsequent tubes can be overridden by the anticoagulant in them.
Plasma separator gel tubes (PSTs)	Green and gray rubber Light green plastic	Contains heparin, which affects coagulation tests and interferes in collection of serum specimens. Causes the least interference in tests other than coagulation tests.
Heparin tubes	Green	Same as PST.
Ethylenediaminetetraacetic acid (EDTA) tubes	Lavender	Causes more carryover problems than any other additive. Elevates sodium and potassium levels. Chelates and decreases calcium and iron levels. Elevates prothrombin time and partial thromboplastin time results.
Oxalate/fluoride tubes	Gray	Sodium fluoride and potassium oxalate elevate sodium and potassium levels, respectively. Comes after hematology tubes because oxalate damages cell membranes and causes abnormal red blood cell morphology.

Alternate Syringe Order of Draw

Because the clotting process is activated the minute that blood starts to fill a syringe, some institutions prefer to use a separate order of draw for syringe collections so that tubes most affected by microclot formation are filled as soon as possible. This order of draw assumes that blood that enters the syringe last is the freshest and least affected by microclot formation. Sterile specimens are still filled first, but are immediately followed by anticoagulant tubes. This alternate syringe order of draw is shown in Box 7-3.

Box 7-3

ALTERNATE SYRINGE ORDER OF DRAW

1. Sterile specimens (i.e., blood cultures)
2. Light blue tops (i.e., coagulation tubes)
3. Lavender tops and plasma preparation tube (PPTs)
4. Green tops and plasma separator tube (PSTs)
5. Gray tops (antiglycolytic tubes)
6. Red tops and serum separator tubes (SSTs)

Key Point ➤ To prevent carryover when this method is used it is important for the phlebotomist to keep the transfer needle above the fill level of the tube so that blood mixed with additive does not contaminate it.

Memory Jogger ➤ An easy way to remember the alternate order of draw for syringe collections is to remember the nonsense jingle "Silly ladies love green and gray roses," where the first letter in each word stands for a tube in the order of draw. "S" for sterile, "L" for light blue coagulation tube, "L" for lavender, "G" for green, "G" for gray, and "R" for red.

NCCLS Skin Puncture Order of Draw

The order of draw for collecting multiple specimens by skin puncture (see Chapter 10) differs from that of venipuncture. Skin puncture blood contains tissue thromboplastin and will begin to clot immediately. It is important to collect specimens quickly to minimize the effects of platelet clumping and microclot formation, which invalidate hematology test results, and to ensure that an adequate amount of specimen is collected before the site stops bleeding. The NCCLS order of draw for collection of skin puncture specimens is:

- EDTA specimens
- Other additive specimens
- Serum specimens

STUDY & REVIEW QUESTIONS

1. Which of the following substances will sterilize a blood collection site?
   a. 0.5% Chlorhexidine gluconate
   b. 70% Isopropyl alcohol
   c. Zephiran chloride
   d. None of the above

2. Containers used for disposing of needles and other sharp objects must be all of the following *except*
   a. clearly marked "biohazard."
   b. disposable.
   c. puncture resistant.
   d. recyclable.

3. You are about to perform routine venipuncture on a patient with no known allergy to antiseptics. Which of the following substances would you use to clean the site?
   a. Antibacterial soap and water
   b. Povidone iodine
   c. 70% Isopropyl alcohol
   d. 5.25% Sodium hypochlorite

4. Needles are color coded according to their
   a. brand.
   b. expiration date.
   c. gauge.
   d. length.

5. Which of the following needles has the smallest diameter?
   a. 19 gauge
   b. 20 gauge
   c. 21 gauge
   d. 23 gauge

6. What causes evacuated tubes to fill with blood automatically?
   a. Arterial pressure
   b. Fist pumping by the patient
   c. Pressure created by the tourniquet
   d. Tube vacuum

Continued

7. The color code that is most often associated with tubes used to collect hematology tests is

   a. green.
   b. light blue.
   c. lavender.
   d. red.

8. Which additive prevents glycolysis?

   a. EDTA
   b. Heparin
   c. Potassium oxalate
   d. Sodium fluoride

9. For which of the following tubes is the blood to additive ratio most critical?

   a. Green stopper
   b. Lavender stopper
   c. Light blue stopper
   d. Red stopper

10. Which of the following tubes or blood containers should be filled last in the recommended order of draw?

    a. Blood culture bottle
    b. Lavender top
    c. Light blue top
    d. Nonadditive red top

11. Which anticoagulant prevents coagulation by inhibiting thrombin formation?

    a. EDTA
    b. Heparin
    c. Sodium citrate
    d. Potassium oxalate

12. Butterfly needles are used to collect specimens from

    a. Difficult veins
    b. Hand veins
    c. Small veins
    d. All the above

CASE STUDY 7-1: PROPER HANDLING OF ANTICOAGULANT TUBES

A phlebotomist named Chi is collecting an SST and two lavender tops (one for a glycohemoglobin and one for a complete blood count [CBC]) on an inpatient named Louise Jones. He fills the SST, lays it down while he places the first lavender top in the tube holder, then picks it up and mixes it as the lavender top is filling. When the lavender top is full he lays it down while he places the second lavender top in the tube holder. The second lavender top fails to fill with blood so he makes several needle adjustments to try to establish blood flow. Nothing works so he decides to try a new tube. The new tube works fine. While it is filling he picks up the first lavender top and mixes it. After completing the draw he labels his tubes, putting the hematology label on the lavender top he collected first. He finishes up with the patient, delivers the specimens to processing, and goes on break. When he returns from break his phlebotomy supervisor tells him to recollect the CBC on Louise Jones because the specimen had a clot in it.

QUESTIONS:
1. What can cause clots in EDTA specimens?
2. What most likely caused the clot in this specimen?
3. Did the problem with the second lavender top contribute to the problem?
4. Would the problem with the second lavender top have been an issue if Chi had handled the first lavender top properly?
5. What can Chi do to prevent this type of thing from happening in the future?

CASE STUDY 7-2: ORDER OF DRAW

Jake, a phlebotomist, is sent to the emergency room (ER) to collect an EDTA specimen for a stat type and cross match on an accident victim. He properly identifies the patient and is in the process of filling the lavender top tube when an ER nurse tells him that the patient's physician wants to add a stat set of electrolytes to the test order. Jake acknowledges her request. He finishes filling the lavender top, and grabs a green top. After completing the draw he takes the specimens straight to the laboratory to be processed immediately.

QUESTIONS:
1. One of the specimens that Jake drew is compromised. Which one is it?
2. Why is the specimen compromised and how may test results be affected?
3. How could Jake have avoided the problem without drawing the patient twice?

■ CASE STUDY 7-3: BUTTERFLY USE AND ORDER OF DRAW

Maria, who was recently hired in her first job as a phlebotomist, has been sent to the intensive care unit to collect a stat hemoglobin and hematocrit and protime on a patient. The patient is an elderly woman. Her left arm has an intravenous line. Maria checks the right arm and finds a small but suitable vein. She decides to use a butterfly with the evacuated tube system and selects a light blue top and a lavender top from her blood collection tray. The patient's nurse asks her how long she thinks it will take because she wants to give the patient a shot in that arm. Maria tells her that she only has two tubes to collect so it shouldn't take long. The nurse leaves. Maria makes a successful venipuncture, fills the light blue top and mixes it gently by inverting it eight times. Then she fills the lavender top. After finishing the draw, properly labeling the tubes and checking and bandaging her patient she returns to the lab. Specimen processing immediately rejects the protime and asks her to recollect it.

QUESTIONS:
1. Why do you think specimen processing rejected the protime?
2. How did the way Maria collected the specimen cause the problem?
3. Why does the lab reject tubes with this problem?
4. What can Maria do differently when she recollects the specimen?

Bibliography and Suggested Readings

Bishop, M., Duben-Engelkirk, J., & Fody, E. (1996). *Clinical chemistry: Principles, procedures, correlations* (3rd ed.). Philadelphia: Lippincott-Raven Publishers.

Burtis, C., Ashwood, E., & Tietz, . (2001). *Fundamentals of clinical chemistry* (5th ed.). Philadelphia: W. B. Saunders.

College of American Pathologists (CAP). (1999.) *So you're going to collect a blood specimen* (8th ed.). Northfield, IL: CAP.

Gottfried, El., & Adachi, M. M. (1997). Prothrombin time (PT) and activated partial thromboplastin time (APTT) can be performed on the first tube. *American Journal Clinical of Pathologists 107*, 681–683.

National Committee for Clinical Laboratory Standards, H1-A4. (December 1996). *Evacuated tubes and additive for blood specimen collection* (4th ed.).Wayne, PA: NCCLS.

National Committee for Clinical Laboratory Standards, H3-A4. (June 1998). *Procedures for the collection of diagnostic blood specimens by venipuncture* (4th ed.). Wayne PA: NCCLS.

National Committee for Clinical Laboratory Standards, M29-A. (December 1997). *Protection of laboratory workers from instrument biohazards and infectious disease transmitted by blood, body fluids and tissue* (Approved guideline). Wayne, PA: NCCLS.

Stevens, M. (1997). *Fundamentals of clinical hematology.* Philadelphia: W. B. Saunders.

8

VENIPUNCTURE SPECIMEN COLLECTION PROCEDURES

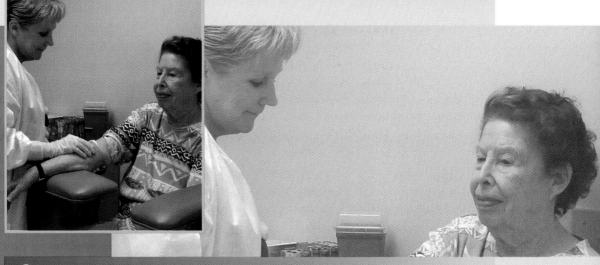

Upon successful completion of this chapter, the reader will be able to:

1 Define the key terms and abbreviations listed at the beginning of this chapter.

2 Describe the test request process, identify the types of requisitions used, and list required requisition information.

3 List and define test status designations, identify status priorities, and describe the procedure to follow for each status designation.

4 Describe proper bedside manner and how to handle special situations associated with patient contact.

5 Explain the importance of proper patient identification and describe what information is verified, how to handle discrepancies, and what to do if a patient's identification band is missing.

6 Describe how to prepare patients for testing, how to answer inquiries concerning tests, and what to do if a patient objects to the test.

7 Describe how to verify fasting and other diet requirements and what to do when diet requirements have not been met.

8 Describe each step in the venipuncture procedure, list necessary information found on specimen tube labels and list the acceptable reasons for inability to collect a specimen.

9 Describe collection procedures when using a butterfly or syringe and the proper way to safely dispense blood into tubes after syringe collection.

10 Describe unique requirements associated with drawing special populations including pediatric, geriatric, and long-term care patients.

INTRODUCTION

Venipuncture (puncture of a vein) is the term used to describe the process of collecting or "drawing" blood from a vein. It is the most common way to collect blood specimens for laboratory testing. The following venipuncture procedures were written to conform to guidelines established by the National Committee for Clinical Laboratory Standards (NCCLS) and include all the steps necessary for a phlebotomist or other qualified health-care provider to obtain an appropriately identified quality blood specimen from a patient's vein. Initial steps covered in this chapter are necessary for all blood collection procedures, including venipuncture, skin puncture, and arterial puncture, and refer to inpatient test collection. Ambulatory or outpatient procedures are the same, if applicable, unless otherwise indicated. Venipuncture steps are listed in Box 8-1 and explained as follows.

Box 8-1

VENIPUNCTURE STEPS

- Receive and accession the test request
- Identify the patient
- Verify diet restrictions
- Prepare the patient for testing
- Assemble equipment and supplies
- Wash hands and put on gloves
- Reassure patient
- Position patient
- Apply tourniquet
- Ask the patient to make a fist
- Select the venipuncture site
- Release tourniquet
- Clean the site
- Verify equipment and tube selection
- Reapply tourniquet
- Pick up and position blood collection equipment
- Remove the cover and inspect the needle
- Anchor the vein
- Insert the needle into the vein
- Fill the tubes
- Withdraw the needle
- Dispose of the puncturing unit

---

continued

continued

- Label the tubes
- Observe special handling instructions
- Check the patient's arm and apply bandage
- Dispose of contaminated materials
- Thank the patient
- Remove gloves and wash hands
- Check specimen collection logs
- Transport the specimen to the lab

THE TEST REQUEST

Initiation of the Test Request

Blood collection procedures begin legally with the test request. All laboratory testing must be requested by a physician or other designated healthcare professional and results must be reported to that person with the exception of certain rapid tests that can be purchased and performed at home by consumers.

In a hospital setting, a **health unit coordinator,** also known as a health unit clerk or secretary, fills out the test request paperwork manually or enters the test orders in a computer under the direction of the patient's nurse. Manual requests must be physically delivered to the laboratory. A computer request is transmitted through a special computer network and a requisition prints in the laboratory. In an outpatient setting, the physician's office may call and inform the lab of the order, or the patient may arrive at the lab with the order in hand from the physician's office. Outpatients who require repeat testing at regular intervals often have what are called "standing" orders filed in the laboratory so that they do not have to have a new physician's order for each visit. A requisition is filled out from the standing order at the time of testing.

 Key Point ➤ Verbal test requests are sometimes used in emergencies; however, the request is usually documented on standard request forms or entered in the computer by the time the phlebotomist arrives to collect the specimen.

Requisitions

The forms on which test orders are entered and sent to the lab are called test **requisitions.** Test requisitions become part of the patient's permanent medical record and require specific information to ensure that the right patient is tested, the physician's orders are met, the correct tests are performed at the proper time under the required conditions, and the patient is billed properly. Required requisition information is listed in Box 8-2. Requisitions come in manual and computer-generated forms.

Box 8-2

REQUIRED REQUISITION INFORMATION

- Ordering physician's name
- Patient's first and last name and middle initial
- Patient's medical record number
- Patient's date of birth or age
- Room number and bed (if inpatient)
- Type of test to be performed
- Date test is to be performed
- Billing information and ICD-9 codes (if outpatient)
- Test status (e.g., timed, fasting, priority)

MANUAL REQUISITIONS

Manual requisitions (Fig. 8-1) come in many different styles and types. Some institutions have separate requisitions for each department, often using different colors for each department so that they can be easily distinguished. Others use one large form with separate sections for the different departments. Some requisitions are a three-part form that serves as a request, report, and billing form. With increased use of computer systems, use of manual requisitions is declining; however, they are typically used as a backup when computer systems fail.

Key Point ➤ As a phlebotomist, you will be responsible for labeling the specimen tubes with the required patient information when a manual requisition is used.

COMPUTER REQUISITIONS

Computer requisitions (Fig. 8-2) normally contain the actual labels that are placed on the specimen tubes immediately after collection. There are a number of different types of computer requisitions. In addition to patient identification and test status information, many indicate the type of tube needed for the specimen and some indicate additional patient information such as "potential bleeder" or "no venipuncture right arm."

Key Point ➤ When a computer-generated label is used you will normally be required to write the time of collection and your initials on the label after collecting the specimen.

Quest Diagnostics
SmithKline Beecham Clinical Laboratories, Now a Part of Quest Diagnostics

SelecTest®
HOSPITAL

85351402-2   6606516-8

BOSWELL MEMORIAL HOSPITAL
10401 W THUNDERBIRD BLVD
SUN CITY, AZ 85351-3004

PXPBR00   623-876-5381

DID YOU REMEMBER...
TO REQUEST OR MARK TEST(S)?
TO PROVIDE ORDER CODE(S) FOR HANDWRITTEN TESTS?

PATIENT INFORMATION - PLEASE PRINT
PRINT NAME (LAST, FIRST, MIDDLE) OR REGISTRATION NO

ROOM #   REGISTRATION #   LAB REFERENCE #

DOB (MM/DD/YYYY)   SEX   PATIENT I.D. #
M ☐ F ☐

REFERRING PHYSICIAN   REF. PHYSICIAN PROVIDER #

Call Results to:(   )   Fax Results to:(   )

Report Comments: ☐ **STAT**

Internal Comments: ☐ **STAT PICK UP**

DATE COLLECTED   TIME   AM/PM   ☐ Fasting (Hours)
☐ Serum ☐ Plasma ☐ Blood ☐ Urine ☐ Frozen ☐ Other

Side margin (vertical): F=FROZEN P=PLASMA B=LIGHT BLUE TOP TUBE L=LAVENDER TOP TUBE G=GRAY TOP TUBE R=RED TOP TUBE Y=YELLOW CAP URINE TUBE U=SCREW CAP URINE BOTTLE S=SERUM SEPARATOR TUBE

REFERRED

FOLD HERE

PANELS		
7352	☐ CARDIOLIPIN ANTIBODIES (IgG, IgA, IgM)	S
4451	☐ CK ISOENZYME PANEL (Total + Isoenzymes)	FS
7940	☐ EBV AB EVAL, COMP (anti-VCA IgM, anti-VCA IgG, anti-VCA IgD, anti-EA(R), anti-EBNA)	S
10306	☐ HEPATITIS PANEL, ACUTE W/REFLEX (HbsAg w/reflex confirm, HC Ab, HA Ab IgM, HbcAb, IgM)	S
7083	☐ IMMUNOGLOBULINS (IgG,IgA,IgM)	S
4411	☐ LDH ISOENZYME PANEL (Total + Isoenzymes)	S
7260	☐ THYROID AUTOANTIBODIES (Thyroglobulin + Peroxidase)	S
7065	☐ VITAMIN B12/FOLIC ACID	1

TESTS		
237	☐ AFP TUMOR MARKER	S
227	☐ ALDOLASE	FS
230	☐ ALDOSTERONE	S
249	☐ ANA W/REFLEX TITER	S
8431	☐ ANCA	S
683	☐ ANGIOTENSIN CONVERT ENZYME	S
4420	☐ C-REACTIVE PROTEIN	S
29256	☐ CA 125	S
5619	☐ CA 15-3	S
4698	☐ CA 19-9	FS
29493	☐ CA 27.29	S
329	☐ CARBAMAZEPINE	1
4661	☐ CARDIOLIPIN IGA AB	S
4662	☐ CARDIOLIPIN IGG AB	S
4663	☐ CARDIOLIPIN IGM AB	S
978	☐ CEA	S
377	☐ CK ISOENZYMES	FS
374	☐ CK, TOTAL	S
351	☐ COMPLEMENT C3	FS
353	☐ COMPLEMENT C4	FS
618	☐ COMPLEMENT, TOTAL (CH50)	FS
367	☐ CORTISOL	S
402	☐ DHEA SULFATE	S
255	☐ DNA AB, NATIVE	S
7849	☐ EBV ANTI-EA (D+R)	S
8564	☐ EBV ANTI-EBNA	S
8474	☐ EBV ANTI-VCA IGG	S

6426	☐ EBV ANTI-VCA IGM	S
427	☐ ERYTHROPOIETIN	S
429	☐ ESTRADIOL	S
457	☐ FERRITIN	S
467	☐ FOLIC ACID, RBC	1
466	☐ FOLIC ACID, SERUM	1
470	☐ FSH	S
4112	☐ FTA-ABS	S
478	☐ GASTRIN	FS
29407	☐ H. PYLORI IGG, QUAL	S
29408	☐ H. PYLORI IGG, QUANT	S
502	☐ HAPTOGLOBIN	S
496	☐ HEMOGLOBIN A1C	L
517	☐ HEMOGLOBIN ELECTROPHORESIS	L
508	☐ HEP A AB - TOTAL	S
512	☐ HEP A IGM AB	S
501	☐ HEP B CORE AB, TOTAL	S
4848	☐ HEP B CORE IGM AB	S
499	☐ HEP B SURFACE AB QUAL	S
8475	☐ HEP B SURFACE AB QUANT	S
498	☐ HEP B SURFACE AG W/REFLEX CONFIRM	S
8472	☐ HEP C VIRUS AB	S
6449	☐ HIV SCR-WB CONF	S
31789	☐ HOMOCYSTEINE	1
539	☐ IMMUNOGLOBULIN A	S
542	☐ IMMUNOGLOBULIN E	S
543	☐ IMMUNOGLOBULIN G	S
545	☐ IMMUNOGLOBULIN M	S
561	☐ INSULIN	FS
597	☐ LDH ISOENZYMES	S
593	☐ LDH, TOTAL	S
599	☐ LEAD (B)	1
6687	☐ LEGIONELLA PNEUMO AB 1-6	S
615	☐ LH	S
606	☐ LIPASE	S
613	☐ LITHIUM	1
7079	☐ LUPUS ANTICOAGULANT	1
6646	☐ LYME DISEASE AB-WB CONF	S
4555	☐ MICROALBUMIN (U)	U
6517	☐ MICROALB/CREAT RATIO	U
2649	☐ MITOCHONDRIAL AB	S
8624	☐ MUMPS VIRUS IGG	S
659	☐ MYCO PNEUMONIAE IGG AB	S
272	☐ NORTRIPTYLINE	1
4847	☐ PREALBUMIN	S
745	☐ PROGESTERONE	S
746	☐ PROLACTIN	S
747	☐ PROTEIN ELECTROPHORESIS	S

754	☐ PROTEIN, TOTAL	S
5363	☐ PSA	S
8847	☐ PT WITH INR	1
8446	☐ PTH, INTACT W/CALCIUM	FS
8837	☐ PTH, INTACT(IRMA) W/CALCIUM	FS
787	☐ RENIN ACTIVITY	1
799	☐ RHEUMATOID FACTOR	S
797	☐ RPR (MONITORING) W/REFLEX TITER	S
36125	☐ RPR (DX) W/REFLEX CONFIRM TP-PA	S
802	☐ RUBELLA IGG AB	S
964	☐ RUBEOLA IGG AB	S
30261	☐ STONE ANALYSIS, KIDNEY	1
30260	☐ STONE ANALYSIS, OTHER	1
34429	☐ T-3, FREE	S
859	☐ T-3, TOTAL	S
861	☐ T-3, UPTAKE	S
867	☐ T-4 (THYROXINE)	S
866	☐ T-4, FREE	S
7924	☐ T-HELPER/SUPPRESSOR RATIO	1
30741	☐ TESTOSTERONE, FREE AND TOTAL	S
873	☐ TESTOSTERONE, TOTAL	S
267	☐ THYROGLOBULIN AB	S
5081	☐ THYROID PEROXIDASE AB	S
891	☐ TRANSFERRIN	S
899	☐ TSH	S
36127	☐ TSH W/REFLEX T-4, FREE	S
916	☐ VALPROIC ACID	1
4439	☐ VARICELLA-ZOSTER IGG AB	S
4128	☐ VDRL, CSF	1
927	☐ VITAMIN B12	S
934	☐ VMA	1

MICROBIOLOGY		
SOURCE:		
8756	☐ C DIFFICILE TOXIN A	1
389	☐ CULTURE, BLOOD	1
690	☐ CULTURE, CHLAMYDIA TRACH	1
4553	☐ CULTURE, FUNGUS	1
2692	☐ CULTURE, HSV (RAPID)	1
2649	☐ CULTURE, HSV WITH TYPING	1
4554	☐ CULTURE, MYCOBACTERIUM	1
395	☐ CULTURE, URINE, RTN	1
689	☐ CULTURE, VIRUS, COMP	1
6919	☐ DNA PROBE, CHL & GC	1
8502	☐ DNA PROBE, CHLAMYDIA	1
8501	☐ DNA PROBE, GC	1
30264	☐ E. COLI SHIGA TOXINS, EIA STOOL	1
681	☐ OVA & PARASITES	1

ADDITIONAL TESTS: (MUST INCLUDE COMPLETE TEST NAME AND ORDER CODE. REFER TO SBCL DIRECTORY OF SERVICES.)

TOTAL TESTS ORDERED ☐

	85351402	85351402
	6606516	6606516
REQHPLA	85351402	85351402
	6606516	6606516

■ FIGURE 8-1 ■

Manual requisition. (Courtesy Sun Health Systems, Sun City, AZ.)

■ FIGURE 8-2 ■

Computer requisition with barcode.

BARCODE REQUISITIONS

Either type of requisition may contain a **barcode** (Fig. 8-2). A barcode is a series of black and white stripes of varying widths corresponding to letters and numbers; the stripes can be grouped together to represent patient names, identification numbers, or laboratory tests. Barcoded manual requisitions normally contain copies of the barcode that can be peeled off and placed on the patient specimens. Computer requisitions typically have the barcode on each label. Barcode information can be scanned into a computer using a special light or laser. Barcode systems allow for fast, accurate processing and their use has been shown to decrease laboratory errors associated with clerical mistakes.

Key Point ➤ Whatever the system used, it is essential that as a phlebotomist you become familiar with the various forms in order to interpret them quickly and accurately.

Receipt of Test Request by the Lab

Computer requisitions usually print out at a computer terminal at the phlebotomist station in the laboratory (Fig. 8-3). Inpatient manual requisitions are sent by courier or pneumatic tube system or are collected during "sweeps" by members of the phlebotomy team. Outpatients are given laboratory requisitions or prescription slips with test orders written on them by their physicians. They are then responsible for taking the requisition or prescription slip to the lab. In this case it is up to laboratory personnel to make certain all the required information is on the requisition provided by the patient or fill out a requisition from the physician's order slip.

Review of the Test Requisition

In an inpatient facility, a phlebotomist is typically in charge of gathering the test requisitions as they are delivered or printed in the lab and sorting them according to date, time, location of the patient, priority of collection, and any other conditions involved in collecting the specimen. When reviewing a requisition, check to see that all required information is present and complete. Verify the tests to be collected, time and date of collection, diet restrictions or other special circumstances that must be met, and priority of test collection. This information is necessary to properly record specimen collection and accession the specimen.

Key Point ➤ To accession a specimen means to take steps to unmistakably connect a specimen and the accompanying paperwork with a specific individual.

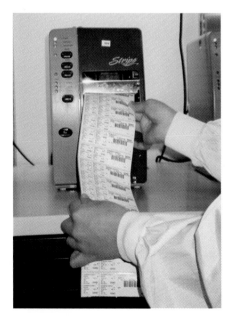

■ FIGURE 8-3 ■

Computer requisitions printing in the laboratory.

Assessment of Test Status and Priority

The status of a test is indicated on the test request. The status designation given to a test may involve specific timing of test collection, conditions under which the specimen is to be collected such as diet restrictions to be followed by the patient, the type of patient involved, or priority of collection according to the patient's condition. Test status designations, priorities, and response times are determined by individual laboratories and may differ somewhat from one laboratory to another. Table 8-1 lists and describes common test status designations and priorities.

INITIATING PATIENT CONTACT

When it is time to collect the specimens, check the requisitions to see that all of the needed equipment is on the blood-collecting tray or cart, arrange the test requests according to priority, and proceed to the first patient's room. Outpatients are generally seated in a waiting room and must be called into the room where specimen collection is performed.

Entering the Patient's Room

Doors to patient rooms are usually open. If the door is closed, knock lightly, open the door slowly, and say something like "good morning," before proceeding into the room. Even if the door is open, it is a good idea to knock lightly to make occupants aware that you are about to enter. Curtains are often pulled when nurses are working with patients or when patients are using bedpans or urinals. Make your presence known to patients before proceeding or opening the curtain to protect their privacy and avoid embarrassing them.

Looking for Signs

It is important to look for signs (Fig. 8-4) containing information concerning your patient. Signs are typically posted on the door to the patient's room or on the wall behind the head of the patient's bed. Signs of particular importance to phlebotomists are signs that signify infection control precautions to follow when entering the room or those that prohibit blood pressures or blood draws from a particular arm. Other commonly encountered signs include those that limit the number of visitors allowed in the room at one time, indicate that fall precautions are to be observed for the patient, or warn that the patient has a severe allergy (e.g., latex, flowers). A sign with a picture of a fallen leaf and a teardrop is sometimes used on obstetric wards to indicate that a patient has lost a baby. A sign with the letters **DNR** means that the patient has a **"Do Not Resuscitate"** order. A DNR order, also called a "no-code," usually means that no code is to be called and no heroic measures are to be taken if the patient stops breathing.

Key Point ➤ A *code* is a way to transmit a message, normally understood by healthcare personnel only, over the facility's public address system. A code uses numbers or words to convey information needed by healthcare personnel to respond to certain situations.

Table 8-1

Common Test Status Designations

Status	Meaning	When Used	Collection Conditions	Test Examples	Priority
STAT (stat)	Immediately (From Latin *statim*)	Test results are urgently needed on critical patients	Immediately collect, test, and report results. Alert staff when delivered to lab. ER stats typically have priority over stats from other areas.	Glucose H & H Electrolytes Cardiac enzymes	First
Med Emerg	Medical Emergency (Replaces STAT)	Critical patients only	Same as STAT	See STAT	First
Timed	Collect at a specific time	Tests where timing is critical for accurate results	Collect as close as possible to requested time. Record actual time collected.	2-hour PP GTT Cortisol Cardiac enzymes TDM Blood cultures	Second
ASAP	As soon as possible	Test results are needed soon to respond to a serious situation, but the patient is not critical	Follow hospital protocol for type of test	Electrolytes Glucose H & H	Second or third, depending on test
Fasting	No food or drink except water for 8–12 hours before specimen collection	To eliminate diet effects on test results	Verify patient has fasted. If patient has not fasted, check to see if specimen should still be collected.	Glucose Cholesterol Triglycerides	Fourth
NPO	Nothing by mouth (from Latin *nulla per os*)	Prior to surgery or other anesthesia procedures	Do not give patient food or water. Refer requests to physician or nurse.	N/A	N/A
Pre-op	Before an operation	To determine whether the patient's condition is suitable for surgery	Collect before the patient goes to surgery	CBC PTT BT	Same as ASAP
Post-op	After an operation	Assess patient condition after surgery	Collect when patient is out of surgery	H & H	Same as ASAP
Routine	Relating to established procedure	Used to establish a diagnosis or monitor a patient's progress	Collect in a timely manner, but no urgency involved. Typically collected on morning sweeps or the next scheduled sweep.	CBC, Chem profile	None

H & H, hemoglobin and hematocrit; PP, post prandial; GTT, glucose tolerance test; TDM, therapeutic drug monitoring; CBC, complete blood count; BT, bleeding time; Chem. profile, chemistry profile.

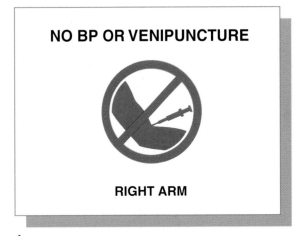

NO BP OR VENIPUNCTURE

RIGHT ARM

A

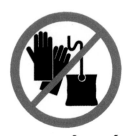

LATEX PRECAUTIONS

PRECAUCIÓN LÁTEX

FORM LTX   Brevis Corp., 3310 South 2700 East, SLC, UT 84109   ©1998 Brevis Corp.

B

■ FIGURE 8-4 ■

Two examples of warning signs. (*A*) "No blood pressures or venipuncture in right arm." (*B*) Latex allergy precautions.   (Courtesy Brevis Corp., Salt Lake City, UT.)

Identifying Yourself

Identify yourself to the patient by stating your name, that you are from the lab, and why you are there (e.g., "Good morning. My name is Joe Smith. I'm from the lab and I'm here to collect a blood specimen if it is all right with you."). If you are a student, communicate this information to the patient as well and ask permission to do the blood draw. This is a part of informed consent and patient rights. The patient has a right to refuse to have blood drawn by a student.

Key Point ➤ Be aware of conflicting permission statements. This often happens with student phlebotomists. For example, when a student asks permission to collect the specimen, a patient may say "yes, but I would rather not." The patient has given permission and taken back that permission in the same statement. In this case it is best if the student does not collect the specimen.

Handling Special Situations

The Patient is Asleep

If the patient is asleep, as is often the case on early morning rounds, wake him or her gently. Try not to startle the patient. (Startling can cause a change in test results.) Nudge the bed rather than the patient. Speak softly but distinctly, and avoid turning on bright overhead lighting, at least until the patient's eyes have adjusted to being open.

Key Point ➤ *Never* attempt to collect a blood specimen from a sleeping patient. Such an attempt may startle the patient and cause injury to the patient or the phlebotomist. In addition, drawing blood from a sleeping patient doesn't allow proper identification to take place, violates the patient's right to informed consent, and could result in a claim of assault and battery.

The Patient is Unconscious

Unconscious patients are often encountered in emergency rooms and intensive care units. When patients are unconscious, next of kin have usually given permission for procedures. If the patient is unconscious, continue to speak to the patient. Identify yourself and inform the patient of your intent just as you would an alert patient. Unconscious patients can often hear what is going on around them even though they are unresponsive.

Key Point ➤ An unconscious patient may be able to feel pain and may move when you insert the needle, so it may be necessary to have someone assist you in holding the arm during the blood draw.

A Physician or Member of the Clergy is with the Patient

If the patient's physician or a member of the clergy is with the patient, don't interrupt. The patient's time with the physician or clergy is private and limited. Proceed to the next patient and come back to that patient later. If the request is for a stat or timed specimen, excuse yourself, explain why you are there, and ask permission to proceed.

Family or Visitors are with the Patient

Often there are family members or visitors in the room when you arrive to collect a specimen. It is best to ask them to step outside the room until you are finished. Most will prefer to do so; however, some family members will insist on staying in the room. Occasionally a family member, especially a spouse, is willing to assist you if needed. It is generally acceptable to let a willing family member help steady the arm or hold pressure over the site while you label tubes.

The Patient is not in the Room

If the patient is not in the room, check at the nurses' station to find out where the patient is. If the patient has been taken to another department such as x-ray, you may be able to collect the specimen while the patient is in the waiting area of that department, before procedures have begun. Follow facility protocol.

Key Point ➤ Every attempt should be made to find the patient, especially if the test is timed.

If the patient cannot be located, is unavailable, or you are unable to obtain the specimen for any other reason, it is the policy of most laboratories that you fill out a form stating that you were unable to obtain the specimen at the requested time and the reason why. The original copy of this form is left at the nurses' station and a copy goes to the lab.

PATIENT IDENTIFICATION

Key Point ➤ **Patient identification** is the most important step in specimen collection. Obtaining a specimen from the wrong patient can have serious, even fatal, consequences, as in the case of specimens for type and crossmatch before blood transfusion. Misidentification of a patient or specimen can be grounds for dismissal of the person responsible and could even lead to a malpractice lawsuit against that person.

Determining the Patient's Name and Date of Birth

When identifying a patient, ask the patient to state his or her name and date of birth. For example, *never* say "Are you Mrs. Smith?" A person who is very ill, hard of hearing, or sedated may say "yes" to anything. Use a "memory jogger" such as having a patient spell an unusual name or comment in some positive way about a name to help you remember that you verified it. The patient's response must match the information on the requisition and the patient's identification bracelet.

Checking the Patient's Identification Bracelet

If the patient's response matches the information on the requisition, proceed to check the patient's **identification (ID)** band (Fig. 8-5) (also called **ID bracelet, arm band,** or **wrist band**). Inpatients are normally required to wear an ID band, usually on the wrist. The typical ID band (Fig. 8-6) lists the patient's name and hospital identification number or **medical record (MR) number.** Additional information includes the patient's birth date or age, room number and bed designation, and physician's name.

The patient's name, MR number, and birth date information on the ID band must match the information on the requisition *exactly.* It is not unusual to have patients with the same

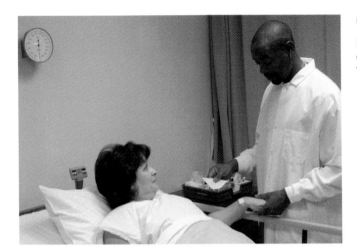

■ FIGURE 8-5 ■

Phlebotomist at bedside checking patient identification band.

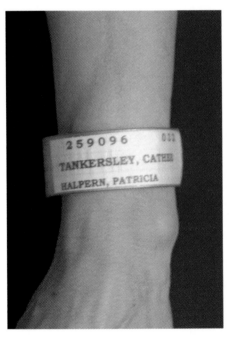

■ FIGURE 8-6 ■

Typical identification bracelet.

or similar names in the hospital at the same time. (Examples are patients with common last names, fathers and sons who have been in accidents, multiple birth babies, and relatives involved in tissue transplant procedures.) There have even been instances in which two unrelated patients shared the same full name and birth date. Two patients will not, however, have the same hospital or medical record number, although it may be similar.

Identification protocol may vary slightly from one healthcare institution to another. Generally, ID information such as room number, bed number, and physician's name are allowed to differ. For instance, occasionally a room number will differ because the patient has been moved. In addition, the name of the ordering physician may be different because it is not unusual for a patient to be under the care of several different physicians at the same time.

How to Handle ID Discrepancies

If there is a discrepancy between the name, MR number, or date of birth on the ID band and the information on the requisition, the patient's nurse should be notified. The specimen should not be obtained until the discrepancy is addressed and the patient's identity is verified.

What to Do if the ID Band is Missing

If there is no ID band on either of the patient's wrists, check to see if it is on an ankle. Intravenous lines in patient's arms often infiltrate the surrounding tissues and cause swelling that necessitates removal of the ID band. When this occurs, especially on a patient with intravenous (IV) lines in both arms, nursing personnel sometimes place the ID band around the ankle. In some instances, an ID band is removed from an IV-infiltrated arm or while other procedures are being performed on the patient and placed on an IV pole or the night table by the patient's bed. An ID band on an IV pole or night table could belong to a patient who previously occupied that bed and should not be used. It is also not unusual for a new patient to occupy a bed before the nursing staff has a chance to attach his or her ID band.

Key Point ➤ *Never* verify information from an ID band that is *not* attached to the patient or collect a specimen from a patient who does not have an ID band. Ask the patient's nurse to attach an ID band before collecting the specimen.

In rare emergency situations in which there is no time to wait for attachment of an ID band, the patient's nurse is allowed to verify the patient's ID and the name or initials of the nurse making the ID verification are written on the requisition. Follow your institution's protocol.

Emergency Room Identification Procedures

It is not uncommon for an emergency room (ER) to receive an unconscious patient with no identification. In many institutions, the phlebotomist is allowed to attach a special three-part identification band, such as a Typenex Blood Recipient ID band (Fenwal Laboratories, a division of Travenol Laboratories, Deerfield, IL), to an unidentified ER patient's wrist. All three parts contain the same number. The first part becomes the patient's ID band. The second part is attached to the specimen. The third part is used if the patient needs a transfusion, and is attached to the unit of blood. Follow your institution's protocol for unidentified patients.

Key Point ➤ *Never* collect a specimen without some way to positively connect that specimen to the patient.

Identification of Infants

Never rely on the name card on the infant's bed for identification purposes. Always check the ID band. Infant ID bands are usually located on an ankle. Newborns may have more than one ID band—one with the infant's information and one with the mother's. Be very careful when identifying as-yet-unnamed newborn infants. They are typically identified by date and time of birth, sex, and the mother's last name. For example, the infant may be identified as "Baby Boy" or "Male Baby" Jones.

 Key Point ➤ Be especially careful when identifying twins or other multiple-birth babies. They are commonly identified, for example, as Jones "Twin A" or "Twin B."

Identification of Young, Mentally Incompetent, or Non-English Speaking Patients

If the patient is young, mentally incompetent, or non-English speaking, ask the patient's nurse, attendant, relative, or friend to identify him or her by name, address, and identification number or birth date. This information must match the information on the test requisition and the patient's ID band if applicable.

Identification of Outpatients

Outpatients often arrive with the order from their doctor in hand. The outpatient area receptionist will verify the patient's identity and fill out the proper lab requisition or generate one via computer. Some labs supply the proper lab forms to physicians who use their services so that the patient arrives with the lab requisition already filled out. A patient may be required to show proof of identification such as a driver's license or other picture ID. Outpatients do not normally have ID bands. However, they may have clinic issued **ID cards** that contain their name and other information identifying them as clinic patients. ID cards are sometimes used to imprint specimen requisitions or labels using an address-o-graph–type machine.

Even though a receptionist has identified the patient, you must personally verify the patient's ID when you call him or her into the blood-drawing area from the waiting room. Simply calling a person's name and having someone respond is not verification enough. Anxious or hard-of-hearing patients may think they heard their name called, when in fact a similar name was called. It is also possible to have two patients in the waiting area with the same name. Ask an outpatient to state his or her name and date of birth and compare it with your requisition before obtaining the specimen.

PREPARING THE PATIENT FOR TESTING

Bedside Manner

Gaining the patient's trust and confidence and putting the patient at ease are important aspects of **bedside manner.** A phlebotomist with a professional manner and appearance will more easily gain a patient's trust. A confident phlebotomist will convey that confidence to the patient and help him feel at ease.

Key Point ➤ A cheerful and pleasant manner and an exchange of small talk with the patient will help to put a patient at ease and divert attention from any discomfort associated with the procedure.

Handling Difficult Patients

Your cheerful, pleasant manner may not be echoed by the patient. Hospitalization or illness is typically a stressful situation for a patient. A patient may be lonely, scared, fearful, or just plain disagreeable and may react in a negative manner toward you. It is important to remain calm and professional and treat the patient in a caring manner under all circumstances.

Explaining the Procedure

Most patients have had a blood test before. A statement of your intent to perform a blood test is usually sufficient for them to understand what is about to occur. To a patient who has never had a blood test, a more detailed explanation may be necessary. Special procedures may require additional information.

If a patient does not speak or understand English, you may have to use sign language or other nonverbal means to demonstrate what is to occur. If this fails, an interpreter must be located.

Speaking slowly and distinctly, using sign language, or writing down information may be necessary for patients with hearing problems.

 Key Point ➤ Regardless of difficulties involved, you must always determine that the patient understands what is about to take place and obtain permission before proceeding. This is part of informed consent.

Handling Patient Inquiry Concerning Tests

Some hospitals will allow the phlebotomist to tell the patient the name of the test or tests to be performed. Others prefer that all inquiries be directed to the patient's physician. Never attempt to explain the purpose of a test to a patient. Because a particular test can be ordered to rule out a number of different problems, any attempt to explain its purpose could mislead or unduly alarm the patient. Handle such inquiries by stating that it is best to have the doctor or nurse explain them.

In cases where bedside testing is being performed (such as glucose monitoring), the patient is often aware of the type of test being performed and may ask about results. Check with the patient's nurse to see if it is acceptable to tell the patient the results.

Handling Patient Objections to Testing

Most patients understand that blood tests are needed in the course of their treatment. Occasionally a patient will object to the procedure. A reminder that the doctor ordered the test as part of his or her care will sometimes convince the patient to cooperate. If not, the patient's nurse may be able to convince the patient to cooperate.

Key Point ➤ Do not attempt to badger the patient into cooperating or restrain a conscious, mentally alert adult patient to obtain a specimen. Remember, the patient *does* have the right to refuse testing.

If a patient truly refuses to cooperate, write on the requisition that the patient has refused to have blood drawn and notify the patient's nurse and the phlebotomy supervisor that the specimen was not obtained because of patient refusal. Depending upon institution policy, you may be required to fill out a special form stating why you were unable to collect the specimen.

VERIFYING DIET RESTRICTIONS

After the patient has been properly identified and has consented to the procedure, verify that any special diet instructions or restrictions have been followed. The most common diet requirement is for the patient to fast (refrain from eating) for a certain period of time, typically overnight such as after the last meal of the day or after midnight until the specimen is collected the following morning.

If you determine that the patient did not fast or otherwise follow diet instructions, notify the patient's nurse (or physician, in the case of an outpatient) so that a decision can be made as to whether or not to proceed with the test.

 Key Point ➤ If you are told to proceed with specimen collection, write "nonfasting" on the requisition and the specimen label.

ROUTINE EVACUATED TUBE SYSTEM (ETS) VENIPUNCTURE

Assemble Equipment and Supplies

Gather blood collection supplies and evacuated tube system components. Routine venipuncture equipment is listed in Box 8-3. Select the required tubes. Check the expiration date on each one to make certain it is not expired. Arrange the tubes in proper order of draw. Screw the needle into the tube holder (Fig. 8-7), making certain that it is securely fastened. Seat the first tube in the holder.

 Key Point ➤ It is sometimes better to assemble blood collection equipment after you have selected the vein and determined the appropriate equipment to use. In this case, equipment assembly can take place after you have cleaned the site and are waiting for it to dry.

Wash Hands and Put On Gloves

Proper hand washing is a very important part of the venipuncture procedure. Wash hands in a downward motion, scrubbing from wrists to fingertips to prevent backflow of contaminated water and soap. Use a circular scrubbing motion with plenty of fric-

---

Box 8-3

ROUTINE VENIPUNCTURE EQUIPMENT

- Alcohol prep pads (or alternate antiseptic if required)
- Povidone-iodine swabs for blood cultures (or alternate antiseptic such as chlorhexidine)
- Nonalcohol-based antiseptic for blood alcohol collections
- Gauze pads (or cotton balls for patients with dermatitis)
- Adhesive bandages or other bandaging materials
- Gloves
- Tourniquet
- Blood collection tubes
- Needle
- Tube holder
- Sharps container
- Permanent marker or pen

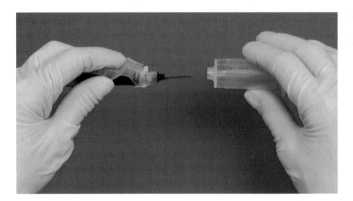

▓ FIGURE 8-7 ▓

Needle and holder assembly.

tion to help dislodge surface debris and bacteria. Pay particular attention to areas between the fingers and around the nails. Rinse hands from wrists to fingertips and dry with a clean paper towel. If the sink does not have an automatic shut off, turn the water off using a clean, dry paper towel. Put on a clean pair of gloves.

Reassure Patient

Reassuring the patient is a part of bedside manner. If the patient is worried about the amount of pain associated with the procedure, be honest and tell him or her that there will be a small amount of discomfort, but it will be of short duration.

Key Point ➤ *Never* tell a patient that it won't hurt. Even children expect to be told the truth.

Explain the importance of holding the arm very still during the procedure. Gain a child's cooperation by having him or her take an active part in the process, such as holding the gauze pad or adhesive bandage. Rewards such as stickers, character badges, or smiley face bandages will help give a child a positive memory of the procedure.

Position Patient

Patients should be either seated or lying down when having blood drawn. They should *never* be standing or seated on a high stool.

Seated Patient

Outpatients are most commonly seated in a special blood-drawing chair (see Chapter 7). When seated, a patient's arm should be supported firmly on a slanted armrest and extended downward in a straight line from the shoulder to the wrist (Fig. 8-8). The arm should *not* be bent at the elbow. Straightening the arm at the elbow helps fix the vein and make it easier to locate. A downward position allows gravity to help the veins enlarge and become more prominent. In addition, a downward position helps assure that blood collection tubes fill from the bottom up, which is necessary to prevent reflux or backflow of tube contents (see Chapter 9) and additive carryover between tubes.

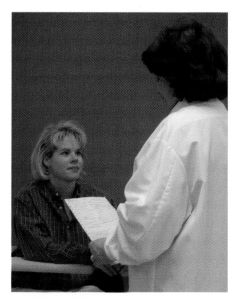

▓ FIGURE 8-8 ▓

Phlebotomist explains procedure to outpatient seated in blood-drawing chair.

Supine Patient

Inpatients normally have blood drawn while supine or lying down. An outpatient in a weakened condition or one who has fainted previously when having a blood test should also have blood drawn lying down. As with the seated patient, the arm should be extended in a straight line from shoulder to wrist and not bent at the elbow. In proper position, the hand should be lower than the elbow. Use a pillow or rolled towel to support and position the arm if necessary.

Other Considerations

BED RAILS

Bed rails may be let down, but be careful not to catch IV lines, catheter bags and tubing, or other patient apparatus. They *must* be raised again when the procedure is finished. Many phlebotomists have learned to collect specimens with bed rails in place so they don't have to worry about forgetting to put them back up when they are finished.

 Key Point ➤ A phlebotomist who lowers a bed rail and forgets to raise it can be held liable if the patient falls out of bed and is injured.

OBJECTS IN THE PATIENT'S MOUTH

Do not allow a patient to eat, drink, chew gum, or have a thermometer, toothpick, or any other foreign object in the mouth during blood collection. Objects in the mouth can cause choking.

Apply Tourniquet

 Key Point ➤ If a patient has prominent veins without the use of a tourniquet, tourniquet application can wait until after the site is cleaned and you are ready to insert the needle.

Apply the tourniquet 3 to 4 inches above the intended venipuncture site. If it is closer to the site, the vein may collapse as blood is withdrawn. If it is too far above the site, it may be ineffective. Apply it tight enough to slow the venous flow without affecting the arterial flow. This allows more blood to flow into the area than out, causing the veins to enlarge, and making them easier to find and penetrate with a needle. A tourniquet that is too tight may prevent arterial blood flow into the area and result in failure to obtain blood. A tourniquet that is too loose will be useless. The tourniquet should feel slightly tight to the patient. It should not be rolled or twisted and it should not be so tight that it pinches, hurts, or causes the arm to turn red or purple. If a patient has sensitive skin or dermatitis, apply the tourniquet over a sleeve or a dry washcloth or gauze wrapped around the arm. *Do not* apply a tourniquet over an open sore. Choose another site. The procedure for tying a latex or vinyl strip tourniquet is shown in Procedures Box 8-1.

Key Point ➤ According to NCCLS, when a tourniquet is used during vein selection, it should be released and not reapplied for at least 2 minutes.

PROCEDURES BOX 8-1

PROCEDURE FOR TYING A LATEX OR VINYL STRIP TOURNIQUET

- Position the tourniquet around the arm (Fig. 8-9, *A*) with each hand grasping one side of the tourniquet a few inches from the end and applying a small amount of tension.
- While maintaining tension, bring the two sides of the tourniquet together, grasping both between the thumb and forefinger of the right hand (Fig. 8-9, *B*).
- Reach over the right hand and grasp the right side of the tourniquet between the thumb and forefinger of the left hand, releasing it from the grip of the right hand. The tourniquet ends will now be held in opposite hands.
- Cross the left end over the right end near the left index finger, grasping both sides together between the thumb and forefinger of the left hand, close to the patient's arm (Fig.8-9, *C*).
- While securely grasping both sides, tuck a portion of the left side under the right side, using either the left middle finger or right index finger, and pull the tucked portion into a loop (Fig. 8-9, *D*).
- The ends of a properly tied tourniquet will point toward the shoulder (Fig.8-9, *E*). A slight tug on the end on the right (the side forming the loop) should easily release it from the patient's arm.

Ask the Patient to Make a Fist

When a patient makes a fist the veins in that arm become more prominent. This makes them easier to locate and enter with a needle.

Key Point ➤ Do not allow the patient to vigorously **pump** (open and close) the fist because it causes hemoconcentration (see Chapter 9) and leads to erroneous test results.

Select the Venipuncture Site

Venipuncture is most commonly performed in the antecubital area of the arm where the median cubital, cephalic, and basilic veins lie fairly close to the surface. Examine this area first. Some veins are easily visible; others will have to be located by feel. A pa-

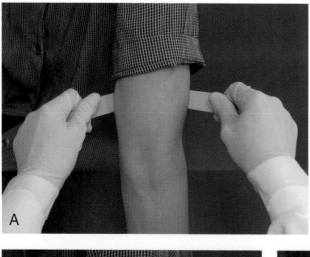

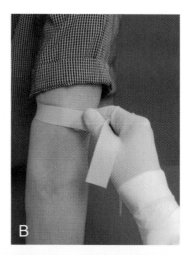

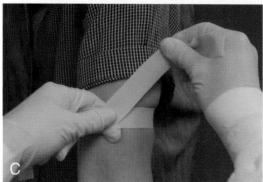

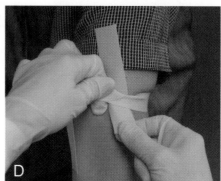

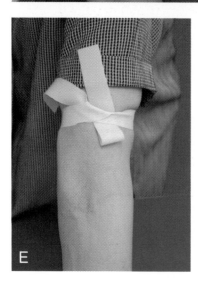

■ FIGURE 8-9 ■

Tourniquet application. (*A*) Proper tourniquet placement with tension applied. (*B*) Both tourniquet sides grasped between thumb and forefinger of the right hand. (*C*) Left side of tourniquet crossed over the right side with both sides held between the thumb and index finger of the left hand. (*D*) Left end of tourniquet tucked under right side, forming loop. (*E*) Properly tied tourniquet.

tient will generally have the most prominent veins in the dominant arm. Place the arm in a downward position forming a straight line from shoulder to wrist and not bent at the elbow. This will help "fix" the veins and gravity will help enlarge them. You may need to place a pillow or rolled towel under the arm of a patient who is lying down to achieve proper positioning.

Use the tip of the index finger to **palpate** (Fig. 8-10, *A*) or feel veins to determine their suitability for venipuncture or to locate veins that cannot be seen. Besides helping to locate veins, palpating helps determine their size, depth, and direction or the path they follow. To adequately palpate a vein, press and release it several times. A vein has a bounce or resilience to it. An artery has a pulse and must be avoided.

Key Point ➤ To avoid inadvertently puncturing an artery, *never* select a vein that overlies or is close to where you feel a pulse.

Do not select a vein that feels hard and cord-like or lacks resilience as it is probably sclerosed or thrombosed (see Chapter 9). These veins roll easily, are hard to penetrate, and may not have adequate blood flow to yield a representative blood sample. Tendons are also hard and lack resilience. Rotating the patient's arm slightly will sometimes help you find a vein or help differentiate a vein from other structures. Dimming the lights and using a transilluminator device or halogen flashlight can help locate veins especially on infants and children.

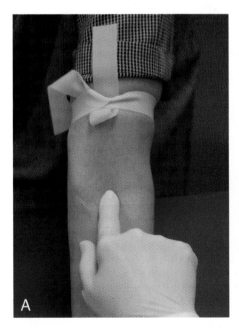 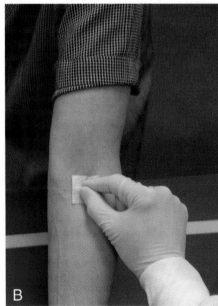

■ FIGURE 8-10 ■

Venipuncture procedure. (*A*) Palpating (feeling) for a vein. (*B*) Cleaning the site (note: the tourniquet has been removed for this procedure). *continued*

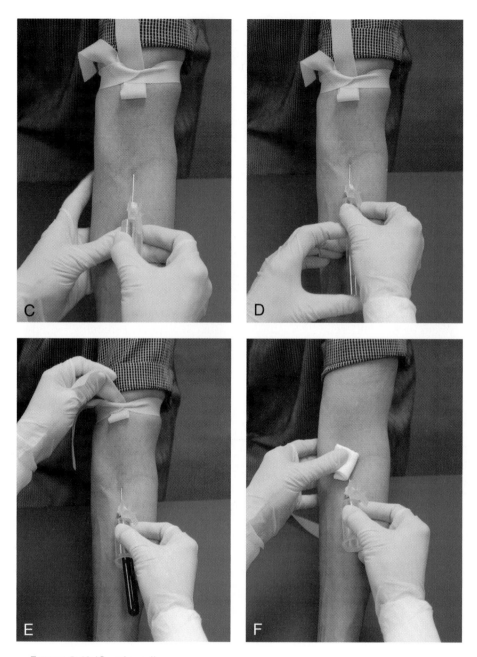

■ FIGURE 8-10 (Continued) ■

(*C*) Entering the vein with the needle while the thumb pulls the skin taut (note: the tourniquet has been retied). (*D*) Positioning the evacuated tube. (*E*) Removing the tourniquet: one hand steadies the tube holder as the tube fills with blood; the other pulls the end of the tucked side of the tourniquet to release it from the patient's arm. (*F*) Placing the gauze before needle removal.

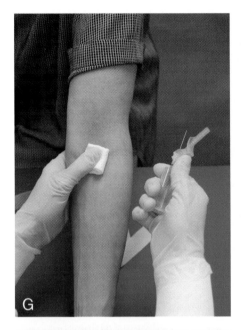

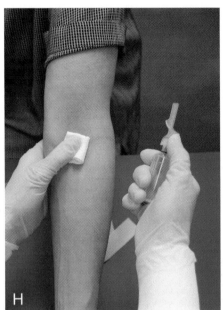

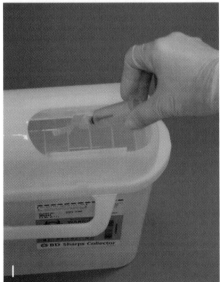

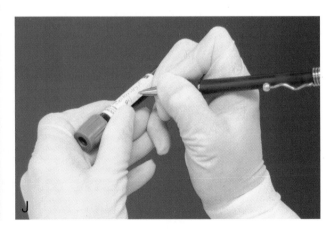

▩ FIGURE 8-10 (Continued) ▩

(*G*) Phlebotomist holding pressure over the venipuncture site. (*H*) Needle with safety shield engaged. (*I*) Discarding the needle and tube holder as a unit. (*J*) Labeling the specimen tube.

If no suitable antecubital vein can be found check the other arm. If no suitable antecubital vein can be found in either arm, check for hand or wrist veins. If a suitable vein still cannot be found, massage the arm from wrist to elbow to force blood into the area or wrap a warm, wet towel around the arm or hand for a few minutes. Warming the site increases blood flow and helps make the veins easier to feel. If you think you feel a vein but are not certain, tap the site sharply a few times. This helps dilate the vein and makes it more prominent.

Key Point ➤ *Do not* manipulate the site excessively because this may change the composition of the blood in the area and cause erroneous test results.

Do not use leg, ankle, or foot veins except as a last resort and after obtaining permission from the patient's physician. Blood flow to the extremities, especially in bedridden patients, is not representative of the general circulation and may yield erroneous results. In addition, venipuncture in the lower extremities can have dangerous consequences such as thrombus (blood clot) formation, especially if the patient has coagulation problems.

When you have found a vein, roll your finger from one side to the other while pressing against it to help judge its size. Its depth is indicated by the degree of pressure required to feel it. The direction of the vein can be determined by palpating above and below where you first feel it.

After you have selected a vein, try to mentally visualize its location. It often helps to note the position of the vein in reference to a freckle, mole, hair, skin crease, superficial surface vein, or imperfection to make relocation easier after cleaning the site. Procedures Box 8-2 shows how to use an alcohol pad to mark the location of a vein.

Release Tourniquet

If the tourniquet was applied during vein selection, release it while you clean the site. This allows the vein to return to normal and minimizes the effect that blockage of the blood flow has on specimen composition.

PROCEDURES BOX 8-2

USING AN ALCOHOL PAD TO MARK THE LOCATION OF A VEIN

- Locate the vein with the nondominant index finger.
- Keeping your finger over the site, use the other hand to align one corner of a clean alcohol pad over the vein, near your finger (Fig. 8-11, *A*).
- Slide the pad away from the site, paralleling the direction of the vein and keeping the corner of the pad pointing in the direction of the vein (Fig. 8-11, *B*).
- Keep the pad far enough away from the site it will not to be in the way or disturbed when cleaning the site (Fig. 8-11, *C*).

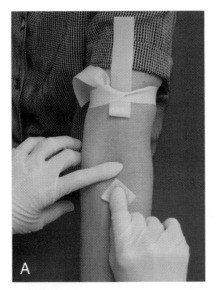
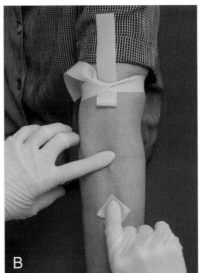
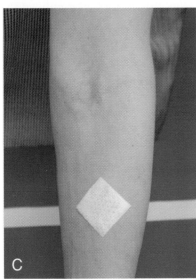

■ FIGURE 8-11 ■

Marking the site with an alcohol pad. (*A*) Align the corner of a clean alcohol pad over the vein located by the index finger. (*B*) Slide the pad away from the site, paralleling the direction of the vein and keeping the corner of the pad pointing in the direction of the vein. (*C*) Alcohol pad pointing in the direction of the vein.

Clean the Site

Cleaning the venipuncture site with an antiseptic (Fig. 8-10, *B*) helps prevent microbial contamination of the specimen and the patient. However, it will *not* sterilize the site. The recommended antiseptic is 70% isopropyl alcohol. Most healthcare institutions use a commercially prepared, sterile, prepackaged alcohol pad referred to as an **alcohol prep pad.**

Clean the site using a circular motion, starting at the center of the site and moving outward in ever-widening **concentric circles.** Use sufficient pressure to remove surface dirt and debris but do not rub so vigorously that you abrade the skin, especially on infants and elderly patients whose skin is thin and more delicate. If the site is especially dirty, clean it again with another alcohol prep pad. *Allow the area to dry* for 30 seconds to 1 minute. The evaporation and drying process helps destroy microbes. In addition, inserting the needle while the alcohol is wet may cause a burning sensation in the patient and hemolysis of the specimen.

- *Do not* contaminate the site by drying the alcohol with unsterile gauze.
- *Do not* introduce airborne contaminants to the site by fanning it with your hand or blowing on it to hasten drying time.
- *Do not* touch the site after cleaning it.

 Key Point ➤ If it is necessary to repalpate the vein, clean the site afterward or decontaminate the gloved finger before touching the site.

Verify Equipment and Tube Selection

Assemble evacuated tube system components if you have not already done so. Choose an appropriate needle according to the age of the patient, the size of the patient's vein, the size of the tubes, and the amount of blood to be collected. Verify that you have selected the correct tubes and other equipment for the requested tests. Tap additive tubes lightly to dislodge any additive that may be adhering to the tube stoppers.

- *Do not* push the tube past the guideline on the holder or loss of vacuum may result.
- *Do not* remove the **needle sheath** (cover) until just before needle insertion.

Place the blood-drawing equipment within easy reach and make certain that the phlebotomy tray is also within easy reach.

 Key Point ➤ *Do not* place the phlebotomy tray on the patient's bed.

Reapply Tourniquet

Reapply the tourniquet, being careful not to touch the cleansed area. Be aware that there are a few tests that must be collected without using a tourniquet.

Pick Up and Position Blood Collection Equipment

Hold the blood-drawing equipment in your dominant hand with the thumb on top of the evacuated tube holder and the fingers underneath. (Some phlebotomists like to position the index finger near the hub of the needle during vein entry; however, the gloved finger *must not* touch the needle.)

Verify that the tube is positioned in the evacuated tube holder. A properly positioned tube is pushed onto the needle just far enough to hold the tube and keep it from falling out of the holder, but not far enough to release the vacuum of the tube. (Most tube holders contain a guideline beyond which the tube should not be pushed.) If the tube tries to prematurely push off of the needle or you have trouble positioning the tube on the needle without losing the vacuum, it is acceptable to wait until the needle is inserted in the patient's vein to put the tube into the holder.

Remove the Cover and Inspect the Needle

Remove the needle cover. Visually inspect the needle tip for obstructions, imperfections, or barbs that could hurt the patient or obstruct blood flow. If any are noted, discard the needle and select a new one.

 Key Point ➤ After the cap is removed, *do not* let the needle touch anything before venipuncture. If it does, remove it and replace it with a new needle.

Anchor the Vein

Grasp the patient's arm with your nondominant hand, placing your thumb 1 to 2 inches below the intended venipuncture site and pulling the skin toward the wrist. This pulls the skin taut, which **anchors** the vein and helps keep it from moving or rolling to the side upon needle entry. (If the vein rolls, the needle may slip beside the vein, not into it.) Use the fingers of your anchoring hand to support the back of the arm in the area of the elbow and pull the skin to the side. It is not uncommon for an apprehensive patient to suddenly pull back the arm as the needle is inserted. If your fingers are wrapped around the arm, the patient is less likely to pull away from your grasp and the needle is more likely to stay in the vein. This is sometimes described as the "L" hold procedure for anchoring the vein.

 Key Point ➤ For safety reasons, *do not* use the two-finger technique (also called the "C" hold) in which the entry point of the vein is straddled by the index finger above and the thumb below. If the patient pulls the arm back when the needle is inserted, there is a possibility that the needle may recoil as it comes out of the arm, springing back into your index finger.

Insert the Needle into the Vein

Have the patient make a fist. (You can sometimes eliminate this step on patients with prominent veins that are easily anchored.) Line the needle up with the vein with the bevel up, pointing the same direction as the venous flow and following the path of the vein. Warn the patient by saying something like "There is going to be a little poke now." Insert the needle into the skin at a 15- to 30-degree angle depending on the depth of the vein. Use one smooth motion to penetrate first the skin and then the vein (Fig. 8-10, *C*).

 Key Point ➤ *Do not* push down on the needle as it is inserted. It is painful to the patient and enlarges the vein opening, increasing the risk of hematoma formation and bruising.

When the needle enters the vein, you will feel a slight "give" or decrease in resistance. Some phlebotomists describe this as a "pop." When you sense this or are otherwise certain that the needle is in the vein, stop advancing it and securely anchor the tube holder.

At this point, some phlebotomists switch to holding the blood-drawing apparatus in their nondominant hand so that tube changes can be made with the dominant hand. This is accomplished by gently slipping the fingers of the opposite hand under the holder and placing the thumb atop the holder as the other hand lets go. Another method is to grasp the holder between the thumb and index finger, with the hand resting on the patient's arm over (but not touching) the needle. Many phlebotomists, particularly those who are left-handed, do not change hands but continue to steady the holder in the same hand and change tubes with the opposite.

Whatever the method, it is important to hold the blood-drawing apparatus steady so there is minimal needle movement. If the holder is not securely anchored, the needle can push through the back of the vein, or pull out of the vein when tubes are changed during the draw. When the tube holder is securely anchored, the knuckles of the anchoring fingers are typically pressed against the patient's arm.

Fill the Tubes

With the tube holder securely anchored, advance the tube onto the needle in the holder (Fig. 8-10, *D*), using your thumb to push the tube while your index and middle fingers grasp the flange of the tube holder. (This procedure is slightly different for self-blunting needles. Follow manufacturer instructions.) Blood should begin to flow freely into the evacuated tube. If not, exert constant forward pressure on the end of the tube in case the rubber needle sleeve is trying to push the tube off of the needle.

As soon as blood flows into the tube, release the tourniquet (Fig. 8-10, *E*) and have the patient release his or her fist, if applicable. Blood should continue to flow and multiple tubes can still be collected. On elderly patients and others with fragile veins that might collapse, or in other difficult draw situations where release of the tourniquet might cause stoppage of blood flow, the tourniquet is sometimes left on until the last tube is filled. *Do not*, however, leave the tourniquet on for more than 1 minute.

 Key Point ➤ Three or four tubes can generally be filled in less than a minute.

Hold the needle steady. Try not to pull up, press down, or move it sideways in the vein. These actions can be painful to the patient and enlarge the hole in the vein, resulting in leakage of blood and hematoma formation.

Maintain the arm and the tube in a downward position so that blood fills the tube from the bottom up and does not contact the needle in the tube holder. This prevents carryover of additives to other tubes by means of blood left on the needle as tubes are changed. It also prevents reflux (flow of blood from the tube back into the vein) and possible adverse patient reaction. Do not change position of the tube or allow back and forth movement of the blood in the tube as this too can cause reflux.

To ensure a proper ratio of additive to blood, let the tube fill until the vacuum is exhausted and blood ceases to flow. Tubes do not fill completely to the top. When blood flow stops, remove the tube, using a reverse twist and pulling motion while bracing the thumb against the flange of the holder. The rubber sleeve will cover the needle and prevent leakage of blood into the tube holder.

If the tube contains an additive, mix it immediately by gently inverting it three to eight times (depending upon the type of additive and manufacturer's recommendations) before putting it down. Lack of or inadequate mixing can lead to clot formation. Nonadditive tubes do not require mixing.

Key Point ➤ *Do not* vigorously mix or shake tubes as this can cause hemolysis (breakage of red blood cells and release of hemoglobin into the serum or plasma.)

If other tubes are to be drawn, place them into the holder and push them all the way onto the needle. Steady the tube holder so that the needle does not pull out or penetrate through the vein as tubes are placed and removed. Be certain to follow the proper order of draw (see Chapter 7).

When the last tube has been filled, remove it from the holder and mix it, if applicable, before removing the needle from the arm. If the tube is still attached when the needle is removed from the arm, the needle will drip blood and cause needless contamination. The chance of bruising is also increased.

Withdraw the Needle

After the last tube has been removed from the holder, fold a clean gauze square in fourths and place it directly over the site where the needle enters the vein (Fig. 8-10, *F*).

Key Point ➤ *Do not* press down on the gauze while the needle is in the vein. It puts pressure on the needle during removal, causing pain, and the needle may slit the vein and the skin as it is withdrawn.

Withdraw the needle in one smooth motion, immediately apply pressure to the site with a gauze pad (Fig. 8-10, *G*) and activate the needle safety device (Fig. 8-10, *H*). Needle-blunting devices are typically activated before the needle is withdrawn from the vein. Follow manufacturer recommendations. Apply pressure to the site for 3 to 5 minutes or until the bleeding stops. Failure to apply pressure or inadequate pressure can result in leakage of blood and hematoma formation. It is acceptable to have the patient hold pressure while you proceed to label tubes, providing the patient agrees to and is fully alert and able to do so.

Key Point ➤ *Do not* bend the arm up. Keep it extended or raised. Studies show that bending the arm increases the chance of bruising by keeping the wound open or disrupting the platelet plug when the arm is lowered.

If the sharps container has been moved out of reach (as sometimes happens in emergencies when others are working on the patient at the same time) and the patient is not able to hold pressure, it is generally acceptable to bend the patient's arm up temporarily while locating the sharps container and disposing of the collection device.

Dispose of the Puncturing Unit

Immediately discard the needle and tube holder in a sharps container (Fig. 8-10, *I*). *Do not* cut, bend, break, or recap needles. *Never* stick the needle into the patient's mattress. Luckily these dangerous actions are less likely with the safety devices now in use.

Label the Tubes

Affix computer labels or barcodes to the specimen tubes or use an indelible pen to label them manually (Fig. 8-10, *J*), if applicable, with the following information as a minimum:

- Patient's name
- Hospital number (if applicable) or date of birth
- Date and time of collection
- Phlebotomist's initials

Include additional pertinent information such as "fasting" or "nonfasting." If using a preprinted computer label, write the date, time, your initials, and other pertinent information on the label. Compare the information on each labeled tube with the patient's ID band and the requisition before leaving the patient.

- *Do not* label tubes before venipuncture.
- *Do not* leave the room before labeling the tubes.
- *Do not* dismiss an outpatient before labeling is completed.
- *Do not* label tubes with a pencil.

Observe Special Handling Instructions

If applicable, follow recommended special handling procedures for each specimen, such as putting it in crushed ice to cool (e.g., ammonia), keeping it warm (e.g., cold agglutinin), or protecting it from light (e.g., bilirubin).

Check the Patient's Arm and Apply Bandage

Examine the patient's arm to see if bleeding has stopped. If it has, apply an adhesive bandage (or tape over several folded gauze squares) over the site. Instruct the patient to leave the bandage on for a minimum of 15 minutes, after which it should be removed to avoid irritation. If the patient is allergic to adhesive bandages, apply paper tape over a clean, folded gauze square. If the patient has sensitive skin or is allergic to the paper tape also, wrap gauze around the arm and place the tape over the gauze or wrap the arm with self-adhering gauze-like material.

Key Point ➤ Some hospitals prefer *not* to bandage the site because bandages tend to irritate the skin and leave a sticky residue that interferes with subsequent venipunctures. Follow hospital protocol.

Instruct an outpatient not to carry a purse or other heavy object or lift heavy objects with that arm for a minimum of 1 hour.

Dispose of Contaminated Materials

Dispose of contaminated materials in the proper biohazard containers. *Do not* leave other materials such as needle caps and wrappers in the patient's room. Check to see that you have your tourniquet and other equipment before exiting the patient's room.

Thank the Patient

Thank the patient for his or her cooperation. This is courteous and helps to leave the patient with a positive feeling about the laboratory.

Remove Gloves and Wash Hands

Remove gloves aseptically by grasping one glove at the wrist and pulling it inside out and off of the hand, ending up with it in the palm of the still-gloved hand. Slip your nongloved fingers under the second glove at the wrist and pull it off of the hand, ending with one glove inside the other with the contaminated surfaces inside. Dispose of them in the manner required by your institution and wash your hands before proceeding to the next patient or back to the lab.

 Key Point ➤ Washing your hands is extremely important in protecting yourself from infection and preventing the spread of infection to others.

Check Specimen Collection Logs

Check the patient's name off of the specimen collection and diet restriction logs at the nursing station if applicable. In an outpatient setting, inform the patient that it is all right to go ahead and eat if no other tests are scheduled that require fasting.

Transport the Specimen to the Lab

Transport specimens to the laboratory in a timely fashion. Enter specimens into the computer system or logbook to document or verify collection. The specimen collection process is not complete until the appropriate patient and specimen collection information is documented.

PROCEDURE FOR INABILITY TO OBTAIN A SPECIMEN

If you are unable to obtain a specimen on the first try, evaluate the problem (procedural errors that result in the failure to establish blood flow are explained in Chapter 9) and try again below the first site, on the opposite arm or on a hand or wrist vein. If the patient's veins are small or fragile it may be necessary to use a butterfly or syringe on the second attempt.

 Key Point ➤ Never probe for a vein. It is painful and can injure the patient.

If the second attempt is unsuccessful, *do not* try a third time. Another phlebotomist should take over. Unsuccessful venipuncture attempts are frustrating to the patient and the phlebotomist. With the exception of stat and other priority specimens, if the second phlebotomist is also unsuccessful, it is a good idea to give the patient a rest and come back at a later time. An outpatient may be given the option of returning another day after consultation with his or her physician.

There are times when a phlebotomist is not able to obtain a specimen from a patient without even attempting venipuncture. Occasionally, a patient will refuse to give permission to draw the specimen. Other times, the patient is unavailable because he or she has gone to surgery or to another testing department such as radiology. The patient may even have already been discharged from the hospital. The following are the most common and generally accepted reasons for inability to obtain a specimen:

- Phlebotomist attempted but was unable to draw blood
- Patient refused
- Patient was unavailable

Whatever the reason, if the specimen cannot be obtained, notify the patient's nurse or physician. In addition, you may be required to fill out a form stating that the specimen was not obtained and the reason why. The original form is delivered to the nurses' station and placed in the patient's chart. The laboratory retains a copy.

BUTTERFLY PROCEDURE

A phlebotomist may elect to use a winged infusion set or butterfly when attempting to draw blood from antecubital veins of infants and small children or when drawing blood from difficult adult veins, such as small antecubital veins or wrist or hand veins.

Identify Patient and Prepare for Specimen Collection

Follow the same identification, permission, and patient preparation procedures as in routine venipuncture. Wash hands and put on clean gloves.

Select Equipment

Butterfly needles are available that can be attached directly to syringes; however, a butterfly needle with a threaded multiple-sample Luer adapter that can be attached directly to an evacuated tube holder is preferred. A 23-gauge needle will easily penetrate small veins and not rupture or "blow" them. Choose small-volume or **pediatric tubes** to collect the specimen. Large-volume tubes may create too much vacuum draw on the vein and cause it to collapse. In addition, large-volume tubes used with a 23-gauge needle may hemolyze the specimen.

Position Patient and Apply Tourniquet

When drawing the specimen from an antecubital vein, proceed as you would a routine venipuncture, being certain to anchor the vein securely. If drawing from a hand or wrist vein, apply the tourniquet to the wrist proximal to the wrist bone. Have the patient either make a fist or bend the fingers slightly. Make certain the hand is well-supported on the bed, a rolled towel, or an armrest.

Choose a Vein and Clean the Site

Choose a vein, release the tourniquet, and clean the site as in routine venipuncture.

Assemble Equipment

Assemble the equipment while the site is drying and the tourniquet is off. Remove the butterfly device from the package. (Retain the package to place the needle in when tying the tourniquet.) The tubing will be coiled somewhat because it was coiled in the package. Extend the tubing its full length and stretch slightly to help keep it from coiling back up. To stretch the tubing, hold it by the tubing near each end, not by the needle or hub as either or both may come loose. Attach the butterfly to the evacuated tube holder and seat the first tube in it.

Reapply Tourniquet and Position Equipment

Reapply the tourniquet. Cradle the tube holder and tubing in the palm of your dominant hand or lay it next to the patient's hand. Hold the wing portion of the needle between your thumb and index finger or fold the wings together upright and grasp them together.

Anchor the Vein

Anchor an antecubital vein in the same manner as routine ETS venipuncture. Anchor a hand vein by pulling the skin taut over the knuckles with the thumb.

Insert the Needle into the Vein

With the needle bevel facing up and lined up with the vein, slide the needle into the vein (Fig. 8-12, *A*) at a shallow angle between 10 and 15 degrees. Be careful not to penetrate all the way through the vein. A "flash" or small amount of blood will appear in the tubing when the needle is in the vein. "Seat" the needle by threading it within the lumen (central area) of the vein slightly so that the needle will not twist out of the vein if you let go of the needle. If the needle tries to twist out of the vein, hold it with the thumb of the opposite hand.

Fill the Tubes

Push the tube to the end of the holder. Release the tourniquet when blood begins to flow into the tube. (Because butterfly draws are usually performed on difficult veins, the tourniquet is sometimes left in place until the last tube is filled, as long as the draw takes less than 1 minute.)

Keep the tube and holder in a downward position so that the tube fills from the bottom up (Fig. 8-12, *B*), as in routine venipuncture. Follow the proper order of draw.

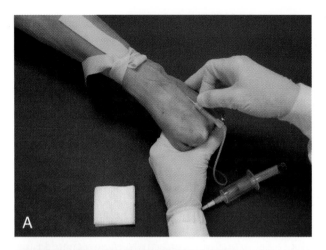

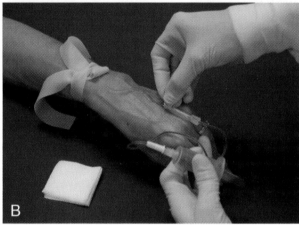

■ FIGURE 8-12 ■

Procedure for using butterfly in a hand vein. (*A*) The wings of the butterfly are held together as the needle is inserted into the vein, while the skin is pulled taut over the knuckles. (*B*) Blood flows through the tubing into the tube when it is advanced onto the needle in the holder.

Withdraw the Needle and Dispose of Collection Equipment

When the last tube has been filled, remove it from the holder. Place gauze over the site (Fig. 8-12, *C*). Remove the needle and activate the safety device per the manufacturer's instructions and apply pressure to the site (Fig. 8-12, *D*).

If the draw was difficult and the tube was not completely filled, it may be placed back in the needle holder and advanced onto the needle to draw the remaining blood out of the tubing, if it is done immediately. Discard the blood collection device in a sharps container.

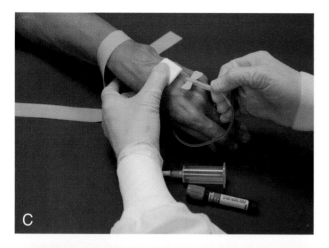

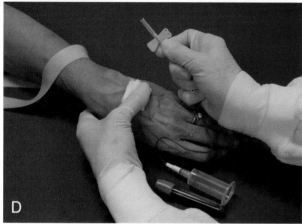

■ FIGURE 8-12 (Continued) ■

(*C*) Gauze is placed over the site and the needle is removed from the vein. (*D*) The needle safety shield is activated as soon as the needle is withdrawn from the vein.

Follow-Up Procedures

Label the tubes and observe specimen-handling requirements. Check the venipuncture site, apply a bandage, and thank the patient. Dispose of contaminated materials in the proper containers, remove gloves, and wash hands. Check specimen collection logs and transport the specimen to the lab. The above follow-up procedures should be carried out in the manner described under routine ETS venipuncture.

SYRINGE PROCEDURE

The preferred method of obtaining venipuncture specimens is the evacuated tube method; however, a needle and syringe or butterfly and syringe may be used if the patient has small, fragile, or weak veins that collapse easily. The vacuum pressure of the evacuated tube may be too great for such veins. This is often the case with elderly patients and newborn infants. When a syringe is used, the pressure can be controlled by pulling slowly on the syringe plunger.

Identify Patient and Prepare for Specimen Collection

When drawing blood by syringe, follow the same identification, permission, and patient preparation procedures as in routine venipuncture. Wash hands and put on clean gloves.

Select Equipment

To comply with Occupational Safety and Health Administration (OSHA) regulations, use a needle-locking syringe (e.g., Luer lock). Choose a syringe and needle size that are compatible with the size and condition of the patient's veins and the amount of blood to be collected.

Position Patient and Apply Tourniquet

When drawing the specimen from an antecubital vein, proceed as you would with a routine venipuncture, being certain to anchor the vein securely. If drawing from a hand or wrist vein, apply the tourniquet to the wrist proximal to the wrist bone. Have the patient either make a fist or bend the fingers slightly. Make certain the hand is well-supported on the bed, a rolled towel, or an armrest.

Choose a Vein and Clean the Site

Choose a vein, release the tourniquet, and clean the site as in routine venipuncture.

Assemble Equipment

Syringes and syringe needles used for blood collection are commonly available in sterile pull-apart packages. The syringe typically comes with the plunger pulled back slightly. Advance the plunger to the end of the syringe before opening the sterile package. Open the packages in an aseptic manner and securely attach the needle to the syringe. *Do not* yet remove the needle cover.

Reapply Tourniquet and Position Syringe

Reapply the tourniquet. Pick up the syringe, holding it as you would ETS equipment. Remove the needle cover and visually inspect the needle for defects.

Anchor the Vein and Insert the Needle

Anchor the vein and slide the needle into the vein (Fig. 8-13, *A*) in the same manner described for routine venipuncture. When the vein has been entered, you will see blood appear in the hub of the needle. Release the tourniquet.

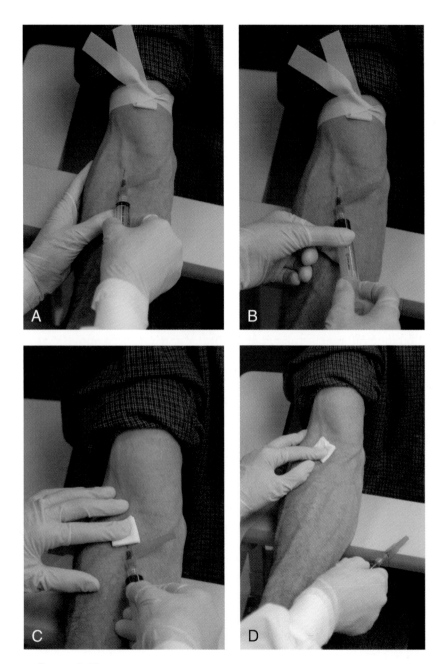

■ FIGURE 8-13 ■

Drawing blood using a needle and syringe. (A) Inserting the syringe needle into the vein. (B) Steadying the syringe with the non-dominant hand and filling it by slowly pulling on the plunger. (C) Placing the gauze and withdrawing the needle from the vein. (D) Activating the safety device while holding pressure over the venipuncture site.

Fill the Syringe

Steady the syringe as you would the evacuated tube holder. (As with evacuated tube venipuncture, some phlebotomists switch hands at this point.) Slowly pull back on the plunger of the syringe and allow the barrel of the syringe to fill with blood (Fig. 8-13, *B*).

Withdraw the Needle and Activate Safety Device

When an adequate amount of blood has been collected, place gauze over the needle entry site, withdraw the needle (Fig. 8-13, *C*) in the same manner described for routine venipuncture, and activate the needle or syringe safety device (Fig. 8-13, *D*).

Transfer Blood to Evacuated Tubes

Syringe Transfer Device

The safest way to transfer blood from a syringe into the evacuated tubes is to use a **syringe transfer device** (Fig. 8-14). A typical syringe transfer device is similar to an ETS tube holder and contains a needle that is similar to the stopper-puncturing end of a multisample needle. The needle is permanently attached to the hub inside the device. The hub of the transfer device can be attached to the tip of a syringe that is filled with blood. An evacuated tube can then be placed in the device and advanced onto the needle. Blood will be safely drawn from the syringe into the tube. Several tubes can be filled as long as there is enough blood in the syringe. The transfer device greatly reduces the chance of accidental needle sticks and confines any aerosol or spraying of the specimen that may be generated as the tube is removed.

Procedure for Using a Syringe Transfer Device

- Remove the safety needle from the syringe and attach the syringe tip to the hub of the transfer device, rotating the syringe clockwise to ensure secure attachment.
- Hold the syringe vertically, with the tip down and the transfer device at the bottom.
- Following the proper order of draw, push the evacuated tube onto the needle within the transfer device until the stopper is penetrated and blood flows into the tube.
- Keep the tube vertical so that it fills from the bottom up to prevent additive contamination of the transfer needle and cross contamination of subsequent tubes. Let the tube fill using the vacuum draw of the tube.

Key Point ➤ *Do not* force the blood into the tube by pushing on the syringe plunger as it can lead to hemolysis of the specimen or cause the tube stopper to pop off of the tube, splashing the contents.

- If you do not wish to fill the tube completely, pull back on the plunger to stop the flow before removing the tube. Remember to mix each tube that contains an additive as it is removed from the transfer device.
- Dispose of the syringe and transfer device as one unit by dropping it into a sharps container.

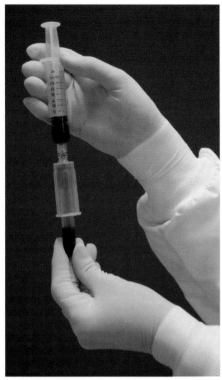

■ FIGURE 8-14 ■

Blood being transferred using a Greiner transfer device attached to a syringe. (Courtesy Greiner Bio-One, Kremsmuenster, Austria.)

Transferring Blood from a Syringe Without a Transfer Device

- If a transfer device is not available, place the required tubes in the proper order of draw in a rack or slot in the phlebotomy tray.

 Key Point ➤ *Never* hold the tubes in your hand if filling them from a syringe without using a safety transfer device.

- Penetrate the stopper of the tube with the syringe needle and allow the vacuum draw of the tube to fill the tube as in the transfer device method. To minimize the chance of hemolysis, slant the needle to the side of the tube so that the blood runs down the side of the tube.
- Carefully withdraw the needle and fill subsequent tubes. Remember to mix additive tubes.
- When the last tube is filled, withdraw the needle, activate the safety device, and drop the entire assembly into a sharps container. If the needle or syringe does not have a safety device, leave the needle in the last tube, and carry it to the sharps container with needle and syringe attached. Withdraw the needle from the tube and drop it into the sharps container with the syringe still attached.

Follow-Up Procedures

Label the tubes and observe specimen-handling requirements. Check the venipuncture site, apply a bandage, and thank the patient. Dispose of contaminated materials in the proper containers, remove gloves, and wash hands. Check specimen collection logs and transport the specimen to the lab. The syringe follow-up procedures identified above should be carried out in the same manner as routine venipuncture.

PEDIATRIC VENIPUNCTURE

Collecting blood by venipuncture from infants and children may be required for tests that require large amounts of blood (i.e., crossmatching and blood cultures) and tests that cannot be performed by skin puncture (i.e., ammonia levels and most coagulation studies).

Venipuncture in children younger than the age of 2 years should be limited to superficial veins and not deep, hard-to-find veins. Normally, the most accessible veins of infants and toddlers are the veins of the antecubital fossa and forearm. Other venipuncture sites are the medial wrist, the dorsum of the foot, the scalp, and the medial ankle. The use of dorsal hand vein technique for neonate blood collection is increasing in popularity.

Challenges

Performing venipuncture on pediatric patients presents special challenges and requires the expertise and skill of an experienced phlebotomist. In addition, every attempt should be made to collect the minimum amount of blood required for testing because of the small blood volume of infants and children. Removal of more than 10% of an infant's blood volume at one time can lead to cardiac arrest. Removal of large amounts of blood over an extended period can lead to anemia and may require the infant to undergo a blood transfusion. (See Appendix D for information on how to calculate blood volume.)

Dealing with Parents or Guardians

If parents or guardians are present, it is important for the phlebotomist to earn their trust before attempting the procedure. A phlebotomist who behaves in a warm and friendly manner and displays a calm, confident, and caring attitude will more easily earn that trust, and limit parental anxiety as well. Give parents the option of staying in the room during the procedure or waiting outside until you are finished.

Dealing with the Child

With older children, it is important to gain their trust as with adults. Remember that children have a wider zone of comfort. Approach them slowly and gain their trust before handling equipment or touching their arms to look for a vein. An adult towering over a child is intimidating. Physically lower yourself to the patient's level. Explain what you are going to do in terms the child can understand and answer questions honestly.

Key Point ➤ *Never* tell a child that it won't hurt. Instead say it will hurt just a little bit, but it will be over quickly.

Help the child to understand the importance of holding still. Give the child a job to do such as holding the gauze or adhesive bandage. Offer the child a reward for being brave. However, *do not* put conditions on receiving the reward, such as "you can only have the reward if you don't cry." Some crying is to be anticipated and it is important to let the child know that it is all right to cry.

 Key Point ➤ It is important to calm a crying child as soon as possible because the stress of crying and struggling can alter blood components and lead to erroneous test results.

Selecting a Method of Restraint

Immobilization of the patient is a critical aspect in obtaining an adequate specimen from infants and children while ensuring their safety. A newborn or young infant can be wrapped in a blanket but physical restraint is often required for older infants, toddlers, and younger children. Older children may be able to sit by themselves in the blood-drawing chair, but a parent or another phlebotomist should help steady the arm.

Toddlers are most easily restrained by having them sit upright on a parent's lap (Fig. 8-15). The arm to be used for venipuncture is extended to the front and downward. The parent places an arm around the toddler over the arm that is not being used. The other

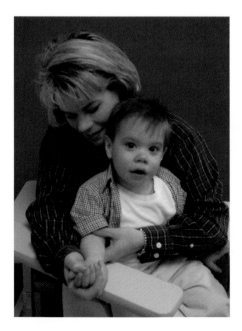

■ Figure 8-15 ■

Seated adult restraining a toddler.

arm supports the venipuncture arm from behind, at the bend of the elbow. This helps steady the child's arm and prevents the child from twisting the arm during the draw.

If the child is drawn while lying down (supine), the parent or another phlebotomist leans over the child form the opposite side of the bed. One arm reaches around and holds the venipuncture arm from behind, the other reaches across the child's body, holding the child's other arm secure against his or her torso.

Equipment Selection

Because infants and children have small blood volumes and small veins, it is important to select the smallest tubes and needles allowed to collect the required specimen. In addition, you may need to use a pediatric-sized tourniquet.

Procedures

Regardless of the collection method, every attempt should be made to collect the minimum amount of blood required for testing because of the small blood volume of the patient. Follow proper identification requirements outlined earlier in the chapter. You may be required to wear a mask, gown, and gloves in the newborn nursery or neonatal intensive care unit.

Antecubital Vein

Venipuncture of an antecubital vein is most easily accomplished using a 23-gauge butterfly needle attached to an evacuated tube holder or syringe. The tubing of the butterfly allows for flexibility if the child struggles or twists during the draw. Using the evacuated tube method of collection is preferred because it minimizes chances of clotted specimens and inadequately filled tubes. However, the smallest tubes available should be used to reduce the risk of creating too much vacuum draw on the vein and causing it to collapse. In difficult draw situations, a small amount of blood can be drawn into a syringe and the blood placed in microcollection containers or bullets rather than tubes.

 Key Point ➤ Laboratory personnel will assume blood in microcollection containers is skin puncture blood. It is important to label the specimen as venous blood because reference ranges for some tests differ depending on the source of the specimen.

Dorsal Hand Vein

Dorsal hand veins are favored sites for venipuncture in neonates (newborns) and infants younger than 2 years of age. Dorsal hand vein venipuncture (Fig. 8-16) is more efficient and less time-consuming than skin puncture because specimens can be collected quickly from a single venipuncture, as opposed to the multiple sticks often required to collect skin puncture specimens. In addition, specimens are less likely to be diluted with tissue fluids or hemolyzed. The procedure for dorsal hand vein venipuncture is shown in Box 8-4.

Box 8-4

DORSAL HAND VEIN VENIPUNCTURE

- Put on mask and gown, if applicable, and gloves.
- Identify the infant.
- Immobilize the infant by wrapping him snugly in a blanket.
- Check for the most visible vein in either hand.
- Encircle the wrist with your thumb underneath and index finger on top. Apply pressure with your index finger to enlarge the vein. (Use of a tourniquet is not necessary.)
- Flex the wrist downward, being careful not to bend it too much or the vein may flatten out and be harder to see. It may also collapse when punctured.
- After selecting the vein, release your grasp and clean the site with alcohol.
- Allow the alcohol to air dry. Select an appropriate needle for the size of the vein. A 23- to 25-gauge transparent hub syringe needle is commonly used.
- Encircle the wrist as before and bend the hand slightly downward. Create pressure on the vein with your index finger.
- Line the needle up parallel to the vein. Slip the needle into the vein at an approximate 15-degree angle with the skin. Advance the needle slowly until blood appears in the hub.
- Fill microcollection tubes or PKU filter paper directly from the hub. Avoid bumping the hub or putting pressure on the needle. Release finger pressure intermittently to encourage blood flow.
- After collecting the specimen, place gauze, withdraw the needle, and apply pressure until bleeding stops. Immediately dispose of the needle in a sharps container.
- Do not apply a bandage because it may tear the skin when removed later.
- Label the specimen in the proper manner and follow any special handling instructions for specimens.
- Discard all used supplies in the proper containers. Remove mask, gown, and gloves and wash hands. Enter collection information in the nursery log book.
- Deliver the specimen to the lab.

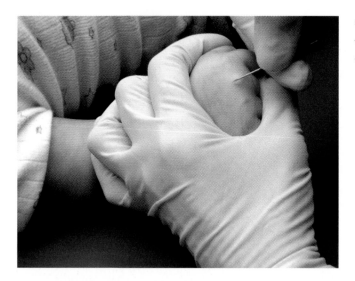

■ FIGURE 8-16 ■

Venipuncture of an infant dorsal hand vein.

GERIATRIC VENIPUNCTURE

According to the National Institute on Aging (NIA), life expectancy has doubled over the last century and there are now more than 35 million Americans age 65 or older. This segment of the population is expected to grow by 137% over the next 50 years and become the major focus in healthcare. Already a major portion of laboratory testing is performed on the elderly. (See Table 8-2 for a list of tests commonly ordered on geriatric patients.)

Although aging is a normal process, it involves physical, psychological, and social changes leading to conditions, behaviors, and habits that may seem unusual to those unaccustomed to working with elderly patients. To feel comfortable working with elderly patients, it is important to understand the aging process and be familiar with the physical limitations, diseases, and illnesses associated with it. It is also important to remember that elderly patients are unique individuals with special needs who deserve to be treated with compassion, kindness, patience, and respect.

Challenges

Physical effects of aging, such as skin changes and hearing and vision problems; mobility issues often related to arthritis and osteoporosis; diseases such as diabetes; and mental and emotional conditions, present challenges not only to the patient, but to a phlebotomist's technical expertise and interpersonal skills as well.

Skin Changes

Skin changes include loss of collagen and subcutaneous fat, resulting in wrinkled, sagging, thin skin with a decreased ability to stay adequately hydrated. Lack of hydration along with impaired peripheral circulation caused by age-related narrowing of blood vessels make it harder to obtain adequate blood flow, especially during skin puncture.

Table 8-2

Tests Commonly Ordered on Geriatric Patients

Test	Typical Indications for Ordering
ANA, RA, or RF	Diagnose lupus and rheumatoid arthritis, which can affect nervous system function.
Complete blood count	Determine hemoglobin levels, detect infection, and identify blood disorders.
Blood urea nitrogen/creatinine	Diagnose kidney function disorders that may be responsible for problems such as confusion, coma, seizures, and tremors.
Calcium/magnesium	Identify abnormal levels associated with seizures and muscle problems.
Electrolytes	Determine sodium and potassium levels critical to proper nervous system function.
ESR	Detect inflammation; identify collagen vascular diseases.
Glucose	Detect and monitor diabetes. Abnormal levels can cause confusion, seizures, or coma or lead to peripheral neuropathy.
PT/PTT	Monitor blood thinning medications; important in heart conditions, coagulation problems, and stroke management.
SPEP, IEP	Identify protein or immune globulin disorders that lead to nerve damage.
VDRL/FTA	Diagnose or rule out syphilis, which can cause nerve damage and dementia.

ANA, antinuclear antibody; RA, rheumatoid arthritis; RF, rheumatoid factor; ESR, erythrocyte sedimentation rate; SPEP, serum protein electrophoresis patterns; IEP, immunoelectrophoresis; VDRL, Venereal Disease Research Laboratory; FTA, fluorescent treponemal antibody.

In addition, aging skin cells are replaced more slowly, causing the skin to lose elasticity and increasing the likelihood of injury. Blood vessels also lose elasticity, becoming more fragile and more likely to collapse, resulting in an increased chance of bruising and failure to obtain blood, respectively.

Key Point ➤ Skin changes make veins in the elderly easier to see; however, sagging skin combined with loss of muscle tone may make it harder to anchor veins and keep them from rolling.

Hearing Impairment

Effects of aging include loss of auditory hair cells resulting in a hearing loss in upper frequencies and trouble distinguishing sounds such as *ch, s, sh,* and *z.* Hearing-impaired patients may strain to hear and have difficulty answering questions and understanding instructions. If you know or have reason to suspect that a patient has a hearing impairment, move closer and face him or her when you speak. Speak clearly and distinctly, but use your normal tone of voice. Never shout; shouting raises the pitch of your voice and makes it harder to understand. Allow the patient enough time to answer questions and always confirm responses to avoid misunderstanding. Repeat information if necessary. Watch for nonverbal verification that your patient understands. Be mindful of nonverbal messages you may be inadvertently sending the patient. Use pencil and paper to communicate if necessary. A relative or attendant often accompanies a patient with a hearing or other communication problem. If this person is included in the conversation, do not speak to him or her directly as if the patient were not present.

Key Point ➤ Although hearing loss is common in the elderly, never assume that an elderly person is hard of hearing.

Visual Impairment

Effects of aging on the eyes include a diminished ability of the lens to adjust causing farsightedness, clouding of the lens or cataract formation resulting in dim vision, and other changes that lead to light intolerance and poor night vision. It is important that the phlebotomy area have adequate lighting without glare. Be aware that you may need to guide elderly patients to the drawing chair or escort them to the restroom if a urine specimen is requested. Provide written instructions in large print. Avoid using gestures when speaking and use a normal tone of voice.

Key Point ➤ A common mistake and one that is irritating to the visually impaired is to raise your voice when speaking to him or her.

Mental Impairment

Slower nerve conduction associated with aging leads to slower learning, slower reaction times, and a diminished perception of pain. Diminished pain reception leads to an increase in injuries. Reduced cerebral circulation can lead to loss of balance and frequent falls. The effects of some medications can make these problems worse. Speak clearly and slowly and give the patient plenty of time to respond. Be especially careful in obtaining patient identification information. Be aware that you may have difficulty verifying patient compliance with diet instructions.

Conditions such as Alzheimer's disease and other forms of dementia may render the patient unable to communicate meaningfully and you may have to communicate through a relative or other caregiver. Some patients with Alzheimer's will exhibit anger and hostility that should not be taken personally. Always approach the patient in a calm and professional manner. Use short, simple statements and explain things slowly. You may require assistance to steady the patient's arm during the draw.

Key Point ➤ Although mental confusion and dementia are common in elderly patients, always assume that an elderly person is of sound mind unless you have information to the contrary.

Effects of Disease

Although the majority of elderly are generally healthy, many are not. Some of the diseases that affect the elderly and the challenges they present to the patient and the phlebotomist include the following.

ARTHRITIS

There are two basic types of arthritis—osteoarthritis and rheumatoid arthritis. Osteoarthritis is a type of arthritis that occurs with aging and also results from joint injury. Although it sometimes affects the spine, hands, and fingers, the hips and knees are most commonly affected and can cause a patient to have difficulties getting in and out of a blood-drawing chair. Rheumatoid arthritis affects connective tissue throughout the body and can occur at any age. Although it primarily affects the joints, connective tissue in the heart, lungs, eyes, kidneys, and skin may also be affected. Inflammation associated with both types of arthritis may leave joints painful and swollen and cause the patient to restrict movement. This may result in the patient being unable or unwilling to straighten an arm or open the hand. Use the opposite arm if it is unaffected. If that is not an option, let the patient decide what position is comfortable. A butterfly needle with 12-inch tubing helps provide the flexibility needed to access veins from awkward angles.

Key Point ➤ Never use force to extend a patient's arm or open a hand.

COAGULATION PROBLEMS

Patients who have coagulation disorders or who take blood-thinning medications as a result of heart problems or strokes are at risk of hematoma formation or uncontrolled bleeding at the blood collection site. Make certain adequate pressure is held over the site until bleeding is stopped. You must hold pressure if the patient is unable to do so. However, do not hold pressure so tightly that the patient is injured or bruised and do not apply a pressure bandage in lieu of holding pressure. If bleeding persists notify the patient's physician or follow your facility's policy.

DIABETES

Many elderly patients have diabetes. Diabetes affects circulation and healing, particularly in the lower extremities, and generally makes venipuncture of leg, ankle, and foot veins off limits. Scarring from numerous skin punctures to check glucose levels along with peripheral circulation problems may make skin puncture collections difficult. Warming the site before blood collection can help encourage blood flow.

PARKINSON'S AND STROKE

Stroke and Parkinson's disease can affect speech. Keep in mind that difficulty speaking does not imply problems in comprehension. However, the frustration it can cause both the patient and the phlebotomist can present a barrier to effective communication. Allow these patients time to speak and do not try to finish their sentences. Tremors and movement of the fingers of Parkinson's patients can make blood collection difficult and the patient may require help to hold still.

PULMONARY FUNCTION PROBLEMS

Changes in pulmonary function related to aging include reduced elasticity of airway tissues and decreased effectiveness of respiratory defense systems. Consequently, the effects of colds and influenza are more severe in the elderly. In addition, weakened chest muscles reduce ability to clear secretions and increase the chance of developing pneumonia. If you have a cold, refrain from drawing elderly patients if possible or wear a mask.

OTHER PROBLEMS

Disease and loss of immune function in the elderly increases chance of infection. Lack of appetite resulting from disease or decreased sense of smell and taste can result in emaciation. Poor nutrition can intensify the effects of aging on the skin, affect clotting ability, and contribute to anemia.

Safety Issues

Although all patients require an unencumbered traffic pattern, geriatric patients may need wider, open areas to accommodate wheelchairs and walkers. Some patients tend to shuffle when they walk so floors should be nonslip surfaces and free of clutter. Dispose of equipment packaging properly and watch for items inadvertently dropped on the floor. Floor mats should stay snug against the floor so that they do not become a tripping hazard for any age patient and employees as well.

Patients in Wheelchairs

Many geriatric patients are wheelchair-bound or are so weak they are transported to the laboratory in wheelchairs. Be careful transporting wheelchair patients (Fig. 8-17) from the waiting room to the blood drawing room. Remember to lock wheels when drawing patients in wheelchairs, assisting them to and from the drawing chair, or after returning them to waiting areas. Do not attempt to lift patients to transfer them from a wheelchair to a drawing chair. It is not part of a phlebotomist's scope of practice and attempting to do so can result in injury to the patient, the phlebotomist, or both.

Key Point ➤ It is generally safest and easiest to draw the patient while in the wheelchair, supporting the arm on a pillow or on a special padded board placed across the arms of the chair.

Blood Collection Procedures

Although the venipuncture steps are basically the same for all patients, extra care must be taken in the following areas when drawing elderly patients.

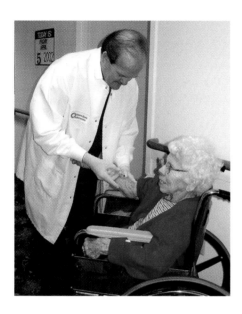

Elderly patient in a wheelchair.

Patient Identification

Be extra careful identifying patients with mental or hearing impairments. Do not rely on nods of agreement or other nonverbal responses. Verify patient information with a relative or attendant if possible.

Equipment Selection

It is often best to use butterfly needles and pediatric or short-draw tubes for venipuncture on the elderly. Although veins may appear prominent, they are apt to roll or collapse easily, making blood collection difficult. Sometimes it is best to select equipment after you have selected the venipuncture site so that you can choose the best equipment for the size, condition, and location of the patient's vein. If the patient's veins are extremely fragile you may have to collect the specimen by syringe or perform finger puncture.

Tourniquet Application

Apply the tourniquet snugly, but loose enough to avoid damage to the patient's skin. It is acceptable to fasten the tourniquet over the patient's sleeve or over a clean dry washcloth wrapped around the arm. A tourniquet that is tied too tightly can cause the vein to collapse when the evacuated tube is engaged or the tourniquet is released.

 Key Point ➤ A tourniquet that is too tight can cause the vein to become so distended that it "blows" or splits open on needle entry, resulting in hematoma formation.

Select Venipuncture Site

Elderly patients, especially inpatients, often have bruising in the antecubital area from previous blood draws. Check the other arm. If both are bruised, select a needle entry point below the bruising to avoid effects of the hemostatic process on the blood specimen and possible erroneous results. In addition, drawing in a bruised area can be painful to the patient. Have the patient make a fist to aid in vein selection; however, be aware that some elderly patients may not be able to make a fist because of muscle weakness.

If no suitable vein can be found, gently massage the arm from wrist to elbow to force blood into the area or wrap a warm, wet towel around the arm or hand for a few minutes to increase blood flow. Avoid heavy manipulation of the arm because that can cause bruising. Have the patient hold the arm down at the side for a few minutes to let gravity help back up blood flow. When a suitable vein has been selected, release the tourniquet to allow blood flow to return to normal while you clean the site and ready your equipment.

Clean the Site

Clean the site in the manner described for routine venipuncture. Be careful not rub too vigorously or you may abrade or otherwise damage the skin. The site may need to be cleaned a second time on some elderly patients who are unable to bathe regularly. Do not make an issue of how dirty it was and embarrass the patient. Simply clean it again as if it were part of your normal procedure.

Perform the Venipuncture

Elderly patient's veins are often tough and have a tendency to roll so it is important to anchor the vein firmly. A firmly anchored vein will be easier to penetrate with the needle. If the skin is quite loose and the vein is poorly fixed in the tissue, it sometimes helps to wrap your hand around the arm from behind and pull the skin taut from both sides rather than stretch the skin below the vein with just your thumb. Because veins in the elderly tend to be close to the surface of the skin, a shallow angle of needle insertion may be required.

Hold Pressure

As discussed earlier in this chapter under "Coagulation Problems," it may take longer for bleeding to stop in elderly patients, especially if they are on anticoagulant therapy. Be certain that bleeding has stopped before bandaging the patient. Remember, if bleeding does not stop, notify the patient's physician or follow laboratory protocol.

DIALYSIS PATIENTS

The kidneys help the body maintain fluid, electrolyte and acid-base balance, and remove waste products from the blood. When they fail to function or do not function properly, waste products such as urea and creatinine build up in the blood and can reach toxic levels. **Dialysis** is a process in which the blood is artificially filtered to remove waste products while maintaining fluid, electrolyte, and acid-base balance. The most common reason for dialysis is end stage renal disease (ESRD), a serious condition in which the kidneys have deteriorated to a point where they fail (no longer function). The most common cause of ESRD is diabetes and the second most common cause is high blood pressure. Patients with ESRD require ongoing dialysis treatments or a kidney transplant.

There are two main types of dialysis—**hemodialysis** and **peritoneal dialysis.** Both types require a time commitment ranging from four 1-hour treatments a week to nightly treatments of up to 12 hours depending upon the method used.

Hemodialysis

In hemodialysis the patient's blood is circulated through a special filtering machine often called an artificial kidney. The procedure is normally performed at special dialysis clinics. Access for dialysis is commonly provided by a permanent fusion of an artery and a vein in the forearm to create what is called an arteriovenous (AV) fistula or shunt. If the patient's veins are too small, as is often the case with elderly or diabetic patients, an artificial material or piece of vein from the thigh is used to connect the artery and vein creating what is called an AV graft. A typical AV fistula or graft appears as a loop just under the skin in the forearm near the wrist. Both have a buzzing sensation called a "thrill" when palpated. During dialysis a special needle attached to tubing is inserted into the fistula or graft to provide blood flow to the dialysis machine.

Key Point ➤ Never take blood pressures or perform routine venipuncture on an arm with an AV fistula or graft. It is the dialysis patient's lifeline and must not be damaged.

Peritoneal Dialysis

In peritoneal dialysis the patient empties a salt and sugar solution called dialysate into the abdominal cavity through a catheter. Waste products pass through the peritoneum or lining of the abdominal cavity into the dialysate. After 4 to 6 hours, depending on the method used, the dialysate is drained from the body, taking the waste products with it. An advantage of peritoneal dialysis is that the patient can perform the procedure and it can take place while he or she sleeps.

LONG-TERM CARE PATIENTS

Long-term care includes a variety of healthcare and social services required by certain patients with functional disabilities who cannot care for themselves, but do not require hospitalization. Long-term care serves the needs of patients of all ages who have debilitating birth defects, spinal cord injuries, mental impairment, and chronic illnesses. Primary recipients, however, are the elderly who can no longer function independently. Long-term care can be delivered to individuals in adult daycare facilities, nursing homes, assisted long-term care facilities, rehabilitation facilities (Fig. 8-18), or even in their own homes.

HOME CARE PATIENTS

Care for the sick at home plays an important role in today's healthcare delivery system. Many individuals who would have been confined to a healthcare institution are now able to remain at home. Numerous studies show that patients are happier and get better sooner or survive longer when they are treated at home. Home care services are provided through numerous agencies and include professional nursing and home health aid services; physical, occupational, and respiratory therapy services; and laboratory services. Laboratory services are often provided by phlebotomists who travel to the patient's home to collect specimens and then deliver them to the laboratory for testing. A home care phlebotomist must have exceptional phlebotomy, interpersonal, and organizational skills; be able to function independently; and be comfortable working in varied situations and under unusual circumstances. A traveling phlebotomist must carry all necessary phlebotomy supplies in his or her vehicle (Fig. 8-19), including sharps containers and biohazard bags for disposing of contaminated items, and containers for properly protecting specimens during transportation. In addition, a home care phlebotomist often provides his or her own transportation.

HOSPICE PATIENTS

Hospice is a type of care designed for patients who are dying. The majority of hospice patients have incurable forms of cancer. Hospice care allows terminally ill patients to spend their last days in a peaceful, supportive atmosphere that emphasizes pain man-

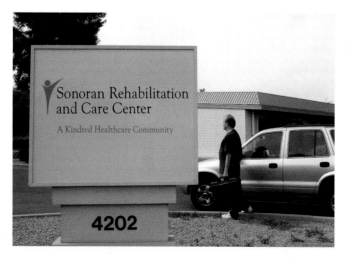

■ FIGURE 8-18 ■

A phlebotomist making a visit to a rehabilitation center.

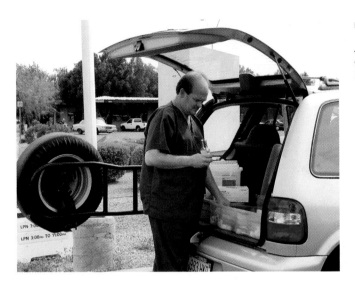

FIGURE 8-19

A traveling phlebotomist getting supplies from the back of his vehicle.

agement to help keep them comfortable. Some individuals are uncomfortable with the subject of death or being around dying patients and react with indifference out of ignorance. It is important for phlebotomists who deal with hospice patients to be able to approach them with care, kindness and respect.

STUDY & REVIEW QUESTIONS

1. Which of the following is required requisition information?
   a. Ordering physician's name
   b. Patient's first and last name
   c. Type of test to be performed
   d. All the above

2. The following test orders for different patients have been received in the lab at the same time. Which test would you collect first?
   a. fasting glucose
   b. STAT glucose in the ER
   c. STAT hemoglobin in the intensive care unit
   d. ASAP complete blood count in the intensive care unit

3. A member of the clergy is with the patient when you arrive to collect a routine specimen. What should you do?
   a. Ask the patient's nurse what to do
   b. Come back later after the clergy member has gone
   c. Fill out a form saying you were unable to collect the specimen and return to the lab
   d. Say, "excuse me; I need to collect a specimen on this patient"

4. If a patient adamantly refuses to have blood drawn, you should
   a. convince the patient to cooperate.
   b. notify the patient's nurse and fill out a failure to obtain specimen form explaining what happened.
   c. restrain the patient and collect the specimen.
   d. write a note to the physician.

5. The most important step in specimen collection is
   a. entering the patient's room correctly.
   b. handling visitors.
   c. identifying the patient.
   d. identifying yourself to the patient.

6. You are sent to collect a specimen on an inpatient. The patient is not wearing an ID band. What do you do?
   a. Ask the patient's name and collect the specimen if it matches the requisition
   b. Ask the patient's nurse to put an ID band on the patient before drawing the specimen
   c. Identify the patient by the name card on the door
   d. Refuse to draw the specimen and return to the lab

Continued

7. The patient is eating breakfast when you arrive to collect a fasting glucose. What is the best thing to do?

   a. Consult with the patient's nurse to see if the specimen should be collected
   b. Draw the specimen quickly before the patient finishes eating
   c. Draw the specimen and write "nonfasting" on the lab slip
   d. Fill out a form saying you were unable to collect the specimen because the patient was eating

8. A tourniquet should be applied

   a. away from open sores.
   b. 8 to 10 inches above the intended venipuncture site.
   c. for at least 2 minutes before releasing.
   d. tight enough to stop all blood flow.

9. After cleaning the venipuncture site with alcohol, the phlebotomist should

   a. allow the alcohol to dry completely.
   b. fan the site to help the alcohol dry.
   c. dry the site with a regular gauze pad or cotton ball.
   d. insert the needle quickly before the alcohol has a chance to dry.

10. Which of the following actions is *not* proper venipuncture technique?

   a. Allow the tubes to fill until the vacuum is exhausted
   b. Fill the tube from the stopper end first
   c. Maintain the tube in a downward position throughout the draw
   d. Remove the tourniquet as soon as blood flows freely into the tube

11. Specimen collection tubes are labeled

   a. at the patient's bedside after collecting the specimen.
   b. at the patient's bedside before the specimen is collected.
   c. in the laboratory after collection.
   d. in the laboratory before the specimen is collected.

12. After penetrating a hand vein with a butterfly needle, the phlebotomist needs to "seat" the needle, meaning

   a. have the patient make a tight fist to keep the needle in place.
   b. keep the skin taut during the entire procedure.
   c. push the needle up against the back wall of the vein.
   d. slightly thread the needle within the lumen of the vein.

Continued

STUDY & REVIEW QUESTIONS (CONTINUED)

13. **Which statement is true of syringe venipuncture?**
    a. A syringe is sometimes used for veins that collapse easily
    b. A syringe is the recommended way to collect most blood specimens
    c. The best way to fill a syringe is to pull the plunger all the way back as soon as blood flow begins
    d. There is no way to tell when the needle is in a vein when using a syringe

14. **Which of the following choices describes proper technique for filling tubes from a syringe?**
    a. Pull back on the syringe plunger to stop the flow of blood if you do not want the tube to fill completely
    b. Hold the collection tube tightly so that it does not slip out of your hand when inserting the syringe needle into the tube stopper.
    c. Hold the syringe horizontally when filling tubes using a transfer device
    d. Slowly push the syringe plunger as the tube fills

15. **What is the best approach to use on an 8-year-old child who needs to have blood drawn?**
    a. Explain what you are going to do in simple terms and ask the child to co-operate
    b. Have someone restrain the child and collect the specimen before he or she has time to think about it
    c. Offer the child a treat or toy, but only if he doesn't cry
    d. Tell the child that it won't hurt and that only babies cry

16. **Which type of patient is most likely to have an AV fistula or graft?**
    a. Arthritic
    b. Dialysis
    c. Hospice
    d. Wheelchair-bound

17. **Which of the following is proper procedure when dealing with an elderly patient?**
    a. Address your questions to an attendant if the patient has a hearing problem
    b. Speak very loudly so that the patient can hear you
    c. Tie the tourniquet extra tightly to make the veins more prominent
    d. Make certain adequate pressure is held over the site until bleeding is stopped

■ CASE STUDY: PATIENT IDENTIFICATION

Jenny works with several other phlebotomists in a busy outpatient lab. This day has been particularly hectic with many patients filling the waiting room. Jenny is working as fast as she can to draw patients. Toward the end of the day, after Jenny finishes drawing what seems like the millionth patient, she mentions how extra busy it has been to a coworker. The coworker says, "Yes it has, but it looks like there is only one patient left." Jenny grabs the paperwork and heads for the door of the waiting room. As her coworker has said, there is only one patient, an elderly woman, sitting there reading a book. The paperwork is for a patient named Jane Rogers. "You must be Jane," Jenny says, glancing at the name on the paperwork. The patient looks up and smiles. "Have you been waiting long?" Jenny says. The patient replies "Not really" and Jenny escorts her to a drawing chair. The patient is a difficult draw and Jenny makes two attempts to collect the specimen. The second one is successful. Jenny places the labels on the tubes, dates and initials them, bandages the patient, and sends her on her way. About 5 minutes later a somewhat younger woman appears at the reception window and says, "My name is Jane Rogers. I just stepped outside to make a phone call and was wondering if you called my name while I was gone." The receptionist notices that the patient's name is checked off the registration log. The receptionist turns around and asks if anyone had called a patient named Jane Rogers. "I already drew her," Jenny says as she walks over to the receptionist window. The woman at the window is not the one Jenny just drew; however, her information matches information on the requisition used to draw that patient.

QUESTIONS:
1. What error did Jenny make in identifying the patient?
2. What assumptions did Jenny make that contributed to her drawing the wrong patient?
3. Who might the other patient that Jenny mistakenly drew have been?
4. How can the error be corrected?

Bibliography and Suggested Readings

Bishop, M. L., Duben-Engelkirk, J. L., & Fody, E. P. (2001). *Clinical chemistry: Principles, procedures, correlations* (4th ed.). Philadelphia: Lippincott Williams & Wilkins.

Becton-Dickinson. Blood transfer device product literature. Franklin Lakes, NJ: BD Vacutainer Systems.

College of American Pathologists (CAP) Publications Committee Phlebotomy Subgroup (1999). *So you're going to collect a blood specimen: An introduction to phlebotomy* (8th ed.). Northfield, IL:

Hosley, J., Jones, A., & Molle-Matthews, E., (1997). Lippincott's *Textbook for medical assistants.* Philadelphia: Lippincott Williams & Wilkins.

National Committee for Clinical Laboratory Standards, H3-A4. (June 1998). *Procedures for the collection of diagnostic blood specimens by venipuncture* (4th ed.).Wayne, PA: NCCLS.

Warren, M., Eason, C., Burch, P., & Pfeiffer-Ewens, J. (2002). *Medical assisting, a commitment to Service.* St. Paul: EMCParadigm.

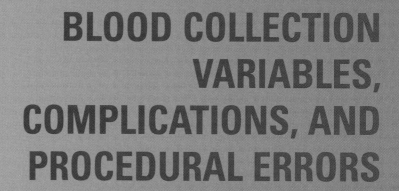

BLOOD COLLECTION VARIABLES, COMPLICATIONS, AND PROCEDURAL ERRORS

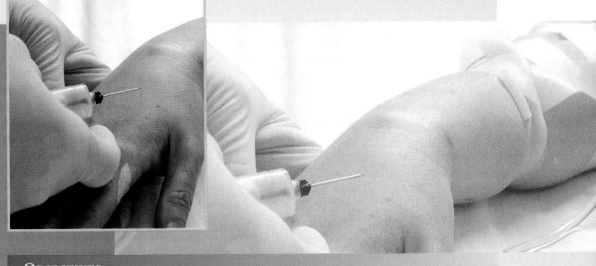

Upon successful completion of this chapter, the reader will be able to:

1 Define the key terms and abbreviations listed at the beginning of this chapter.

2 List and describe physiologic variables that influence basal state and name the laboratory tests affected by each one.

3 List problem areas to avoid in site selection and describe causes for concern and procedures to follow when encountering each.

4 Identify and describe various vascular access devices.

5 List blood collection complications and procedural errors that affect the patient or the quality of the specimen and describe how to handle or avoid them.

6 Identify and describe the procedural errors that lead to failure to draw blood and explain how to handle them.

INTRODUCTION

Each blood collection situation is unique. A competent phlebotomist must not only possess the technical skills necessary to collect a quality specimen, but must also understand the numerous patient variables, complications, and procedural errors that can affect the integrity of the specimen or the health and safety of the patient to avoid or reduce any negative impact. This chapter covers numerous factors that must be considered before blood collection is attempted.

PHYSIOLOGIC VARIABLES THAT INFLUENCE SPECIMEN COMPOSITION

Basal State

Basal state refers to the condition of the body early in the morning when a patient is still at rest and **fasting** (approximately 12 hours after the last intake of food). Collecting a basal state specimen minimizes or eliminates the effects of diet, exercise, and other controllable factors on test results and also provides the ideal specimen for establishing **reference ranges** or normal values for laboratory tests on inpatients.

 Key Point ➤ Outpatient specimens are not basal state specimens and may have slightly different normal values.

Factors That Influence Basal State

Age

Values for numerous blood components vary considerably depending upon the age of the patient. For example, red blood cell (RBC) and white blood cell (WBC) values are higher in newborns than adults.

Some physiologic functions such as kidney function decrease with age in adults. For example, creatinine clearance, a kidney function test, is directly related to the age of the patient, which must be used in calculating test results.

Altitude

Decreased oxygen content of the air at higher altitudes causes the body to produce more RBCs to fulfill the body's oxygen requirements; the higher the altitude, the greater the increase. Thus RBC counts and related determinations such as hemoglobin (Hgb) and hematocrit (Hct) will have higher normal ranges at higher elevations.

Dehydration

Dehydration (a decrease in total body fluid) that occurs with persistent vomiting or diarrhea, for example, causes **hemoconcentration,** a condition in which blood components that cannot easily leave the blood stream become concentrated as a result of the smaller plasma volume. Hemoconcentration falsely increases some blood components such as RBCs, enzymes, iron, calcium, and sodium. In addition, it is often difficult to obtain a blood specimen from a dehydrated patient.

Diet

Blood composition is significantly altered by ingestion of food. Glucose (blood sugar) levels increase dramatically with the ingestion of sugar-laden substances but return to normal within 2 hours if the patient has normal carbohydrate metabolism.

Ingestion of fatty substances, including many fast food items, butter, and cheese, increases lipid content in the blood, a condition called **lipemia.** Normal serum is clear, light yellow and normal plasma is clear to slightly hazy light yellow. Lipemia causes the serum or plasma to appear cloudy white or turbid and the specimen is described as being **lipemic.**

Memory Jogger ➤ To associate lipemic with fat, think of a "fat lip" or visualize a fat white cloud because fat makes the specimen cloudy.

Lipemia may be present for anywhere from 1 to 10 hours or more. In fact, accurate testing of triglycerides (a type of lipid) requires a 12-hour fast. In addition, some chemistry tests cannot be performed on lipemic specimens because the cloudiness interferes with the testing procedure.

Key Point ➤ When a test requires a fasting specimen but the serum or plasma sample is lipemic, it is a clue that the patient was not fasting.

Some laboratory tests are affected by ingestion of certain foods, which must be eliminated from the diet for several days before the test specimen is collected. For example, some methods that detect occult (hidden) blood in stool specimens also detect similar substances in meat and certain vegetables. Therefore a special diet that eliminates these foods must be followed for several days before the specimen is collected.

Fluid intake can also affect blood composition. Excessive fluid intake may cause decreased Hgb levels and alter electrolyte balance. Consumption of caffeine has been demonstrated to affect cortisol levels. Recent alcohol ingestion may also affect test values, especially glucose values.

Key Point ➤ Requiring a patient to fast or follow a special diet eliminates most dietary influences on testing.

Diurnal (Daily) Variations

Many blood constituents exhibit **diurnal** (daily) variations or normal fluctuations throughout the day. Factors that play a role in diurnal variations include activity, eating, daylight and darkness, and being awake or asleep. White blood counts, eosinophil counts, and iron levels are lower in the morning than in the afternoon. Cortisol, insulin, potassium, and testosterone levels are highest in the morning. Diurnal variations can be large. For example, cortisol levels and iron levels can differ by 50% or more between 8 AM and 4 PM.

 Key Point ➤ Tests influenced by diurnal variation are often ordered as timed tests, and it is important to collect them as close to the time ordered as possible.

Drug Therapy

Many drugs alter physiologic functions. In most instances, the effect is desired. In some individuals, however, there are unwanted physiologic effects called side effects or sensitivities. For example, thiazide diuretics often cause increased calcium levels and may cause low potassium levels. Chemotherapy drugs often cause a decrease in the cells of the blood, especially WBCs and platelets. Numerous drugs are toxic to the liver, causing an increase in liver enzymes such as serum glutamic-oxaloacetic transaminase (aspartate transaminase), alkaline phosphatase, and lactate dehydrogenase (LDH/LD). Steroids and diuretics can cause pancreatitis and an increase in serum amylase and lipase values.

 Key Point ➤ It is not uncommon for physicians to monitor levels of certain blood components to check for side effects while a person is receiving drug therapy.

Drugs may also interfere with the performance of the test in the laboratory, causing false increases or decreases in test results. Many lab test procedures are based on fluorescent, chromogenic (color-producing), peroxide-generating, or reagent-binding reactions. A drug may compete with the test reagents for the substance being tested causing a false-negative or false low result, or the drug may enhance the reaction, causing a false-positive or false high result. An acronym used for substances that interfere with the testing process is **CRUD,** which stands for "compounds reacting unfortunately as desired." The College of American Pathologists (CAP) has developed guidelines for reducing interference from drugs that are known to interfere with testing procedures.

 Key Point ➤ According to CAP, drugs known to interfere with blood tests should be stopped or avoided 4 to 24 hours before obtaining the blood sample for testing. Drugs known to interfere with urine testing should be avoided for 48 to 72 hours before urine sample collection.

It is up to the physician to recognize or eliminate drug interferences; however, it is helpful to the technician or technologist performing the test in the laboratory if the phlebotomist notes on the lab slip when he or she observes medication being administered just before blood collection.

Exercise

The effect of exercise on blood composition depends upon the duration and intensity of the activity and the physical condition of the patient. However, even moderate muscular activity will elevate levels of a number of blood components, such as lactic acid, creatinine, protein, and certain enzymes. Levels of these substances return to normal soon after the activity is stopped, with the exception of enzymes such as creatine kinase and LDH, which may remain elevated 24 hours or more.

 Key Point ➤ Athletes generally have higher resting levels of skeletal muscle enzymes, and exercise produces less of an increase.

Fever

Fever affects the levels of a number of hormones. Hypoglycemia caused by fever increases insulin levels followed by a rise in glucagon levels. Fever also increases cortisol levels and may disrupt its normal diurnal variation.

Gender

A patient's gender or sex has a determining effect on the concentration of numerous blood components. Most differences are apparent only after sexual maturity. Differences are reflected in separate normal values for male and female patients. For example, RBC, Hgb, and Hct normal values are higher for males than females.

Jaundice

Jaundice, also called **icterus,** is a condition characterized by increased bilirubin in the blood and deposits of yellow pigment in the skin, mucous membranes, and sclera or whites of the eyes giving the patient a yellow appearance. Serum, plasma, or urine specimens that contain high levels of bilirubin have an abnormal deep yellow to yellow-brown color and the specimen is referred to as "icteric." The abnormal color may interfere in the color reactions of a number of chemistry tests including chemical reagent strip analyses on urine.

 Key Point ➤ Jaundice in a patient may indicate liver inflammation caused by a hepatitis virus such as hepatitis B or hepatitis C virus.

Position

A patient's body position both before and during venipuncture influences blood composition. Going from a supine (lying down on the back) position to standing causes the water or plasma portion of the blood to filter into the tissues, resulting in a decrease in plasma volume and an increase in nonfilterable elements, or substances such as proteins, iron, calcium, and blood cells, that cannot easily pass through the walls of the blood vessels. For example, the RBC count on a patient who has been standing for approximately 15 minutes will be higher than the basal state RBC on the same patient.

Key Point ➤ Calling outpatients into the drawing room and having them sit in the drawing chair while paperwork related to the draw is readied can help minimize effects of posture changes on the specimen.

Pregnancy

Pregnancy causes physiologic changes in many body systems. Consequently, results of a number of laboratory tests must be compared to normal ranges established for pregnant populations. For example, body fluid increases, which are normal during pregnancy, have a diluting effect on the red blood cells, leading to lower red blood counts.

Smoking

Nicotine affects a number of blood components. The extent of the effect depends upon the number of cigarettes smoked. Patients who smoke before specimen collection may have increased cortisol levels and white blood counts. Chronic smoking often leads to decreased pulmonary function and increased hemoglobin levels.

Key Point ➤ Skin puncture specimens may be difficult to obtain from smokers because of impaired circulation in the fingertips.

Stress

Emotional stress in the form of fear or anxiety has been shown to cause short-lived elevations in WBC counts, decreases in serum iron, and increases in adrenal hormone values. For example, studies on crying infants demonstrated marked increases in WBC counts. Counts returned to normal within 1 hour after crying stopped. For this reason, it is best if complete blood count (CBC) or WBC specimens are obtained after the infant has been sleeping or resting quietly for at least 30 minutes. If a specimen is collected while an infant is crying, it should be noted on the report.

The field of **psychoneuroimmunology (PNI)** deals with the study of interactions between the brain, the endocrine system, and the immune system. PNI studies have demonstrated that receptors on the cell membrane of WBCs can sense stress in a person and react by stimulating an increase in cell numbers.

Temperature and Humidity

Environmental factors such as temperature and humidity affect test values by influencing the composition of body fluids. Acute heat exposure causes interstitial fluid to move into the blood vessels and decrease the glomerular filtration rate. This increases plasma volume and influences its composition. Extensive sweating without fluid replacement, on the other hand, can cause hemoconcentration. Ambient temperature and humidity and other environmental factors associated with geographic location are accounted for when establishing normal or reference values.

 Key Point ➤ Temperature and humidity in the laboratory are closely monitored to ensure proper functioning of equipment and to maintain specimen integrity.

SITE SELECTION VARIABLES THAT INFLUENCE SPECIMEN COMPOSITION

Physical Problem Areas to Avoid in Site Selection

Burns, Scars, and Tattoos

Avoid burned, scarred, or tattooed areas. Veins are difficult to palpate or penetrate in these areas. Healed burn sites and other areas with extensive scarring may have impaired circulation and yield erroneous test results. Newly burned areas are painful and susceptible to infection. Tattooed areas may have impaired circulation, are more susceptible to infection, and contain dyes that can interfere in testing.

Damaged Veins

Some patient's veins feel hard and cord-like, and lack resiliency because they are occluded or obstructed. These veins may be **sclerosed** (hardened) or **thrombosed** (clotted) from the effects of inflammation, disease, or the irritation of chemotherapy drugs. Scarring caused by numerous venipunctures, as occurs in regular blood donors and people with chronic illnesses, can also harden veins. Such damaged veins are difficult to penetrate with a needle, yield erroneous test results because of impaired blood flow, and should be avoided.

 Key Point ➤ Draw below (distal to) the damaged area or choose another site.

Edema

Edema is swelling caused by the abnormal accumulation of fluid in the tissues. Edema sometimes results when intravenous (IV) fluids infiltrate the tissues surrounding an IV site.

 Key Point ➤ Phlebotomists on early morning rounds in hospitals are often the first ones to notice infiltrated IVs and they should alert the appropriate personnel to the problem.

Edematous areas should be avoided as blood collection sites. Veins are hard to palpate in theses areas and specimens may be contaminated with tissue fluids resulting in inaccurate test results. In addition, edematous tissue is often fragile and easily injured by tourniquet and antiseptic application. Choose another site if possible.

Hematomas

A **hematoma** is identified by a swelling or mass of blood (often clotted) caused by blood leaking from a blood vessel during or after venipuncture. A large bruise eventually spreads over the surrounding area. Never perform a venipuncture in the area of a hematoma. A venipuncture made through a hematoma is painful to the patient and can result in collection of a specimen that is contaminated with hemolyzed blood from outside the vein and unsuitable for testing. A venipuncture performed in the immediate area surrounding a hematoma is also painful and the slowdown of blood flow to the area because of the obstruction by the hematoma and the effects of hemostasis may lead to inaccurate test results on the specimen.

Key Point ➤ If there is no alternative site, it is acceptable to perform the venipuncture distal to or below the hematoma to ensure the collection of free-flowing blood.

Mastectomy

A patient's physician should be consulted before drawing blood from an arm on the same side as a mastectomy (breast removal). **Lymphostasis** (stoppage of lymph flow) can occur when lymph nodes have been removed as part of the procedure. Lymphostasis leaves the area susceptible to infection and can also change the composition of blood in the area, leading to erroneous test results. In addition, application of a tourniquet to that arm may cause injury. If the patient has had a mastectomy on both sides, the patient's physician should be consulted to determine a suitable site. Generally, the side of the most recent mastectomy is the one avoided.

Vascular Access Areas and Devices to Avoid in Site Selection

IV Sites

It is preferred that blood specimens not be drawn from an arm with an **intravenous (IV)** line (Fig. 9-1). Drawing a specimen from an IV arm may result in dilution of the blood with the IV fluid, causing erroneous results, especially if the specimen is drawn above the IV. When a patient has an IV in one arm, blood specimens should be collected from the opposite arm. If a patient has IVs in both arms or if the other arm is unavailable for other reasons, it is preferred that the specimen be collected by skin puncture. Many specimens (i.e., CBCs) can be easily collected by skin puncture. However, if the specimen is one that cannot be collected by skin puncture (i.e., a coagulation specimen), it may be collected below the IV (Fig. 9-2), but never above, using the procedure in Box 9-1.

> **Box 9-1**
>
> ## PROCEDURE FOR COLLECTING A SPECIMEN FROM AN ARM WITH AN INTRAVENOUS LINE
>
> 1. Ask the patient's nurse to turn off the intravenous (IV) line for at least 2 minutes before collection.
> 2. Apply the tourniquet distal to the IV line and perform the venipuncture in a different vein than the one with the IV line.
> 3. Ask the nurse to restart the IV line after the specimen has been collected.
> 4. State on the requisition form that the specimen was collected from an arm with an IV line. It is also helpful to indicate the type of IV fluid being administered.

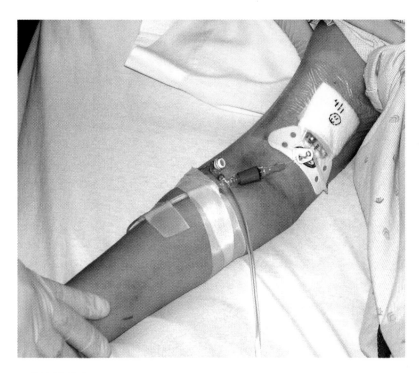

▪ FIGURE 9-1 ▪

Patient's arm with an intravenous (IV) line.

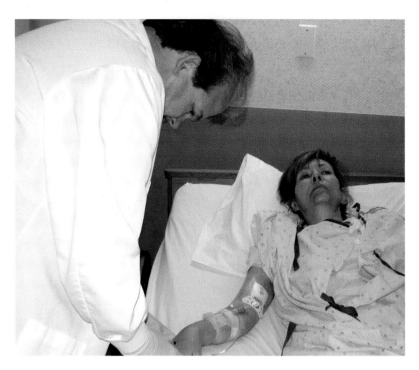

■ FIGURE 9-2 ■

A phlebotomist correctly collects a coagulation specimen from a hand vein below the site of an intravenous (IV) line.

Previously Active IV Sites

Previously active venipuncture sites present a potential source of error in testing. Blood specimens should not be collected from known previous IV sites within 24 to 48 hours of the time that the IV was discontinued.

Arterial Lines

An intra-arterial line or catheter is most commonly located in the radial artery and is used to provide continuous measurement of a patient's blood pressure. It is also used for collection of blood gas specimens.

Arteriovenous Shunts or Fistulas

An **arteriovenous shunt** or **fistula** (Fig. 9-3) is created by a surgical procedure that fuses a vein and artery together permanently. The connection is close to the surface of the skin and the loop created can usually be easily seen and felt. It is commonly created to provide access for dialysis. Never apply a blood pressure cuff or tourniquet to or perform venipuncture on an arm with a shunt.

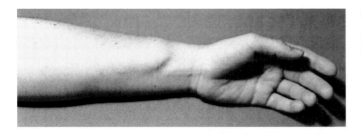

Internal arteriovenous (AV) shunt (fistula).

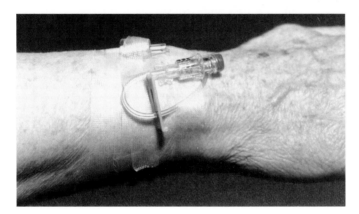

Peripheral heparin lock with extension tubing added for accessibility.

Heparin or Saline Locks

A **heparin** or **saline lock** (Fig. 9-4) is a special winged needle set or **cannula** that can be left in a patient's vein for up to 48 hours. It is commonly located in the lower arm above the wrist and is used to administer medication and draw blood. Because it is flushed with heparin or saline periodically or after use to keep it from clotting, a 5 mL discard tube should be drawn before collection of blood specimens. Drawing coagulation test specimens from heparin locks is not recommended. Only specially trained personnel should draw blood from a heparin lock.

Vascular Access Devices

A **vascular access device (VAD),** also called an **indwelling line,** consists of tubing inserted into a main vein or artery. VADs are used primarily for administering fluids and medications, monitoring pressures, and drawing blood.

Key Point ➤ Only specially trained personnel should access VADs to draw blood. However, the phlebotomist may assist by transferring the specimen to the appropriate tubes.

Most indwelling lines are routinely flushed with heparin or saline to reduce risk of thrombosis. A small amount of blood must be drawn from the line and discarded before a blood specimen can be collected to ensure that it is not contaminated with the flush solution. The amount of blood discarded depends upon the dead space volume of the line. Two times the dead space volume is discarded for noncoagulation tests and six times (normally about 5 mL) is generally recommended for coagulation tests.

CENTRAL VENOUS CATHETERS

A **central venous catheter (CVC)** (Fig. 9-5), also called a **central venous line,** is a line inserted into a large vein such as the subclavian and advanced into the superior vena cava, proximal to the right atrium. The exit end is surgically tunneled under the skin to a site several inches away in the chest. Several inches of tubing protrude from the exit site, which is normally covered with a transparent dressing. There are a number of different types of CVCs, including Broviac, Groshong, and Hickman (Fig. 9-6).

IMPLANTED PORTS

A subcutaneous vascular access device, also called an **implanted port** (Fig. 9-7), is a small chamber that is attached to an indwelling line. The chamber is surgically implanted under the skin in the upper chest or arm. The device is located by palpating the skin. Access is gained by inserting a special noncoring needle through the skin into the self-sealing septum (wall) of the chamber. The site is not normally covered with a bandage when not in use.

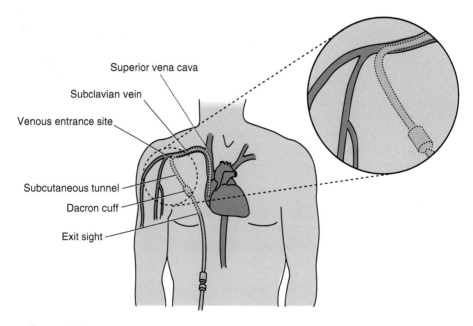

■ FIGURE 9-5 ■

Central venous catheter (CVC).

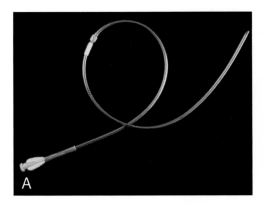
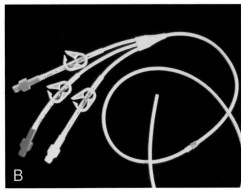

■ FIGURE 9-6 ■

Central venous catheters. (*A*) Groshong. (*B*) Hickman.   (Courtesy Bard Access Systems, Inc., Salt Lake City, UT.)

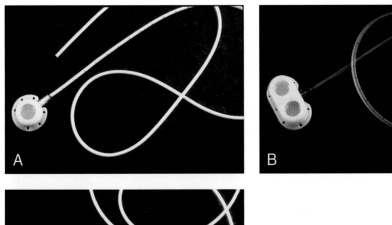

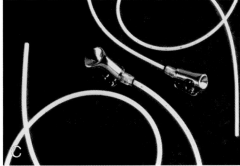

■ FIGURE 9-7 ■

Implanted ports. (*A*) Single port. (*B*) Double port. (*C*) CathLink implanted port.   (Courtesy Bard Access Systems, Inc., Salt Lake City, UT.)

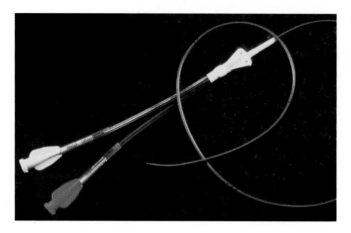

■ FIGURE 9-8 ■

Groshong peripherally inserted central catheter. (Courtesy Bard Access System, Inc., Salt Lake City, UT.)

PERIPHERALLY INSERTED CENTRAL CATHETERS

A **peripherally inserted central catheter (PICC)** (Fig. 9-8) is inserted into the peripheral venous system (veins of the extremities) and threaded into the central venous system (main veins leading to the heart). It does not require surgical insertion. PICCs are commonly placed in either the basilic or cephalic vein with the exit just above the antecubital area. Because a PICC tends to collapse on aspiration, drawing blood from a PICC is not recommended.

COMPLICATIONS AND PROCEDURAL ERRORS ASSOCIATED WITH BLOOD COLLECTION

The phlebotomist must be aware of complications associated with blood collection procedures. Complications may affect the patient, the integrity of the specimen, or both. Some complications are unavoidable; others can be avoided by employing proper collection technique or can be minimized by the alert response of a knowledgeable phlebotomist.

Complications Related to Patient Conditions

Allergies to Antiseptics and Adhesives

Occasionally, a patient is allergic to the antiseptic used in skin preparation before venipuncture or skin puncture. In this case, an alternate antiseptic should be used.

Some patients are allergic to the glue used in adhesive bandages. Usually paper tape placed over a folded gauze square can be used instead. If the patient is also allergic to paper tape, the area can be wrapped with bandaging material such as Coban that sticks to itself, eliminating the need for tape.

Allergies to Latex

Increasing numbers of individuals are developing allergies to latex. Most are seemingly minor and involve irritation or rashes from physical contact with latex products such as gloves. Others are so severe that being in the same room where latex materials are used can set off a life-threatening reaction. If a patient is known to have a severe allergy to latex, there may be a warning sign on the patient's door. It is important that no items made of latex be brought into the room. This means the phlebotomist must wear nonlatex gloves, use a nonlatex tourniquet, and use nonlatex bandages when in the room, whether collecting blood from the patient or the patient's roommate.

Excessive Bleeding

Normally, a patient will stop bleeding from the venipuncture site within a few minutes. Some patients, particularly those on anticoagulant therapy, may take longer to stop bleeding. Pressure must be maintained over the site until the bleeding stops. If the bleeding continues after 5 minutes, notify the nurse. Do not leave until bleeding has stopped or the nurse takes charge of the situation.

Fainting (Syncope)

Some patients become faint at the thought of or sight of their blood being drawn, especially if they are ill. The medical term for fainting is **syncope (sin' ko-pe).**

> *Memory Jogger* ➤ To remember that syncope means fainting, pick the word cope out of syncope. If the body can't cope, the patient faints.

A patient who feels faint, has a history of fainting, or mentions feeling weak from illness of extended fasting should be asked to lie down for the procedure. Inpatients who are already lying down rarely faint during blood draws. Outpatients are more likely to faint, because they are usually sitting up during venipuncture. See Box 9-2 for steps to follow if a patient starts to faint during venipuncture.

Box 9-2

STEPS TO FOLLOW WHEN A PATIENT FEELS FAINT

1. Remove the tourniquet and withdraw the needle as quickly as possible.
2. Talk to the patient to divert attention away from the procedure and to help keep him or her alert.
3. Have the patient lower his or her head and breathe deeply, while physically supporting the patient to prevent injury in case of collapse.
4. Loosen a tight collar or tie if possible.
5. Apply a cold compress or washcloth to the forehead and back of the neck.
6. Call for the designated first aid personnel if the patient does not respond.

A patient who is weak or pale following a blood draw may faint and should lie down until recovered. A patient who recovers from a fainting episode must stay in the area for at least 15 minutes and be instructed *not* to drive a vehicle for at least 30 minutes. The incident should be documented according to facility policy in case of future litigation.

Nausea/Vomiting

A patient who becomes nauseous should be reassured and made as comfortable as possible. A feeling of nausea often precedes vomiting, so it is a good idea to give the patient an emesis basin to hold as a precaution. Ask the patient to breathe slowly and deeply. Apply a cold, damp washcloth or other cold compress to the patient's forehead. If the patient vomits, provide tissues or a washcloth to wipe his or her face. Give the patient water to rinse out his or her mouth unless he or she is scheduled for surgery or other procedures in which water is not allowed. Notify the patient's nurse or appropriate first aid personnel.

Obesity

Obese patients often present a challenge to the phlebotomist. Veins on obese patients may be deep and difficult to find. Proper tourniquet selection and application is the first step to a successful venipuncture. Conventional latex tourniquets may be too short to fit around the arm without rolling and twisting. A long length of Penrose drain tubing or a long Velcro closure strap often works better than a latex strap. A blood pressure cuff can also be used.

Obese patients who have a double crease in the antecubital area often have an easily palpable median cubital vein between the two creases. If this is not the case, another site to try is the cephalic vein. To locate the cephalic vein, the patient's arm is rotated so that the hand is prone. In this position, the weight of excess tissue often pulls downward, making the cephalic vein easy to feel and penetrate with a needle.

Petechiae

Petechiae are small, nonraised red spots that appear on the patient's skin when a tourniquet is applied. These spots are a result of a defect of the capillary walls or platelet defects. They are *not* an indication that the phlebotomist has used incorrect procedure. However, they are an indication that the venipuncture site may bleed excessively.

Seizures/Convulsion

In the rare event that a patient has a seizure or goes into convulsions while the phlebotomist is drawing a blood specimen, it is important to remove the needle as quickly as possible. Try to hold pressure over the site without completely restricting the patient's movement. Do not try to put anything into the patient's mouth. Try to prevent the patient from injuring him or herself without completely restricting movement of the extremities. Notify the appropriate first aid personnel.

Complications and Procedural Errors That Adversely Affect the Patient

Hematoma Formation

Hematoma formation is the most common complication of venipuncture. It is caused by blood leaking into the tissues during or after venipuncture and identified by swelling at or near the venipuncture site. A hematoma is painful to the patient, results in unsightly bruising, and can cause compression injuries to nerves that lead to lawsuits. If a hematoma starts to form during blood collection, the phlebotomist should immediately release the tourniquet, withdraw the needle, and hold pressure over the site for a minimum of two minutes. Cold compresses are sometimes used to relieve pain and reduce swelling. See Box 9-3 for situations that can result in hematoma formation.

Box 9-3

SITUATIONS THAT MAY TRIGGER HEMATOMA FORMATION

1. The vein is fragile or too small for the needle size.
2. The needle penetrates all the way through the vein.
3. The needle is only partly inserted into the vein.
4. Excessive or blind probing is used to locate the vein.
5. The needle is removed while the tourniquet is still on.
6. Pressure is not adequately applied after venipuncture.

Inadvertent Arterial Puncture

The chance of inadvertent arterial puncture is rare, especially if proper vein selection and other venipuncture procedures are followed. It is most often associated with deep or blind probing, especially in the area of the basilic vein because it is in close proximity to the brachial artery. (This is one of the reasons that the basilic vein is the last choice for venipuncture.) If accidental puncture of an artery is suspected, it is important to hold pressure over the site for a full 5 minutes after the needle is removed. A phlebotomist can usually recognize arterial blood by its bright red color or the fact that it spurts or pulses into the tube.

 Key Point ➤ An inadvertently collected arterial specimen can usually be submitted for testing, rather than redrawing the patient. However, the specimen should be labeled as arterial because some test values are different for arterial specimens. Consult laboratory protocol.

Iatrogenic Anemia

Iatrogenic is an adjective used to describe an adverse condition brought on by the effects of treatment. Blood loss as a result of removal for testing purposes is called iatrogenic blood loss. Removal of blood on a regular basis or in large quantities can lead to anemia in some patients, especially infants. One of the primary reasons for blood transfusion in neonatal intensive care unit patients is to replace iatrogenic blood loss. Blood loss to a point where life cannot be sustained is called **exsanguination.** Life is threatened if more than 10% of a patient's blood volume is removed at one time or over a short period. Coordination between nurses, physicians, and the laboratory to minimize duplication in orders, batching test orders to minimize the number of times a patient is drawn, following quality assurance procedures to minimize redraws, and collecting minimum required specimen volumes especially from infants can minimize iatrogenic blood loss.

Infection

Infection at the site after venipuncture is rare, but not unheard of. Using proper aseptic technique including: not touching the site after it has been cleaned, minimizing the time between removing the needle cap and venipuncture, not opening adhesive bandages ahead of time, and reminding the patient to keep the bandage on for at least 15 minutes after specimen collection should minimize the risk of infection.

Nerve Damage

Poor site selection, inserting the needle too deeply or quickly, movement by the patient as the needle is inserted, and excessive or blind probing while performing a venipuncture can lead to injury of a main nerve (such as the median cutaneous nerve), causing permanent damage. Injuries such as this may result in a lawsuit. Following national guidelines for site selection and venipuncture technique minimizes the risk of problems. If initial needle insertion does not result in successful vein entry and proper redirection of the needle does not result in blood flow, the needle should be removed and venipuncture attempted at an alternate site, preferably the opposite arm.

Key Point ➤ Extreme pain, numbness of the arm, and pain that radiates down the arm are signs of nerve involvement and require immediate removal of the needle.

Pain

A small amount of pain is associated with routine venipuncture and skin puncture. Putting the patient at ease before blood collection helps relax him or her and seems to make the procedure less painful. Warning the patient before needle insertion will avoid a startle reflex by the patient. A stinging sensation upon venipuncture can be avoided by allowing the alcohol to dry completely before needle penetration. Excessive, deep, or blind probing with the needle can be very painful to the patient and should never be attempted. Marked or extreme pain, numbness of the arm, or pain that radiates down the arm as a result of venipuncture indicates nerve involvement and requires immediate removal of the needle. If the pain persists after needle removal, the laboratory pathologist or the patient's physician should be consulted. Follow your healthcare facility's protocol.

Key Point ➤ If extreme pain occurs, the venipuncture should be terminated immediately even if there are no other signs of nerve involvement.

Reflux of Anticoagulant

In rare instances, it is possible for blood to **reflux** (backflow) or flow back into the patient's vein from the collection tube during the venipuncture procedure. Some patients have had adverse reactions to tube additives, particularly ethylenediaminetetraacetic acid, attributed to reflux. Reflux can occur when the contents of the collection tube are in contact with the needle while the specimen is being drawn. To prevent reflux reactions, keep the patient's arm in a downward position so that the collection tube remains below the venipuncture site and fills from the bottom up, not from the tube stopper end. This will prevent the needle from being in contact with the blood in the tube. Back-and-forth movement of the contents of the tube should also be avoided until the tube is removed from the evacuated tube holder. An outpatient can be properly positioned by asking him or her to lean forward and extend the arm downward over the arm of the drawing chair. Raising the head of the bed, extending the patient's arm over the side of the bed, or supporting the arm with a rolled towel can be used to achieve proper inpatient positioning.

Vein Damage

Properly performed, occasional venipunctures will not impair the **patency** (state of being freely open) of a patient's veins. Numerous venipunctures in the same area over an extended period, however, will eventually cause a buildup of scar tissue and increase the difficulty of performing subsequent venipunctures. Blind probing and improper technique when redirecting the needle can also damage veins and impair patency.

Procedural Errors That Affect Specimen Quality

Sometimes the quality or integrity of a specimen can be compromised by the methods (techniques) used in collection. A poor-quality specimen will generally yield poor-quality results and affect the care of the patient. However, the fact that the quality of the specimen has been compromised is not always apparent to the phlebotomist or other laboratory personnel. Consequently, it is very important for the phlebotomist to be aware of the following pitfalls of collection.

Hemoconcentration/Venous Stasis

Certain conditions, such as prolonged tourniquet application, cause **venous stasis** or stagnation of the normal blood flow. When venous stasis occurs, some of the plasma and filterable components of the blood pass through the walls of the blood vessels into the tissues. This decreases the plasma volume in the blood vessels and causes **hemoconcentration,** an abnormal increase or concentration of nonfilterable blood components such as RBCs, enzymes, iron, and calcium. Vigorous hand pumping, probing, long-term IV therapy, and sclerosed or occluded veins can also cause hemoconcentration.

Key Point ➤ To minimize the effects of hemoconcentration, release the tourniquet within 1 minute of applying it and do not allow the patient to continuously make and release a fist.

Hemolysis

Hemolysis results from the destruction of RBCs and the liberation of hemoglobin into the fluid portion of the specimen, causing the serum or plasma to be pink (slight hemolysis) to red (gross hemolysis) in color. The specimen is described as being "hemolyzed." Hemolyzed specimens may be the result of patient conditions such as hemolytic anemia, liver disease, or transfusion reactions, but they are more commonly the result of procedural errors in specimen collection. Because hemolysis will affect certain tests, such as enzymes, potassium, and RBC counts, a hemolyzed specimen as a result of procedural error will most likely need to be redrawn. Box 9-4 lists procedural errors that can cause hemolysis.

Box 9-4

PROCEDURAL ERRORS THAT RESULT IN SPECIMEN HEMOLYSIS

1. Mixing additive tubes too vigorously or using rough handling during transport.
2. Drawing blood from a vein that has a hematoma.
3. Pulling back the plunger on a syringe too quickly.
4. Using a needle with too small of a bore for venipuncture.
5. Using too large of a tube when using a small-diameter butterfly needle.
6. Frothing of the blood caused by improper fit of the needle on a syringe.
7. Forcing the blood from a syringe into an evacuated tube.
8. Failure to wipe away the first drop of blood (which may contain alcohol residue) from a skin puncture.
9. Excessive squeezing of the site when obtaining a skin puncture specimen.

Partially Filled Tubes

It is important to fill anticoagulant and other additive tubes until the vacuum is exhausted to obtain the proper ratio of blood to additive for which the tube was designed. Specimens collected in tubes that have not been filled until the vacuum is exhausted are called "short draws." Although in some cases the specimen may be accepted for testing by the laboratory, a partially filled tube will not have the proper blood to additive ratio and test results on the specimen may be inaccurate. In addition, never pour two partially filled additive tubes together in order to fill one tube because this will also affect the blood-to-additive ratio.

The blood-to-anticoagulant ratio is especially critical for light blue sodium citrate tubes used for coagulation studies. Most laboratories will not accept partially filled tubes for coagulation tests. If the tube is not filled properly, the specimen must be recollected.

 Key Point ➤ Never fill a light blue stopper first when a butterfly is used with the evacuated tube system of collection. Air in the tubing is drawn into the first tube collected and prevents proper filling. Collect a few milliliters of blood into a plain red stopper first to eliminate the problem.

Inadvertent partial filling of tubes may result from loss of vacuum and may indicate that a tube is cracked or has been dropped. Cracked tubes present a safety hazard because they may leak or break with further handling.

 Key Point ➤ Never use a tube that has been dropped. Discard it instead.

Partial vacuum tubes that are the same size as standard fill tubes but are designed to contain a smaller amount of blood are available and should be used in situations where it is difficult to obtain larger amounts of blood. These tubes are sometimes referred to as "short draw" tubes, but they are designed to contain the proper additive-to-blood ratio even though they contain less blood (Fig. 9-9).

Specimen Contamination

There are a number of ways a phlebotomist may inadvertently contaminate a specimen. One way is to use the wrong antiseptic to clean the site before specimen collection. For example, using alcohol to clean the site can contaminate an ethanol (blood alcohol) specimen. Using povidone–iodine (e.g., Betadine) to clean a skin puncture site can contaminate the specimen with povidone–iodine and cause erroneously high levels of uric acid, phosphate, and potassium.

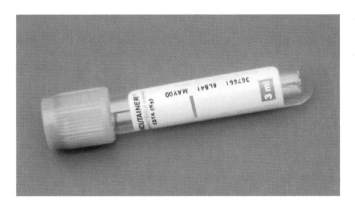

▪ FIGURE 9-9 ▪

"Short draw" tubes for partial filling.

Using the correct antiseptic, but not allowing it to dry, can also cause contamination. For example, contamination of blood cultures can occur if the antiseptic is not dry when the needle is inserted into the vein or into the culture bottles. Traces of the antiseptic in the culture media may inhibit growth of bacteria and cause false-negative blood culture results. Alcohol that is not dry when a skin puncture is performed can cause hemolysis of the specimen and affect test results.

Microbial contamination of blood cultures can result from improperly cleaning the site or culture bottles or from touching the site after it has been prepped (cleaned).

Powder from gloves can contaminate blood films on slides and blood specimens collected by skin puncture, especially blood spots on filter paper used to collect neonatal screening specimens.

Fingerprints, urine from wet diapers, and alcohol residue all have been cited as sources of contamination of filter paper containing newborn screening samples.

Procedural Errors That Lead to Failure to Draw Blood

Failure to draw blood can be caused by a number of procedural errors. Being aware of these errors and how to correct them may determine whether you obtain blood on the first try or have to repeat the procedure. If you fail to obtain blood, remain calm so that you can clearly analyze the situation and check the following.

Tube Position and Vacuum

Check the tube to see that it is properly seated and the needle in the tube holder has penetrated the tube stopper. Reseat the tube to make certain the needle sleeve is not pushing the tube off of the needle. Tubes can lose vacuum during shipping and handling, when they bump one another in trays, if they are dropped, or if they are pushed too far onto the needle before venipuncture. In addition loss of tube vacuum can occur during venipuncture procedures if the needle bevel is not completely under the skin or the bevel backs out of the skin slightly. When this happens a short hissing sound is often heard and there may be a spurt of blood into the tube before the blood flow stops. If you suspect that a tube has lost its vacuum, try a new one.

Needle Position

Improper needle position is a common cause of failure to obtain blood. A seasoned phlebotomist uses visual cues to help determine if the needle is correctly positioned in the vein(Fig. 9-10). Try first to visually determine if any of the following common problems with needle position or insertion have occurred. Some are harder to discern than others. Eliminate the ones that you can and try the remedy for the others to see if one works.

BEVEL AGAINST THE VEIN WALL

Blood flow can be impaired if the needle bevel is up against either the upper or lower wall of the vein (Fig. 9-10, *B* and *C*). This is very hard to determine. Remove the tube from the holder to release vacuum and pull the needle back slightly. Rotating the bevel slightly may also help. If blood flow is established, this was probably the case.

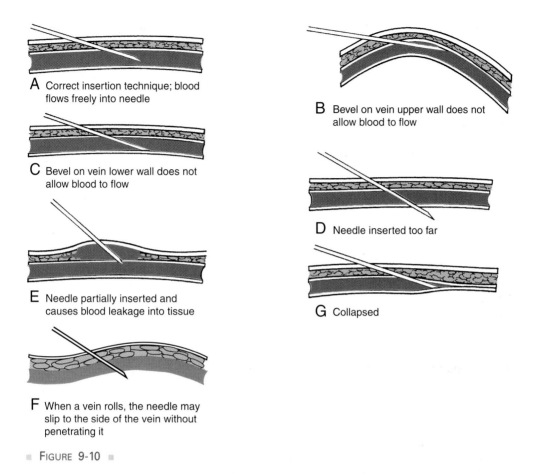

A Correct insertion technique; blood flows freely into needle

B Bevel on vein upper wall does not allow blood to flow

C Bevel on vein lower wall does not allow blood to flow

D Needle inserted too far

E Needle partially inserted and causes blood leakage into tissue

G Collapsed

F When a vein rolls, the needle may slip to the side of the vein without penetrating it

■ FIGURE 9-10 ■

Proper and improper needle positioning. (*A*) Needle correctly positioned in a vein; blood flows freely into the needle. (*B*) Bevel on the upper wall of the vein prevents blood flow. (*C*) Bevel on the lower wall of the vein prevents blood flow. (*D*) Needle inserted too deep penetrates through the vein. (*E*) Partially inserted needle causes blood to leak into tissue. (*F*) Needle slipped beside the vein, not into it; caused when a vein rolls to the side. (*G*) Collapsed vein prevents blood flow.

Key Point ➤ Tube vacuum may hold the vein wall against the needle bevel. Do not rotate the bevel of the needle without first removing the tube and pulling the needle back slightly or the vein may be injured.

NEEDLE TOO DEEP

The needle may have gone in too deep and penetrated all the way through the vein (Fig. 9-10, *D*). This can happen on needle insertion or as the tube is pushed onto the needle if the tube holder is not held steady. If this is the case, withdrawing the needle slightly should establish blood flow. If the needle position is not corrected quickly, blood will leak into the tissues and form a hematoma.

NEEDLE NOT DEEP ENOUGH

If the needle is not completely inserted into the vein (Fig. 9-10, *E*), blood may fill the tube very slowly. By pushing the needle gently into the vein, correct blood flow should be established. Partial needle insertion can also cause blood to leak into the tissue and start to form a hematoma. If this occurs, immediately remove the tourniquet, withdraw the needle, and hold pressure over the site.

BESIDE THE VEIN

Veins are fairly tough and if a vein is not anchored well, it may roll (move away) slightly and the needle may slip to the side of the vein instead of penetrating it (Fig. 9-10, *F*). Often the needle ends up to the side and slightly under the vein. If this happens, slip the tube off of the needle to preserve the vacuum, withdraw the needle slightly until just the bevel is under the skin, anchor the vein securely, and redirect the needle into the vein. If redirection is unsuccessful, do not search or probe for the vein. Discontinue the draw and choose a new site.

Key Point ➤ When phlebotomists "miss" veins, they often tell the patients that they have "veins that roll." This leads patients to mistakenly believe that there is a problem with their veins when more likely the problem is the phlebotomist's technique.

UNDETERMINED

If you cannot determine the position of the needle and the above solutions do not help, you may have to use your fingers to relocate the vein. Remove the tube from the needle and withdraw the needle until the bevel is just under the skin. Clean your gloved finger with alcohol and feel the arm above the point of needle insertion to try to determine needle position and the location of the vein. *Do not* feel too close to the needle; this is painful to the patient.

After you have relocated the vein, redirect the needle into the vein and proceed with the venipuncture. If you cannot relocate the vein, remove the needle and hold pressure over the site.

Key Point ➤ *Do not* blindly probe the arm in an attempt to locate a vein. Probing is painful to the patient and may cause damage to nerves and other tissues. It can also lead to inadvertent puncture of an artery.

Collapsed Vein

Sometimes the vacuum draw of a tube or the pressure created by pulling on a plunger of a syringe can be too much for a vein, causing it to collapse temporarily (Fig. 9-10, *G*) and blood flow to cease. Another reason for vein collapse is that the tourniquet is tied too tightly or too close to the venipuncture site. In this case blood cannot be replaced as quickly as it is withdrawn and the vein collapses. In addition, veins sometimes collapse when the tourniquet is removed during the blood draw.

This is often the case in elderly patients whose veins are fragile and collapse more easily.

 Key Point ➤ Stoppage of blood flow when the tourniquet is removed does not necessarily mean that the vein has collapsed. It may be that the needle is no longer positioned properly and a slight adjustment is needed to reestablish blood flow.

A clue that a normally visible vein has collapsed is that it disappears as soon as the needle penetrates it or when the tourniquet is removed. To reintroduce tourniquet pressure, grasp the ends of the loose tourniquet with one hand and twist them together. That may be enough to reestablish blood flow. If the tourniquet cannot be retightened, use your finger to apply pressure to the vein several inches above the needle. Remove the tube from the needle and wait a few seconds for the blood flow to reestablish. Try using a smaller volume tube or if using a syringe, pull more slowly on the plunger. If the blood flow does not reestablish, you will have to withdraw the needle and attempt a second venipuncture at another site.

STUDY & REVIEW QUESTIONS

1. Values for this test are normally highest in the morning.
   a. Cortisol
   b. White blood count
   c. Iron (Fe)
   d. Eosinophil count

2. What tests may be affected most if the patient is not fasting?
   a. CBC and protime
   b. Glucose and triglycerides
   c. RA and cardiac enzymes
   d. Blood culture and thyroid profile

3. Drugs known to interfere with urine tests should be stopped
   a. 4 to 24 hours before the test.
   b. 24 to 36 hours before the test.
   c. 48 to 72 hours before the test.
   d. not at all; drugs do not interfere with urine tests.

4. Veins that feel hard and cordlike when palpated are called
   a. collapsed veins.
   b. fistulas.
   c. sclerosed veins.
   d. young venules.

5. A hematoma may result from all of the following *except*
   a. the needle bevel is only partly inserted into the vein.
   b. not enough pressure is applied to the site after venipuncture.
   c. the tourniquet is released before needle withdrawal.
   d. the needle has penetrated all the way through the vein.

6. Small, red spots that appear on a patient's arm when the tourniquet is applied are called
   a. edema.
   b. hematoma.
   c. hemolysis.
   d. petechiae.

7. When fingers and hands of the patient are swollen with excess fluids, the condition is called
   a. atherosclerosis.
   b. edema.
   c. hemoconcentration.
   d. syncope.

8. A fistula is
   a. always a congenital problem.
   b. part of a dialysis machine.
   c. a good source of arterial blood.
   d. the fusion of a vein and artery.

Continued

STUDY & REVIEW QUESTIONS *(CONTINUED)*

9. Failure to obtain a blood specimen may be caused by all of the following *except*

   a. the needle bevel has penetrated through the opposite wall of the vein.
   b. the needle bevel is against the vein wall.
   c. the needle bevel is centered in the lumen of the vein.
   d. the needle bevel is only partly inserted into the vein.

10. A phlebotomist needs to collect a plasma specimen for a protime test. The patient has IVs in both arms. Both IVs are located below the antecubital area. What should the phlebotomist do?

   a. Collect the specimen above the IV that is located closest to the wrist area.
   b. Collect the specimen below an IV after it has been shut off for 2 minutes.
   c. Collect the specimen by finger puncture.
   d. Collect the specimen from the IV.

■ CASE STUDY 9-1: PHYSIOLOGIC VARIABLES AND SITE SELECTION

Charles is a phlebotomist who works in a physician's office laboratory. One morning shortly after the drawing station opens he is asked to collect blood specimens for a CBC and a glucose test from a very heavyset woman who appears quite ill. The patient tells Charles that she vomited all night and was unable to eat or drink anything. She also mentions that she has had a mastectomy on the left side and the last time she had blood collected she was stuck numerous times before the phlebotomist was able to successfully collect the specimen.

QUESTIONS:
1. What physiologic variables may be associated with the collection of this specimen and how should they be dealt with?
2. What complications might Charles expect and how should he prepare for them?
3. How should Charles go about selecting the blood collection site?
4. What options does Charles have if he is unable to select a proper venipuncture site?

■ CASE STUDY 9-2: PROCEDURAL ERRORS

A phlebotomist named Sara is in the process of collecting a protime and CBC from a patient. The needle is in the patient's vein. As Sara pushes the first tube onto the needle in the tube holder there is a spurt of blood into the tube and she hears a hissing sound. Then the blood stops flowing. She repositions the needle but is not able to establish blood flow.

QUESTIONS:

1. Why did blood spurt into the tube and then stop?
2. What clues are there to determine what the problem is?
3. What can Sara do to correct the problem?

■ CASE STUDY 9-3: COMPLICATIONS AND PROCEDURAL ERRORS

Erica is a recent phlebotomy program graduate who was hired less than a month ago by a major hospital in her first job as a phlebotomist. Her first 3 months of employment are a probationary period and she is determined to do a good job. This morning she has been asked to collect a stat CBC and electrolytes from a patient in an intensive care unit. The patient is responsive and cooperative but has difficulty breathing. The patient's nurse mentions that she will hook up his oxygen therapy as soon as the phlebotomist is finished with him. He has an IV in his left hand. Erica palpates the right antecubital area. She can feel the median cubital vein but it is deep. The basilic vein is visible and prominent so she decides to use it to collect the specimen. When she inserts the needle into the arm, the vein rolls and her needle ends up beside the vein and slightly under it. She redirects the needle and the vein rolls again. The patient winces in pain but says nothing. Noticing the look of pain on the patient's face Erica asks him if it hurts. The patient says yes and tells her that the pain is radiating down his arm and his fingers are tingling. Erica asks him if he would like her to remove the needle. The patient replies, "No, you've got to get the specimen," so Erica tries again to redirect the needle. Finally, blood spurts into the tube and a hematoma starts to form quickly. At first Erica thinks that she may have hit an artery, but the specimen is normal in color so Erica dismisses the thought. She quickly collects the specimens, covers the site with gauze and asks the patient to hold pressure while she labels the tubes. When finished she thanks the patient and delivers the stat specimens to the laboratory.

QUESTIONS:

1. What site selection variables were associated with the collection of this specimen and were they properly handled?
2. What complications and procedural errors were involved and were they handled properly?

Bibliography and Suggested Readings

Bishop, M. L., Duben-Engelkirk, J. L., & Fody, E. P. (2000). *Clinical chemistry: Principles, procedures, correlations* (4th ed.). Philadelphia: Lippincott Williams & Wilkins.

Burtis, C. A., & Ashwood, E.R. (2001). *Tietz Fundamentals of clinical chemistry* (5th ed.) Philadelphia: W. B. Saunders.

Byrne, C. J., & Saxton, D. (1986). *Laboratory tests: Implications for nursing care.* San Francisco: Addison-Wesley.

Dale, J.C. Pre-analytical variables in laboratory testing. *Laboratory Medicine,* September 1998.

National Committee for Clinical Laboratory Standards, H21-A3. (1998). *Collection, transport, and processing of blood specimens for coagulation testing and general performance of coagulation assays* (3rd ed.). Wayne, Philadelphia: NCCLS.

National Committee for Clinical Laboratory Standards, H3-A4. (June 1998). *Procedures for the collection of diagnostic blood specimens by venipuncture* (3rd ed.). Wayne, PA: NCCLS.

National Committee for Clinical Laboratory Standards, H4-A4 (September 1999*). Procedures and devices for the collection of diagnostic blood specimens by skin puncture* (3rd ed.). Wayne, PA: NCCLS.

10

SKIN PUNCTURE EQUIPMENT AND PROCEDURES

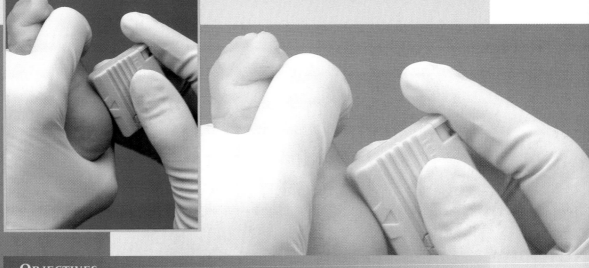

Upon successful completion of this chapter, the reader will be able to:

1 Define the key terms and abbreviations listed at the beginning of this chapter.

2 List and describe the various types of equipment needed to perform skin puncture.

3 State the composition of skin puncture blood, identify which tests have different reference values when collected by skin puncture methods, and name tests that cannot be performed by skin puncture.

4 State indications for performing skin puncture on adults, infants, and children.

5 Describe the proper procedure for selecting a skin puncture site and indicate precautions associated with site selection.

6 Describe the proper procedure for collecting skin puncture specimens from adults, infants, and children.

7 List the order of draw for collecting skin puncture specimens.

8 Describe the procedure for making both routine and thick blood smears and reasons for making them at the collection site.

9 Explain the clinical significance of capillary blood gas, neonatal bilirubin, and newborn screening tests, and describe how specimens for these tests are collected.

INTRODUCTION

Skin puncture, also called dermal or capillary puncture involves penetrating the capillary bed in the dermis of the skin with a lancet or other sharp device or laser in order to collect a blood specimen. With the advent of point-of-care instruments and the trend toward laboratory instrumentation capable of testing small volumes of specimen, many more laboratory tests can be collected by skin puncture now than in the past. The ability to test small volumes of specimen is especially important in pediatrics where removal of large quantities of blood can have serious consequences. Skin puncture is most commonly performed on the fingers of adults and children older than the age of 2 years and the heels of infants.

SKIN PUNCTURE EQUIPMENT

In addition to general blood collection equipment described in Chapter 7, the following special equipment may be required for skin puncture procedures.

Lancets

A **lancet** is a sterile, disposable, sharp-pointed or bladed instrument used to pierce the skin to obtain drops of blood used for testing. Lancets selected for skin puncture must not be capable of puncturing to a depth that penetrates bone. In addition, they must have safety features such as permanently retractable blades to reduce the chance of accidental sharps injuries. A number of companies manufacture safety skin puncture devices in a range of lengths and depths to accommodate various situations and sample requirements. Different lancet devices are available for finger puncture (finger sticks) and heel puncture (heel sticks).

Finger Stick Lancets

Lancets specifically designed for finger puncture include Vacutainer Brand Genie lancets (Fig. 10-1, *A*) available in several different color-coded widths and depths (Becton Dickinson, Franklin Lakes, NJ), and Tenderlett lancets (Fig. 10-1, *B*) available in toddler, junior, and adult versions (International Technidyne Corp., Edison, NJ).

Laser Lancet

A revolutionary new device (Fig. 10-1, *C*), the Lasette *plus* (Cell Robotics, Albuquerque, NM) perforates the skin with a laser instead of a conventional sharp instrument. The laser produces a small hole in the capillary bed by vaporizing water in the skin. Because there is no sharp instrument involved, there is no risk of accidental sharps injury and there is no need for sharps disposal. A special insert that is discarded after each use prevents cross-contamination between patients. The Lasette is cleared by the Food and Drug Administration (FDA) for use on the fingers of adults and children 5 years of age and older. In a clinical setting, the use of the Lasette on children younger than 5 years of age is subject to a physician's discretion.

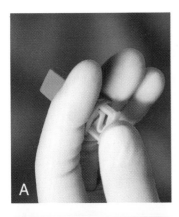

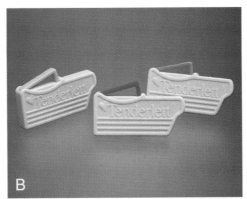

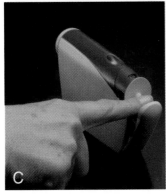

■ FIGURE 10-1 ■

Several types of finger puncture lancets. (*A*) Vacutainer Brand Genie Lancets. (Becton Dickinson, Franklin Lakes, NJ.) (*B*) Tenderlett Toddler, Junior, and Adult lancet devices. (Courtesy of ITC, Edison, NJ.) (*C*) Lasette laser lancet device. (Cell Robotics, Albuquerque, NM.)

Heel Stick Lancets

Special heel puncture lancets include the QuikHeel Lancet (Fig. 10-2, *A*) in infant and preemie versions (Becton Dickinson, Franklin Lakes, NJ), and the Tenderfoot (Fig. 10-2, *B*) toddler, newborn, preemie, and micro-preemie heel incision devices (ITC, Edison, NJ).

Collection Devices

Microcollection Containers

Microcollection containers or tubes (Fig. 10-3) are special small plastic tubes used to collect the tiny amounts of blood obtained from skin punctures. They are often referred to as "bullets" because of their size and shape. Some come with plastic capillary tubes to facilitate specimen collection. Most have color-coded bodies or stoppers that indicate the presence and type (or absence) of an additive, and markings for minimum and maximum fill levels measured in microliters (μL) such as 250 μL and 500 μL, respectively. Some manufacturers print lot numbers and expiration dates on each tube. Color coding typically corresponds to venipuncture blood collection tubes. Examples of microcollection tubes include Microtainers (Becton Dickinson, Franklin Lakes, NJ) shown in Fig. 10-3, *A;* MiniCollect Capillary Blood Collection tubes (Fig. 10-3, *B*)

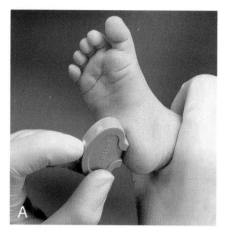
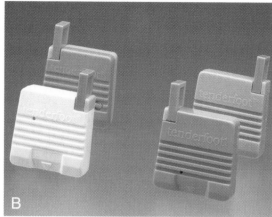

■ FIGURE 10-2 ■

Several types of heel puncture lancets. (*A*) BD QuikHeel infant lancet, also available in a preemie version. (Becton Dickinson, Franklin Lakes, NJ.) (*B*) Tenderfoot toddler, newborn, preemie, and micro-preemie heel incision devices. (Courtesy ITC, Edison, NJ.)

(Greiner Bio-One, Kremsmünster, Austria); Capiject Capillary Blood Collection Tubes (Fig. 10-3, *C*) (Terumo, Somerset, NJ); and Samplette (Fig. 10-3, *D*) Micro Blood Collection Tubes (Tyco Healthcare, Kendall, Mansfield, MA).

Key Point ➤ Sometimes venous blood obtained by syringe during difficult draw situations is put into microcollection containers. When this is done it is important to label the specimen as venous. Otherwise it will be assumed to be a skin puncture specimen, which may have different normal values.

Microhematocrit Tubes

Microhematocrit tubes (Fig. 10-4) are disposable, narrow-bore plastic or plastic-clad glass capillary tubes that fill by capillary action and typically hold 50 to 75 μL of blood. They are primarily used for hematocrit (packed cell volume) determinations although they are sometimes used to collect other skin puncture specimens. Microhematocrit tubes come coated with ammonium heparin for hematocrit specimens and other tests requiring plasma collected by skin puncture, or plain for collecting serum specimens by skin puncture or performing manual hematocrit tests using blood from a lavender top.

Ammonium-heparin–coated tubes have a red band at one end of the tube; plain tubes have a blue band. Smaller microhematocrit tubes designed for use with special microcentrifuges such as those available from StatSpin, Inc. (Norwood, MA), require as little as 9 μL of blood and are often used in infant and child anemia screening programs and pediatric clinics.

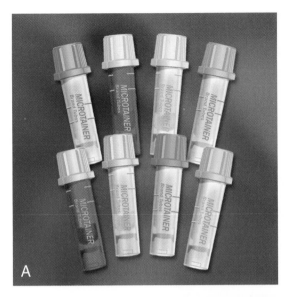

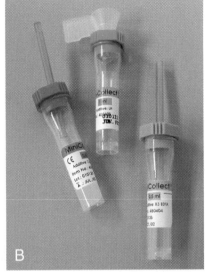

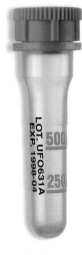

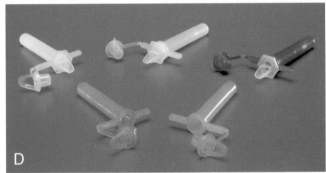

■ FIGURE 10-3 ■

Examples of microcollection containers. (*A*) Microtainers. (Becton Dickinson, Franklin Lakes, NJ.) (*B*) MiniCollect Capillary Blood Collection Tubes. (Courtesy Greiner Bio-One, Kremsmuenster, Austria.) (*C*) Capiject Capillary Blood Collection tubes. (Terumo, Somerset, NJ.) (*D*) Samplette capillary blood collectors. (Courtesy Tyco Healthcare, Kendall, Mansfield, MA.)

Plastic/Clay Sealant

Plastic or **clay sealants** are commonly used to seal one end of microhematocrit tubes and tubes for chemistry determinations or both ends of capillary blood gas specimens. Sealants come in small trays. Traditionally, the dry end of a capillary tube was inserted into the clay to plug it. Because of safety concerns, it is now recommended that sealing methods be used that do not require manually pushing the tube into the sealant.

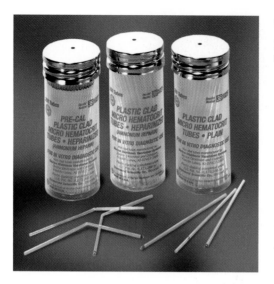

■ FIGURE 10-4 ■

Microhematocrit tubes. (Courtesy Becton Dickinson, Franklin Lakes, NJ.)

Capillary Blood Gas Collection Equipment

Capillary blood gas collection equipment (Fig. 10-5) is used to collect blood gas specimens by skin puncture. The following special equipment, often assembled together in kit form, is commonly used:

Collection tubes: **Capillary blood gas collection tubes** vary according to volume requirements for different testing methods and instrumentation. Tubes of 100 mm in length with a capacity of 100 μL are most common. A color-coded band identifies the type of anticoagulant that coats the inside of the tube; it is usually green, indicating sodium heparin.

Stirrers: **Metal stirrers** (often referred to as **"fleas"**) are inserted into the tube after collection of a capillary blood gas specimen to aid in mixing the anticoagulant.

Magnet: A **magnet** is required to aid in mixing capillary blood gas specimens after collection. The magnet often has a hole in the center so that it can be slipped over the capillary tube. It then is moved back and forth along the tube length, pulling the metal stirrer with it and mixing the anticoagulant into the blood specimen.

Plastic/clay sealant: **Plastic** or **clay sealants** are commonly used to seal both ends of capillary blood gas tubes to maintain specimens under anaerobic conditions.

Plastic caps: **Plastic end caps** or **closures** are available in place of clay to seal microcollection tubes. Capillary blood gas collection tubes often come with their own caps.

Micropipet Dilution System

A **micropipet dilution system** serves as both a collection device and a dilution unit for the blood sample. Components of this disposable system are a sealed plastic reservoir that contains a premeasured amount of diluting fluid; a detachable glass, self-filling capillary

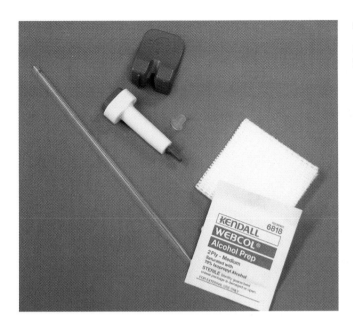

FIGURE 10-5

Capillary blood gas collection equipment.

pipet; and a pipet shield, which also serves as a device to puncture the reservoir covering or diaphragm before adding the sample.

Warming Devices

Warming the area before skin puncture increases blood flow as much as seven times the normal amount. This is especially important when performing heel sticks on newborns. Several **heel-warming devices** (Fig. 10-6) are commercially available. To avoid burning the patient, the devices provide a uniform temperature that does not exceed 42°C. A towel or diaper dampened with warm tap water can also be used to wrap a hand or foot before skin puncture. However, care must be taken not to get the water so hot that it scalds the patient.

SKIN PUNCTURE PRINCIPLES

Composition of Skin Puncture Blood

Blood obtained through skin puncture is a mixture of arterial blood (from arterioles), venous blood (from venules), and capillary blood, along with **interstitial** and **intracellular fluids** from the surrounding tissues. It contains a higher proportion of arterial blood than venous blood because arterial blood enters the capillaries under pressure. Composition of skin puncture blood, therefore, more closely resembles arterial blood than venous blood. This is especially true if the area has been warmed because warming increases arterial flow into the area.

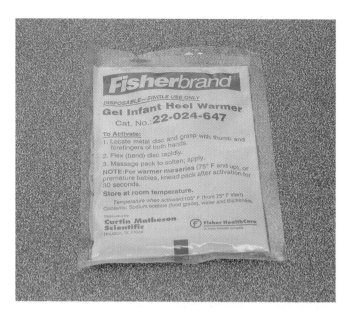

■ FIGURE 10-6 ■

Infant heel warmer.

Reference Values for Skin Puncture Blood

Because skin puncture blood differs in composition from venous blood, **reference (normal) values** for certain tests are different for skin puncture blood. The most notable differences are for glucose, which is higher in skin puncture blood; and total protein, calcium, and potassium, which are lower in skin puncture blood.

 Key Point ➤ Although potassium values are normally lower in properly collected skin puncture specimens, levels may be falsely elevated if there is tissue fluid contamination or hemolysis of the specimen.

Tests That Cannot Be Performed by Skin Puncture

Although today's technology allows many tests to be performed on very small quantities of blood, and a wide selection of devices are available to make collection of skin puncture specimens relatively safe and easy, some tests cannot be performed on skin puncture specimens. These include most erythrocyte sedimentation rate methods, coagulation studies that require collection of a plasma specimen, blood cultures, and tests that require large volumes of serum or plasma.

Indications for Performing Skin Puncture

Adults

Skin puncture is performed on adults when there are no accessible veins, to save veins for other procedures such as chemotherapy, when the patient has thrombotic or clot-forming tendencies, and for certain bedside and home-testing procedures such as glucose monitoring.

Key Point ➤ Skin puncture is generally *not* appropriate for patients who are dehydrated or have poor circulation to the extremities from other causes such as shock as specimens may be hard to obtain and may not be representative of blood elsewhere in the body.

Infants and Children

Skin puncture is the preferred method of obtaining blood from infants and children. Obtaining blood from infants and children by venipuncture is difficult and may damage veins and surrounding tissues. In addition, an infant or child can be injured by the restraining method used while performing the venipuncture. Because infants and young children have such a small blood volume, removing the larger quantities of blood typical of venipuncture or arterial puncture can lead to anemia. Large quantities removed rapidly can cause cardiac arrest.

 Key Point ➤ Skin puncture blood is the preferred specimen for some tests, such as screening tests for **phenylketonuria (PKU)** and several other inherited diseases.

Skin Puncture Site Selection Criteria

General Criteria

A skin puncture site should be warm, pink or normal color, and free of scars, cuts, bruises, or rashes. *Do not* choose a site that is cold, **cyanotic** (bluish in color), or **edematous** (swollen).

Infants

The heel is the recommended site for collection of skin puncture specimens on infants younger than 1 year of age. However, it is important that the puncture be performed in an area of the heel where there is little risk of puncturing the bone. Puncture of the bone can cause painful **osteomyelitis** (os'te-o-mi'el-i'tis) or bone inflammation as a result of infection, and **osteochondritis** (os'te-o-kon-dri'tis), inflammation of the bone and cartilage. Additional punctures through inflamed previous puncture sites may spread the infection.

Studies have shown that the **calcaneus** (kal-ka'ne-us) or heel bone of small or premature infants may be as little as 2.0 mm below the skin on the **plantar** (bottom) **surface** of the heel and half that distance at the **posterior curvature** (back) of the heel. Punctures deeper than this may cause bone damage. The vascular or capillary bed is typically located between 0.35 and 1.6 mm beneath the skin surface (Fig. 10-7) so punctures less than 2.0 mm deep will provide adequate blood flow without risking bone injury. Pain fibers increase in abundance below the capillary bed so deeper punctures are also more painful.

For these reasons, guidelines were developed to determine the safest areas and the optimal depth for performing heel puncture. According to the guidelines recom-

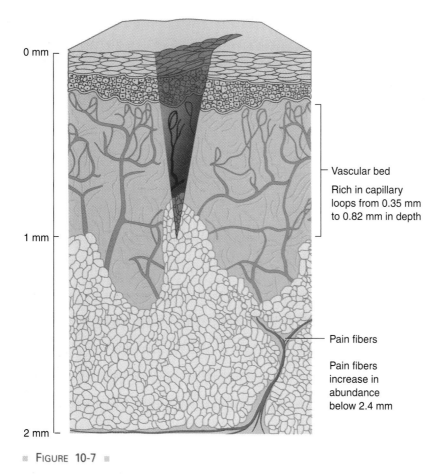

0 mm

Vascular bed

Rich in capillary
loops from 0.35 mm
to 0.82 mm in depth

1 mm

Pain fibers

Pain fibers
increase in
abundance
below 2.4 mm

2 mm

■ FIGURE 10-7 ■

Cross section of full-term infant's heel showing lancet penetration depth needed to access
the capillary bed.

mended by NCCLS document H4-A4, to avoid puncturing bone, the only safe areas for
heel puncture are on the plantar surface of the heel, medial to an imaginary line extending from the middle of the great (big) toe to the heel or lateral to an imaginary line
extending from between the fourth and fifth toes to the heel (Fig. 10-8). Punctures in
other areas risk bone, nerve, tendon, and cartilage injury. Skin puncture precautions
are summarized as follows:

- *Do not* puncture deeper than 2.0 mm.
- *Do not* puncture through previous puncture sites.
- *Do not* puncture the area between the imaginary boundaries.
- *Do not* puncture the posterior curvature of the heel.
- *Do not* puncture in the area of the arch as nerves, tendons and cartilage may be
  injured.
- *Do not* puncture areas of the foot other than the heel.

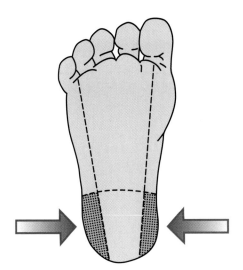

■ FIGURE 10-8 ■

Infant heel. Shaded areas indicated by arrows represent recommended safe areas for heel puncture.

> *Memory Jogger* ➤ One way to remember that the safe areas for heel puncture are the medial or lateral plantar surfaces of the heel is to think of the phrase, "Make little people happy." Using the first letter of each word, "M" stands for medial, "L" stands for lateral, "P" stands for plantar, and "H" stands for heel.

Older Children and Adults

The recommended site for skin puncture on adults and older children is the palmar surface of the **distal segment** (end segment) of the middle or ring finger of the non-dominant hand. The puncture should be made in the central, fleshy portion of the finger, slightly to the side of center and perpendicular to the **whorls** (grooves) of the fingerprint (Fig. 10-9).

- *Do not* puncture the side or very tip of the finger. The distance between the skin surface and the bone is half as much at the side and tip as it is in the central portion of the end of the finger.
- *Do not* puncture parallel to the grooves of the fingerprint. A puncture parallel to or along the lines of the fingerprint will cause blood to run down the finger rather than form a rounded drop, which makes collection difficult.
- *Do not* puncture the index finger. The index finger is more calloused and, therefore, harder to poke than the other fingers. Also, the patient will use that finger more and will notice the pain longer.
- *Do not* puncture the fifth or little finger. The amount of tissue between skin surface and bone is the thinnest in this finger.
- *Do not* puncture fingers of infants and very young children. The amount of tissue between skin surface and bone is so small that bone injury is very likely.

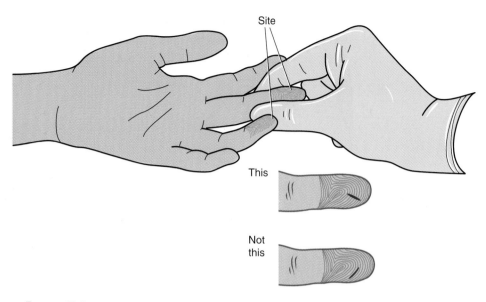

Site

This

Not
this

■ FIGURE 10-9 ■

Recommended site and direction of finger puncture.

SKIN PUNCTURE PROCEDURE

The following procedure was written to conform to NCCLS guidelines and includes the steps necessary for a phlebotomist or other qualified healthcare provider to safely obtain a quality blood specimen from an infant's heel or an adult or older child's finger.

Identify the Patient

Follow identification and preparation procedures outlined in Chapter 8.

Assemble Equipment

1. 70% isopropyl alcohol prep pads
2. Sterile gauze pads
3. Sterile safety lancet or automated skin puncture device
4. Warming device (if applicable)
5. Collection devices (capillary tubes, microtainers, slides, etc.)

Warm the Site

Blood flow can be increased up to seven times the normal amount by warming the site before skin puncture. Because warming primarily increases arterial flow into the area, the specimen obtained will be referred to as an **arterialized** specimen. When collecting pH or blood gas specimens by skin puncture, warming is an essential part of the procedure.

Warming can be accomplished by wrapping the site for a minimum of 3 minutes with a washcloth, towel, or diaper that has been moistened with comfortably warm water (no warmer than 42°C or 108°F), or using a commercial heel warming device.

Clean the Site

Clean the site with 70% isopropanol. *Do not* use povidone-iodine to clean skin puncture sites because it greatly interferes with a number of tests, most notably bilirubin, uric acid, phosphorous, and potassium.

Memory Jogger ➤ Remember the tests affected by povidone-iodine by associating them with the word "**BURPP**," where "**B**" stands for bilirubin, "**UR**" stands for uric acid, and the two "**Ps**" stand for phosphorous and potassium.

After cleaning, allow the site to air dry to ensure maximum antiseptic action and minimize the chance of alcohol contamination of the specimen. Alcohol residue, in addition to causing a stinging sensation, causes rapid hemolysis of red blood cells. Alcohol residue has also been shown to interfere with glucose testing.

Prepare the Puncture Device

Use a new, sterile puncture device for each patient, and prepare it in view of the patient or guardian. Open the package or remove protective covering in an aseptic manner. Do not allow the blade slot opening to rest or brush against any nonsterile surface.

Perform Skin Puncture

Finger Puncture (Finger Stick)

Support the arm on a firm surface and have the patient extend the hand palm up. Select and clean the site (Fig. 10-10, *A*) and allow it to air dry.

Grasp the finger firmly between your thumb and index finger and perform the puncture (Fig. 10-10, *B*) perpendicular to the whorls (lines or ridges) of the fingerprint. This will allow the blood to form a bead or drop that is easily collected. A puncture along the lines or parallel to the fingerprint will allow the blood to run down the finger and make collection difficult.

Heel Puncture (Heel Stick)

Grasp the foot firmly, but gently. Encircle the heel by wrapping the index finger around the arch and the thumb around the bottom (Fig. 10-11). Wrap the other fingers around the top of the foot. Puncture the heel perpendicular to the lines of the footprint (or per manufacturer instructions) using a recommended heel puncture device.

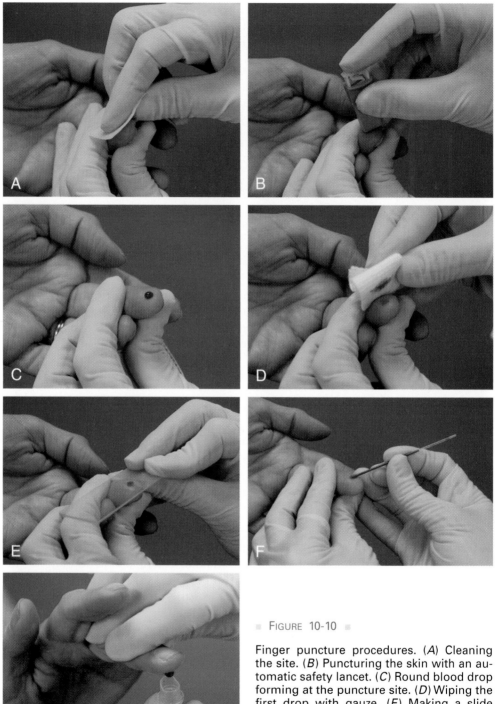

■ FIGURE 10-10 ■

■ FIGURE 10-10 ■

Finger puncture procedures. (*A*) Cleaning the site. (*B*) Puncturing the skin with an automatic safety lancet. (*C*) Round blood drop forming at the puncture site. (*D*) Wiping the first drop with gauze. (*E*) Making a slide from the skin puncture by touching the slide to the drop of blood. (*F*) Collecting skin puncture blood in a capillary tube. (*G*) Collecting skin puncture blood in a microtainer.

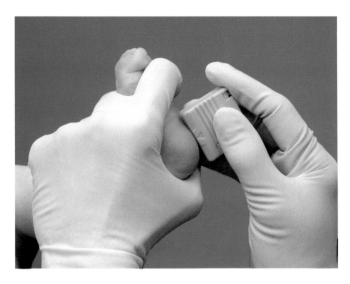

Infant heel puncture using Tenderfoot automatic incision device. (Courtesy ITC, Edison, NJ.)

Finger Puncture and Heel Puncture

Continue both heel sticks and finger sticks in the following manner:

- Dispose of the puncture device promptly in a sharps container.
- Apply gentle pressure toward the site.
- Wipe away the first drop of blood (Fig. 10-10, C) with a dry piece of gauze (Fig. 10-10, D). (The first drop is usually contaminated with excess tissue fluid.) This also gets rid of any remaining alcohol residue that could hemolyze the specimen and also keep the blood from forming a well-rounded drop.
- Position the site downward to enhance blood flow and continue to apply gentle intermittent pressure to tissue surrounding a heel puncture site or proximal to a finger puncture site to keep the blood flowing freely.

 Key Point ➤ *Do not* squeeze, milk, or massage the site vigorously or use strong repetitive pressure. Such activities introduce excess tissue fluid into the specimen and may also cause hemolysis of the specimen.

- Proceed to collect the blood using devices appropriate for the type of test to be performed. Collect slides (Fig. 10-10, E), platelet counts, and other hematology specimens first to avoid the effects of platelet aggregation (clumping). Collect other anticoagulant containers next. Collect serum specimens last.
- Touch the collection device to the drop of blood formed on the surface of the skin. Capillary pipets (Fig. 10-10, F) will fill by capillary action. When filled, seal the dry end of a capillary pipet with clay or other suitable sealant.
- Touch the "scoop" of a microcollection tube (Fig. 10-10, G) to the drop of blood and let the drop of blood run down the walls of the tube. *Do not* use a scooping motion against the surface of the skin. Scraping the scoop against the skin activates platelets and may also cause hemolysis. Tap the tube gently now and then

to encourage the blood to settle to the bottom of the tube. Cover microcollection containers with the cap or cover provided and mix additive tubes by gently inverting them 8 to 10 times. Give the tube a quick shake to remove excess blood from around the cap or cover.

- After collecting the specimen, apply pressure to the site with a clean gauze until bleeding stops. Keep the site elevated while pressure is applied. Bandage the site if the patient is an older child or adult.

Key Point ➤ *Do not* apply bandages to infants and children younger than 2 years old. They may become a choking hazard to the infant or child. In addition, bandages may stick to the paper-thin skin of newborns and tear the skin when removed.

- Label the specimens with the appropriate information (see Chapter 8). Labels can be directly affixed to microcollection containers. Microhematocrit tubes can be placed in a plain red top tube and identifying information written on the tube label. Follow laboratory protocol.
- Follow special specimen handling requirements if indicated.
- Thank the patient.
- Dispose of contaminated gauze in a biohazard container and remove all equipment from the area.
- Remove gloves and wash hands.
- Transport the specimen to the lab.

SPECIAL SKIN PUNCTURE PROCEDURES

Routine Blood Film (Smear) Preparation

A blood smear is required to perform a manual **differential**, either as part of a complete blood count or to confirm abnormal results of a machine generated differential or platelet count. Two blood smears are normally prepared and submitted for testing. Although a common practice in the past, today blood smears are rarely made at the bedside. They are typically made in the hematology department either by hand or using an automated machine that makes a uniform smear from a single drop of blood from the EDTA specimen tube.

Key Point ➤ Blood smears prepared from EDTA specimens should be made within 1 hour of collection to eliminate cell distortion caused by the anticoagulant.

A few special tests require evaluation of a blood film or smear made from a fresh drop of blood from a fingertip. An example is a leukocyte alkaline phosphatase (LAP) stain or score, which usually requires four fresh **peripheral** (skin puncture or venous) **blood smears.** Skin puncture collection of peripheral smears is preferred. In addition, some hematologists prefer blood smears from blood that has not been in contact with anticoagulant. When collected with other skin puncture specimens, blood smears should be collected first to avoid effects of platelet clumping.

- Select two clean glass **slides,** free of cracks or chipped edges.
- Wipe away the first drop of blood in the normal manner. Touch the slide to the second drop in such a manner that the drop ends up 1/2 to 1 inch from the end of the slide or on the clear area of the slide just next to the frosted area, if applicable. The drop should be about 1 to 2 mm in diameter and centered on the slide.
- To make a smear manually from an anticoagulated blood specimen, the tube of blood must first be mixed for a minimum of 2 minutes to ensure a uniform specimen. A capillary tube or pipet is then used to dispense a drop of blood from the specimen tube onto the slide. A device called DIFF-SAFE (Fig. 10-12) (Alpha Scientific, Malvern, PA) allows a slide to be made from an EDTA tube without removing the tube stopper. The device is inserted through the rubber stopper of the specimen tube and is then pressed against the slide to deliver a uniform drop of blood.
- Hold the blood drop slide in the nondominant hand between the thumb and forefinger with the blood drop at the thumb end, grasp the blood drop end between the thumb and forefinger, or place the slide on a flat surface and hold it steady with the index finger of the nondominant hand. Use the dominant hand to rest a second (or spreader) slide in front of the drop at approximately a 30-degree angle (Fig. 10-13, A) with the first slide. The spreader slide is held at one end between the thumb and index finger in either a vertical or horizontal position.
- Pull the spreader slide back to the edge of the blood drop. Stop the spreader slide as soon as it touches the drop and allow the blood to spread along its entire width (Fig. 10-13, B).
- As soon as the blood has spread its entire width, push the spreader slide forward (away from the thumb) in one smooth motion, carrying it the entire length and

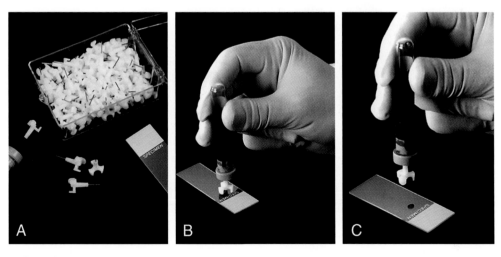

■ FIGURE 10-12 ■

(A) DIFF-SAFE blood delivery device. (B) Applying blood drop to slide using DIFF-SAFE device. (C) Blood drop on slide. (Courtesy Alpha Scientific, Malvern, PA.)

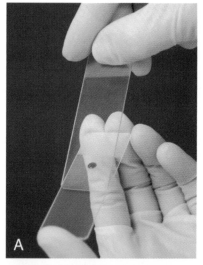

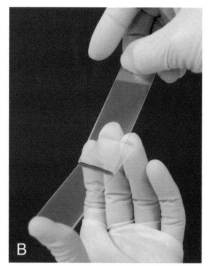

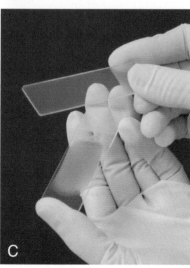

■ FIGURE 10-13 ■

Blood smear preparation. (A) Drop of blood on slide with pusher slide placed in front. (B) Pusher slide with drop of blood spreading to its edges. (C) Completed blood smear.

all the way off the end of the blood drop slide. *Do not* push down on the spreader slide. Let the weight of the spreader slide carry the blood and make the smear.

- Place the drop of blood for the second smear on the spreader slide from the first smear. Use the slide containing the first smear as the spreader slide for the second smear. This way, two smears can be made using only two slides.
- Allow the blood films to dry naturally. *Never* blow on a slide to dry it because red blood cell distortion may result.
- Label frosted blood slides by writing the patient information in pencil on the frosted area. *Do not* use ink because it may dissolve during the staining process. If attaching patient identification labels, place them over the frosted end or in the space left at the blood drop end of slides that are not frosted.

Key Point ➤ Use caution when handling blood smears because they are considered biohazardous or infectious until they are stained or fixed.

Making a good blood smear is a skill that takes practice to perfect. Improperly made blood smears will not contain a normal, even distribution of blood cells and may produce erroneous results. An acceptable smear (Fig. 10-13, *C*) will cover about one-half to three-fourths of the surface of the slide and have no holes, lines, or jagged edges. It will have the appearance of a **feather** in that there will be a smooth gradient from thick to thin when held up to the light. The thinnest area of a properly made smear, often referred to as the "feather," is one cell thick and is the most important area because that is where a differential is performed.

Smears that are uneven, too long (cover the entire length of the slide), too short, too thick, or too thin are not acceptable. Adjusting the size of the blood drop or the angle of the spreader slide can normally be used to control the length and thickness of the smear.

Fingerprints, dirt on the slide, or fat globules and lipids in the specimen can result in holes in the smear. A chipped pusher slide, a blood drop that has started to dry, or uneven pressure as the smear is made can cause the smear to have ragged edges. Table 10-1 lists common problems associated with routine blood smear preparation.

Thick Blood Smear Preparation

Thick blood smears are most often requested to detect the presence of **malaria,** which is caused by four species of parasitic sporozoan (types of protozoa) organisms called plasmodia. These organisms are transmitted to humans by the bite of infected female anopheles mosquitoes. Symptoms of malaria include serial bouts of fever and chills at

Table 10-1

Common Problems Associated with Routine Blood Smear Preparation	
Problem	**Probable Cause**
Absence of feather	Spreader slide lifted before the smear was completed
Holes in the smear	Dirty slide, fat globules in the blood, blood contaminated with glove powder
Ridges or uneven thickness	Too much pressure applied to spreader slide
Smear is too thick	Blood drop too big, spreader slide angle too steep, patient has high red blood cell count
Smear is too short	Blood drop too small, spreader slide angle too steep, spreader slide pushed too quickly, patient has high red blood cell count
Smear is too long	Blood drop too large, spreader slide angle too shallow, spreader slide pushed too slowly, patient has a low hemoglobin value
Smear is too thin	Blood drop too small, spreader slide angle too shallow, patient has a low hemoglobin value
Streaks or tails in feathered edge	Blood drop started to dry out, edge of spreader slide dirty or chipped, spreader slide pushed through blood drop, uneven pressure applied to spreader slide

regular intervals, related to the multiplication of certain forms of the organism within the red blood cells and the consequent rupture of those cells. The progressive destruction of red blood cells in certain types of malaria causes severe anemia.

Malaria is diagnosed by the presence of the organism in a peripheral blood smear. Diagnosis often requires the evaluation of both regular and thick blood smears. Presence of the organism is observed most frequently in a thick smear; however, identification of the species requires evaluation of a regular blood smear. Malaria smears may be ordered stat or at timed intervals and are most commonly collected just before the onset of fever and chills.

To prepare a thick smear, a very large drop of blood is placed in the center of a glass slide and spread with the corner of another slide or coverslip until it is the size of a dime. The smear is allowed to dry for a minimum of 2 hours before staining with fresh diluted Giemsa stain. The water-based Giemsa stain lyses the red blood cells and makes the organism easier to see.

Capillary Blood Gases (Arterialized Skin Puncture Blood Gases)

Because arterial punctures can be hazardous to infants and young children, blood gas analysis on infants and young children is sometimes performed on arterialized skin puncture (capillary) specimens.

Skin puncture blood is less desirable for blood gas analysis not only because of its partial arterial composition, but also because it is temporarily exposed to air during collection, which can alter test results. Proper collection technique is essential to minimize this exposure.

Capillary blood gas specimens are collected from the same sites as routine skin puncture specimens. Warming the site for 5 to 10 minutes before skin puncture helps increase blood flow and arterializes the specimen. Capillary blood gas collection procedure is shown in Box 10-1.

Box 10-1

CAPILLARY BLOOD GAS SPECIMEN COLLECTION PROCEDURE

1. Assemble equipment and supplies.
2. Select and warm the site.
3. Perform the skin puncture following routine skin puncture procedures.
4. Wipe away the first drop and collect the blood in a special heparinized glass capillary tube. Collect the blood carefully to prevent introduction of air bubbles into the capillary tube while obtaining the specimen. (Exposure of the blood to air for as little as 10 seconds can cause erroneous results.) Fill the capillary tube completely.

continued

5. After collecting the specimen, immediately seal one end of the tube with clay or a special cap.
6. Depending on the type of equipment used, place a small magnetic mixing bar or several magnetic "fleas" into the capillary tube.
7. Quickly seal the opposite end and mix the specimen by running a magnet from one end of the tube to the other several times. (This procedure mixes the heparin with the specimen to prevent clotting.)
8. Label the specimen and immediately place it horizontally in a mixture of ice and water to prevent changes in pH and blood gas values.
9. Transport the specimen to the lab immediately.

Neonatal Bilirubin Collection

Neonates (newborns) are commonly tested to detect and monitor increased bilirubin levels caused by overproduction or impaired excretion of bilirubin. Overproduction of bilirubin occurs from accelerated red blood cell hemolysis associated with hemolytic disease of the newborn (HDN). Impaired excretion is often the result of temporary abnormal liver function commonly associated with premature infants. High levels of bilirubin result in jaundice (yellow skin color).

Bilirubin can cross the blood-brain barrier in infants, accumulating to toxic levels that may cause permanent brain damage or even death. A transfusion may be needed if levels increase at a rate equal to or greater than 5.0 mg/dL per hour or when levels exceed 18.0 mg/dL. Bilirubin breaks down in the presence of light and jaundiced infants are often placed under special ultraviolet (UV) lights to lower bilirubin levels.

 Key Point ➤ Turn off the UV light when collecting a bilirubin specimen to prevent it from breaking down bilirubin in the specimen as it is collected.

Proper collection of bilirubin specimens is crucial to the accuracy of results. Specimens are normally collected by heel puncture. They must be collected quickly to minimize exposure to light and must be protected from light during transportation and handling. Specimens are often collected in amber-colored microcollection containers (Fig. 10-14) to reduce light exposure. Specimens must be collected carefully to avoid hemolysis, which could falsely decrease bilirubin results. Because determination of the rate of increase in bilirubin levels depends on accurate timing, specimens should be collected as close as possible to the time ordered.

Newborn Screening

Newborn screening is performed to test for the presence of genetic, or inherited, diseases such as phenylketonuria (fen'il-kee'to-nu'ree-ah) or PKU, hypothyroidism, galactosemia, homocystinuria, maple syrup urine disease, and sickle cell. In the

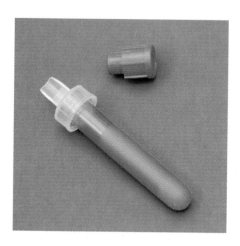

■ FIGURE 10-14 ■

Amber-colored microcollection container used to protect a bilirubin specimen from effects of ultraviolet light.

United States, newborn screening to detect PKU and hypothyroidism are required by law.

PKU

PKU results from a defect in the enzyme that converts the amino acid phenylalanine to tyrosine. Phenylalanine accumulates in the blood and is slowly metabolized by an alternate pathway resulting in increased phenylketones in the urine. Because phenylalanine is not being metabolized properly, phenylalanine can rise to toxic levels. PKU cannot be cured but it can normally be treated with a diet low in phenylalanine. If left untreated or not treated early, PKU can lead to brain damage and mental retardation. PKU testing requires the collection of two specimens, one shortly after an infant is born and another after the infant is 10 to 15 days old. The incidence of PKU in the United States is approximately 1 in 14,000 births.

Hypothyroidism

Congenital hypothyroidism occurs at the rate of approximately 1 in 4,000 births and is the result of insufficient levels of thyroid hormones. Some forms of neonatal hypothyroidism are not inherited but temporarily acquired when the mother has the condition. Newborn screening tests detect both inherited and noninherited forms. In the United States and Canada, the newborn screening test for hypothyroidism measures total thyroxine. Positive results are confirmed by measuring thyroid-stimulating hormone levels. Supplying the missing thyroid hormone treats the disorder.

Collection Procedure

Blood samples for PKU, hypothyroidism, and other newborn screening tests are commonly collected by absorption onto a special filter paper that is part of the test requisition. The filter paper contains printed circles that must be filled with blood (Fig. 10-15). The circles are filled by touching the paper to drops of blood obtained by heel puncture. A large drop of blood must be applied from one side of the paper only and blood must soak completely through to the other side.

Key Point ➤ Blood should *not* be smeared, touched, applied more than once, or layered with successive drops in the same collection circle, nor should the filter paper be contaminated by touching it with gloves or any other object or substance.

The specimen should be allowed to air dry in an elevated horizontal position away from heat or sunlight. Specimens should not be hung to dry or stacked together before or after the drying process. Hanging may cause the blood to migrate and concentrate towards the low end of the filter paper. Stacking may result in cross-contamination between specimens.

■ FIGURE 10-15 ■

Newborn screening specimen forms. (*A*) Initial specimen form. (*B*) Second specimen form.
(Courtesy Daniel Gray, State of New Mexico Scientific Laboratory, Albuquerque, NM.)

STUDY & REVIEW QUESTIONS

1. Which of the following is NOT needed for skin puncture?

   a. Gauze pad
   b. Lancet
   c. Microcollection device
   d. Povidone-iodine pad

2. Skin puncture blood contains

   a. arterial blood.
   b. interstitial fluids.
   c. venous blood.
   d. all of the above.

3. The concentration of this substance is higher in capillary blood than in venous blood.

   a. Blood urea nitrogen
   b. Carotene
   c. Glucose
   d. Total protein

4. A blood test that cannot normally be performed by skin puncture is

   a. CBC.
   b. erythrocyte sedimentation rate.
   c. potassium.
   d. thyroid panel.

5. Skin puncture is typically performed on adults when:

   a. patients have thrombotic tendencies.
   b. there are no accessible veins.
   c. veins need to be saved for other procedures.
   d. all the above.

6. A proper skin puncture site should *not* be

   a. cyanotic.
   b. edematous.
   c. swollen.
   d. all the above.

Continued

7. The least hazardous area of an infant's foot on which to perform skin puncture is the

   a. arch.
   b. central area of the heel.
   c. posterior curvature of the heel.
   d. medial or lateral plantar surface of the heel.

8. It is necessary to control the depth of lancet insertion during heel puncture to avoid

   a. puncturing a vein.
   b. excessive bleeding.
   c. bone injury.
   d. bacterial contamination.

9. A lancet selected for heel puncture should not be capable of puncturing deeper than

   a. 1.5 mm.   c. 2.5 mm.
   b. 2.0 mm.   d. 3.0 mm.

10. Which of the following is *not* proper skin puncture procedure?

   a. Clean the site thoroughly with povidone-iodine
   b. Puncture perpendicular to the grooves of the fingerprint
   c. Use firm pressure to keep the blood flowing freely
   d. Wipe away the first drop of blood

11. When collecting skin puncture tests, which of the following should be collected first?

   a. CBC
   b. Electrolytes
   c. Glucose
   d. Phosphorus

12. When making a routine blood smear, the "pusher slide" is normally used at a

   a. 15-degree angle.   c. 45-degree angle.
   b. 30-degree angle.   d. 60-degree angle.

■ CASE STUDY: DIFFICULT SKIN PUNCTURE

A phlebotomist is sent to collect a complete blood count specimen on a 5-year-old pediatric patient. The patient has an intravenous line in the left forearm. The right arm has no palpable veins so the phlebotomist decides to perform skin puncture on the middle finger of the right hand. This is the phlebotomist's first job and although he is quite good at routine venipuncture, he has not performed very many skin punctures. The child is uncooperative and her mother tries to help steady her hand during the procedure. The phlebotomist is able to puncture the site, but the child pulls her hand away. Blood runs down the finger. The phlebotomist grabs the patient's finger and tries to fill the collection device with the blood as it runs down the finger. The child continues to try to wriggle the finger free. The phlebotomist finally fills the container to the minimum level. When the specimen is tested, the platelet count is abnormally low. A slide is made and platelet clumping is observed. A new specimen is requested. Hemolysis is later observed in the first specimen.

QUESTIONS:
1. How might the circumstances of collection have contributed to the platelet clumping in the specimen?
2. What could have caused the hemolysis?
3. What factors may have contributed to the specimen collection difficulties?

Bibliography and Suggested Readings

Bishop, M. L., Duben-Engelkirk, J. L., & Fody, E. P. (2000). *Clinical chemistry: Principles, procedures, correlations* (4th ed.). Philadelphia: Lippincott Williams & Wilkins.

Harmening, D. (2002) *Clinical hematology and fundamentals of hemostasis* (4th ed.). Philadelphia: F.A. Davis

Lotspeich-Steininger, C. A., Stiene-Martin, E. A., & Koepke, J. A. (1998). *Clinical hematology: Principles, procedure, correlations* (2nd ed.). Philadelphia: Lippincott-Raven.

National Committee for Clinical Laboratory Standards, H4-A4. (September 1999). *Procedures and devices for the collection of diagnostic blood specimens by skin puncture* (4th ed.). Wayne, PA: NCCLS.

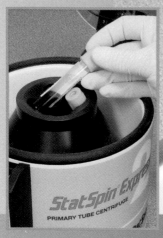

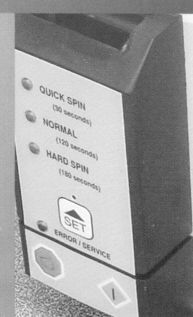

IV

Special Procedures

11

SPECIAL COLLECTIONS AND POINT-OF-CARE TESTING

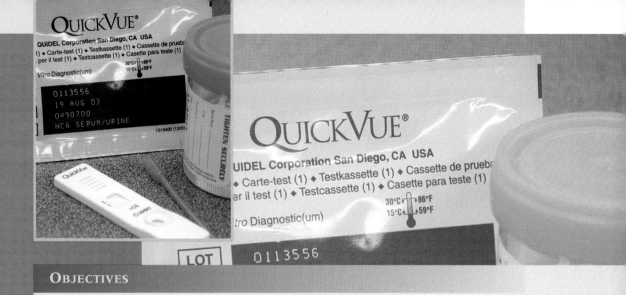

Upon successful completion of this chapter, the reader will be able to:

1 Define the key terms and abbreviations listed at the beginning of this chapter.

2 Explain the principle behind and list any special equipment required and the steps involved for each of the special collection procedures.

3 Describe patient identification and specimen labeling procedures, and identify the type of specimen required for blood bank tests.

4 Explain and state the importance of sterile technique in the collection of blood cultures and identify the reasons why a physician might order them.

5 Identify and describe how to properly collect coagulation specimens.

6 Describe chain of custody procedures and identify the tests that may require them.

7 State the importance of peak and trough levels in therapeutic drug monitoring.

8 Define point-of-care testing (POCT), identify and explain the principle behind the tests commonly performed as POCT, and list special equipment required and the steps involved for POCT tests.

SPECIAL COLLECTIONS

Introduction

Blood specimens for most laboratory tests can be collected using routine venipuncture or skin puncture procedures. Some tests, however, require special or additional collection procedures. Collecting specimens for these tests may require special preparation, equipment, handling, or timing. The following sections describe some of the most commonly encountered special blood test procedures.

Blood Bank Specimens

Specimen Requirements

Blood bank tests require a plain (no serum separator gel) red stopper tube or a lavender or pink top EDTA tube. Strict procedures must be followed when identifying the patient and labeling the specimen. It is important to observe facility-specific procedures because specimens with incomplete or inaccurate information are not accepted by blood banks. Any error in specimen identification resulting from incorrect procedures will unnecessarily delay patient treatment and could cause a patient a fatal transfusion reaction.

Labeling Requirements

Blood bank specimens require the following identification information:

1. Patient's full name (including middle initial)
2. Patient's hospital identification number (or social security number for outpatients)
3. Patient's date of birth
4. Date and time of collection
5. Phlebotomist's initials
6. Room number and bed number (optional)

Blood Type and Crossmatch Requirements

A type and screen determines a patient's blood type (A, B, AB, or O) and Rh (Rhesus) factor (positive or negative). When required, a crossmatch is performed using the patient's type and screen results to help select a donor unit of blood. Patient's plasma or serum and donor red cells are mixed to determine the **compatibility** of blood used in a transfusion. A transfusion of incompatible blood can be fatal because of **agglutination** (clumping) and **lysis** (rupturing) of the red blood cells within the patient's circulatory system. For this reason, hospitals require *strict* identification and labeling procedures when obtaining specimens for type and screens and crossmatches.

Special Identification Systems

There are a variety of blood bank identification systems available. One procedure requires the attachment to the patient's wrist of a special identification (ID) bracelet such as the Typenex Blood Recipient Identification Band 1 (Fenwal Biotech Division, a division of Travenol Laboratories, Chicago, IL) or the Securline Blood Bank

(Precision Dynamics Corporation, San Fernando, CA). In this procedure, the patient's identity is confirmed and the information written on a self-carbon adhesive label on the special bracelet, which contains a unique ID number. The adhesive label is peeled from the bracelet, leaving the carbon copy of the information, including the unique ID number, on the bracelet. The adhesive label is placed on the specimen drawn from the patient as seen in Figure 11-1. Additional ID number labels from the bracelet are sent to the lab with the specimen to be used in the crossmatch process and eventually attached to the unit of blood or other blood products used for transfusion. Figure 11-2 shows how the additional numbered labels are attached to the patient's specimen.

Before the transfusion is given, the nurse *must* match the numbers on the patient's identification bracelet with the numbers on the unit of blood. Some facilities may require the unique number and patient name to be brought to the blood bank when picking up the blood products. This is used as an additional identification check.

An example of a computer transfusion identification system is the MedPoint Transfusion (formerly Immucor I-TRAC plus) System. The MedPoint Transfusion (Bridge Medical Inc., Solana Beach, CA) is a portable bedside barcode scanning system that provides electronic verification and tracing of the blood transfusion process (Fig.11-3). The hardware includes a portable data terminal and printer. This computerized system provides positive identification of each transfusion recipient from blood bank specimen collection to transfusion by providing unique matching of scanned barcoded data at time of transfusion, and uses barcodes to ensure information integrity for the entire transfusion process. MedPoint Transfusion standardizes operation procedures for blood transfusion processes and improves productivity by allowing one transfusionist to use MedPoint Transfusion's electronic verification as the second check before blood transfusion. MedPoint also offers two other software modules, one for medication administration and another for specimen identification and tracking.

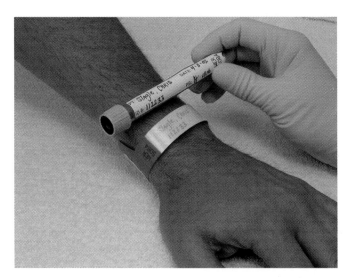

■ FIGURE 11-1 ■

A phlebotomist compares a blood bank tube with a blood bank identification bracelet.

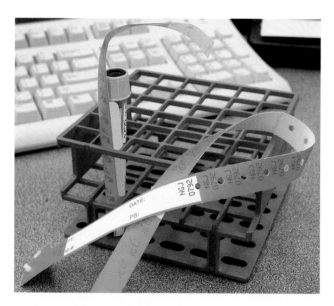

■ FIGURE 11-2 ■

Securline Blood Bank recipient identification band with additional numbers from band shown on blood sample. (Precision Dynamics Corporation, San Fernando, CA.)

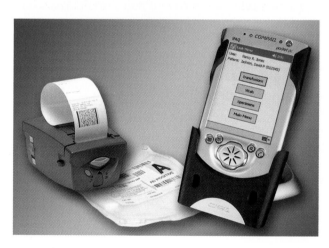

■ FIGURE 11-3 ■

Bridge Medical Medpoint transfusion system. (Bridge Medical, Solona CA.)

Blood Donor Collection

Blood donor collection involves collecting blood in amounts referred to as units to be used for transfusion purposes rather than for diagnostic testing. Donor collection requires special training and exceptional venipuncture skills. Facilities that provide blood donor services are called blood banks. Blood banks follow guidelines of the American Association of Blood Banks (AABB) and the US Food and Drug Administration (FDA).

Key Point ➤ Anyone wishing to donate blood must be interviewed to determine eligibility to donate blood and to obtain information for the records that must be kept on all blood donors.

DONOR ELIGIBILITY

To donate blood, a person must be within the ages of 17 and 66 years and weigh at least 110 lb. Minors must have written permission from their parents. Adults older than age 66 years may be allowed to donate at the discretion of the blood bank physician. A brief physical examination and a complete medical history are needed to determine the patient's state of health. This information is needed each time a person donates, no matter how many times a person has donated before. All donor information is strictly confidential. In addition, the donor must give written permission for the blood bank to use his or her blood.

PROCEDURE

Donor units are normally collected from a large antecubital vein. The vein is selected in a similar manner as for routine venipuncture. Skin preparation involves a two-step cleaning process with a povidone-iodine preparation in a similar manner to blood culture collection. The collection unit is a sterile, closed system consisting of a bag to contain the blood connected by a length of tubing to a sterile needle. A 16- to 18-gauge, thin-wall needle is most commonly used. The bag fills by gravity and must be placed lower than the patient's arm. The collection bag contains an anticoagulant, typically a citrate phosphate dextrose (CPD) solution, and is placed on a mixing unit as the blood is being drawn. The unit is normally filled by weight but generally contains around 450 mL when full. Only one needle puncture can be used to fill a unit. If the unit only partially fills and the procedure must be repeated an entire new unit must be used.

LOOKBACK PROGRAM

A unit of blood can be separated into several components: red blood cells, plasma, and platelets. All components of the unit must be traceable to the donor for federally required **lookback** programs. A lookback program requires notification to all blood recipients when a donor for a blood product they have received has turned positive for a transmissible disease.

AUTOLOGOUS DONATION

Autologous donation is the process by which a person donates blood for his or her own use. This is done for elective surgeries in which it is anticipated that a transfusion will be needed. Using one's own blood eliminates many risks associated with transfusion, such as disease transmission and blood or plasma incompatibilities. Although blood is normally collected several weeks before the scheduled surgery, the minimum time between donation and surgery can be as little as 72 hours. To be eligible to make an autologous donation, a person must have a written order from a physician.

CELL SALVAGING

During some surgical procedures, the patient's blood is perioperatively salvaged and reinfused. Before reinfusion it is recommended to test the washed salvaged blood for residual-free hemoglobin to determine the integrity of the blood. If the free hemoglobin is too high it indicates that too many red cells have hemolyzed during the blood

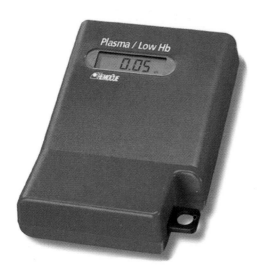

HemoCue Plasma/Low Hb. (HemoCue, Inc. Mission Viejo, CA.)

salvaging and is of no value and could cause renal dysfunction if reinfused. The HemoCue Plasma/Low Hemoglobin analyzer (Fig.11-4) offers a free hemoglobin point-of-care test.

Blood Cultures

Blood cultures are ordered by a physician when there is **fever of unknown origin (FUO)** or reason to suspect **bacteremia** (bacteria in the blood) or **septicemia** (pathogenic bacteria in the blood). Blood cultures help determine the presence and extent of infection and indicate the type of organism responsible and the antibiotic to which it is most susceptible. After septicemia is diagnosed and treatment is initiated, blood cultures are useful in assessing the effectiveness of antibiotic therapy.

Collecting blood cultures in a timely fashion is important because cultures are commonly ordered immediately before anticipated fever spikes and immediately after. Bacteria are most likely to be present in the blood stream at these times.

Blood culture specimens are collected in special tubes or bottles (Fig. 11-5) containing nutrient media that encourage the growth of any organisms present in the blood. Blood cultures are commonly collected in sets of two: one **anaerobic** (without air) and one **aerobic.** Anaerobic culture bottles are filled first when a syringe is used to collect the blood. When a butterfly collection set is used to collect the specimen, some clinicians prefer to have the aerobic bottle filled first because the air in the tubing will be drawn into the first specimen collected. When more than one set is ordered for the same time, the second set should be obtained from a separately prepared site on the opposite arm. However, in some cases, "second-site" blood cultures are more useful when drawn 30 minutes apart. If timing is not specified on the order, follow laboratory protocol.

Skin antisepsis is the most important part of the blood culture collection procedure. Failure to follow sterile technique can introduce skin surface bacteria into the blood culture bottle and interfere with interpretation of results. The laboratory must

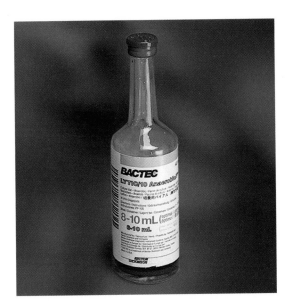

■ FIGURE 11-5 ■

Bactec blood culture bottle. (Courtesy Becton Dickinson, Franklin Lakes, NJ.)

report all microorganisms isolated from blood cultures. It is up to the patient's physician to determine whether the organism is clinically significant or merely a contaminant. If an organism is misinterpreted as pathogenic, it could result in inappropriate treatment.

Sterile technique methods for blood culture collection vary slightly from one laboratory to another. However, most methods require the use of 10% povidone or 1% to 2% tincture of iodine compounds in the form of swabsticks or special cleaning pad kits such as benzalkonium chloride (Fig. 11-6) to clean the collection site. The procedure for one commonly accepted site cleaning method follows.

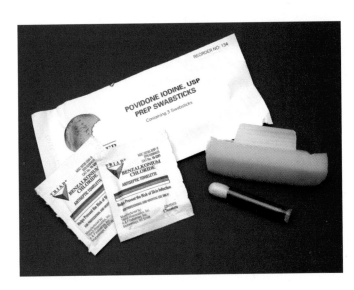

■ FIGURE 11-6 ■

Three types of blood culture cleaning supplies. *Left,* Povidone-iodine swabsticks (The Purdue Frederick Co., Norwalk, CT). *Center,* Benzalkonium chloride (Triad Disposables Inc., Brookfield, WI.). *Right,* Frepp/ Sepp povidone-iodine cleaning kit components. (Medi-Flex Inc., Overland Park, KS.)

Key Point ➤ When preparing the skin on neonates do not scrub aggressively because this may be too harsh and cause the skin to tear.

Collection Procedure

1. After selecting the venipuncture site, release the tourniquet (if applicable) and scrub the site with a 70% alcohol prep pad for a minimum of 30 seconds. This is done to rid the site of excess dirt and surface debris.
2. Next use a 1% to 2% tincture of iodine for 30 seconds or a povidone-iodine swabstick (Fig. 11-7) for 60 seconds to cleanse the site, beginning in the center and moving outward in concentric circles (Fig. 11-8) without going over any area more than once. Cover an area 3 to 4 inches in diameter. Allow the site to air dry. Note that antisepsis does not occur instantly. The cleaning time and drying phase allow time for the antiseptic to be effective.

   Touching or palpating the site after it has been prepared is not recommended. However, if the patient has difficult veins and the necessity to repalpate is an-

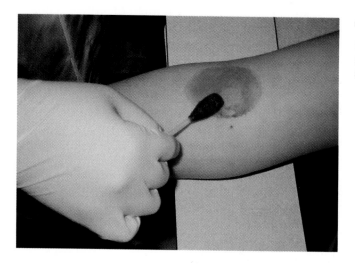

▓ FIGURE 11-7 ▓

Cleaning a blood culture site using a povidone-iodine swabstick.

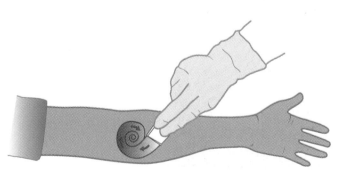

▓ FIGURE 11-8 ▓

Pattern of concentric circles used when cleaning a blood culture site.

ticipated, the phlebotomist's gloved finger should be cleaned in the same manner as the venipuncture site.

3. Remove the protective flip-top covering the rubber septum and clean the tops of the blood culture containers with a 70% alcohol or iodine. A manufacturer may recommend that iodine be used to prep the septum because it will provide a visual confirmation ensuring the septum was cleaned before specimen collection. Others suggest that a clean alcohol prep pad be placed on top of each bottle. Blood culture containers equipped with plastic caps can be cleaned with 70% isopropyl alcohol after removing the cap and covered with an alcohol pad until ready to inoculate. Prepare venipuncture equipment, being careful to handle all equipment in an aseptic manner.

4. Reapply the tourniquet, taking care not to touch the prepped (prepared) area in the process. Perform the venipuncture.

5. Blood culture bottles have a vacuum, but it is not measured as in evacuated tubes. Therefore it is important to mark the minimum and maximum fill (normally 5-10 mL) on the side of the bottles' fill lines to ensure enough, but not too much, blood enters the bottle.

6. Broth inoculation can occur several different ways. Blood may be collected directly into blood culture media when using specially designed holders with a butterfly (Fig. 11-9). Connect the special adapter to the luer connector of the butterfly collection set. Fill the aerobic vial first as the butterfly tubing has air in it. Avoid backflow by keeping the culture bottle or tube lower than the collection site and preventing the culture media from contacting the stopper or needle during blood collection. Pediatric bottles are normally filled with 1 to 3 mL of blood. Mix each container after removing it from the needle holder.

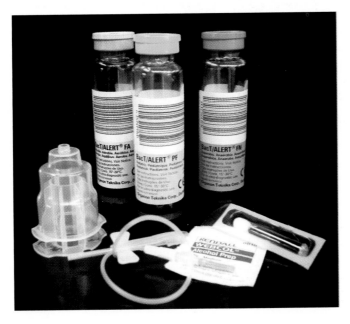

■ FIGURE 11-9 ■

BacT/Alert (bioMerieux, Durham, NC) blood culture supplies, including a specially designed holder for a butterfly needle.

After filling both containers, and collecting any other tests, remove the needle from the patient's arm and hold pressure over the site.

 Key Point ➤ The order of draw is important as it assures the culture or sterile tubes will not be contaminated with carryover from other tubes. Sterile tubes are always to be collected first.

7. When the syringe method is used, the blood must be transferred to the bottles after the draw is completed. The practice of changing needles before this transfer is no longer recommended. Several recent studies have shown that changing needles has little effect on reducing contamination rates and may actually increase risk of needlestick injury to the phlebotomist. To help prevent accidental needlesticks when using a transfer set or needle and syringe, the culture bottle should *not* be held in the phlebotomist's hand during the inoculation process. In addition, when delivering blood to the bottles, direct the flow along the side of the container. Allow the blood to be drawn from the syringe by the vacuum of the container. Never push the plunger to expel the blood into the vial. This can hemolyze the specimen and cause aerosol formation when the needle is removed. If a transfer safety device is not available to transfer blood from the syringe into the bottle and a needle must be used, use extreme caution upon blood transfer.

8. If blood is collected into an intermediate collection tube, a sodium polyanethol sulfonate (SPS), yellow top, is acceptable. Other anticoagulants such as citrate, heparin, EDTA, and oxalate may be toxic for bacteria and are not recommended. Use of SPS tubes is discouraged for three reasons. First, the additional SPS used in the collection tube will be added to the blood culture bottles increasing the final concentration of SPS. Second, the extra step of transferring blood from the intermediate tube to blood culture bottles allows another opportunity for contamination. Third, transferring of blood increases the exposure risk of laboratory staff.

9. After collecting the specimen, clean the iodine from the patient's skin with an alcohol pad; iodine left on the skin can be irritating. Label the specimen containers with required identification information, including the site of collection (e.g., right arm). Some facilities may also request the phlebotomist to include the amount of blood added to the bottle on the specimen label.

10. The practice of routinely dividing blood drawn for culture into both aerobic and anaerobic bottles has come into question because microbial recovery may be increased if all blood drawn were inoculated into two aerobic bottles. Therefore, it has been suggested that if patients are prone to anaerobic infections they should have both aerobic and anaerobic bottles collected and that all other patients should have two aerobic bottles inoculated.

Antimicrobial Neutralization Products

It is not unusual for patients to be on **antimicrobial** (antibiotic) **therapy** at the time blood culture specimens are collected. Presence of the antimicrobial agent in the patient's blood can inhibit the growth of the microorganisms in the blood culture bottle. In such cases, the physician may order blood cultures to be collected in an **antimi-**

crobial removal device (ARD) (Becton Dickinson) **or fastidious antimicrobial neutralization (FAN)** (bioMerieux) bottles. The ARD contains a resin that removes antimicrobials from the blood. The FAN contains an activated charcoal, which neutralizes the antibiotic. The blood can then be processed by conventional technique without the risk of inhibiting the growth of microorganisms. These bottles should be delivered to the lab for processing as soon as possible.

Coagulation Specimens

There are several important things to remember when collecting specimens for coagulation tests.

- Until recently it was customary to draw a "clear" or "discard" tube before collecting a light blue top if it was the first or only tube collected. A few milliliters of blood were drawn into a plain red top tube to clear the needle of tissue thromboplastin picked up as it penetrated the skin. This clearing tube was discarded if it was not needed for other tests. New studies have shown that a "clear" tube is not necessary when collecting a light blue top for a prothrombin time (PT) or a partial thromboplastin time (PTT). A "clear" tube is required for other coagulation tests (i.e., Factor VIII) because NCCLS recommends that they still be the second or third tube drawn.
- Sodium citrate–containing tubes for coagulation studies must be filled until the vacuum is exhausted to obtain a *9:1 ratio of blood to anticoagulant.* Even when the tubes are properly filled, this ratio is altered if the patient has an abnormally high or low hemoglobin level. In such cases, laboratory personnel may request collection of the test in a special tube that has had the volume of anticoagulant adjusted accordingly.
- Do not use light blue top tubes designed for fibrin degradation (FDP) or fibrin split products (FSP) for other coagulation tests. FDP/FSP tubes have a different additive and a different fill volume.

Key Point ➤ It is mandatory that all anticoagulated tubes be gently inverted 3 to 8 times, depending on manufacturers' instructions, immediately after collection to keep microclots from forming, which would invalidate test results.

- *Never* pour two partially filled tubes together because the anticoagulant to blood ratio will be greatly increased.
- Cooling on ice during transport may be required for some tests to protect the coagulation factors. Some coagulation factors V and VIII are not stable and these assays need to be performed in a timely manner or the specimen needs to be centrifuged and the plasma frozen.

If a coagulation specimen must be drawn from an indwelling catheter, NCCLS recommends drawing and discarding 5 mL of blood or six times the dead space volume of the catheter before collecting the specimen. If heparin has been introduced into the line, it should be flushed with 5 mL saline before drawing the discard blood and collecting the specimen.

Paternity/Parentage Testing

Paternity testing is performed to determine the probability that a specific individual fathered a particular child. Generally, results of paternity testing can exclude the possibility of paternity, rather than prove paternity. Paternity testing may be requested by physicians, lawyers, child support enforcement bureaus, or, rarely, individuals. Tests performed usually include ABO and Rh typing, along with human leukocyte antigen typing. Paternity testing generally requires special chain-of-custody protocol and specific identification procedures, which usually include fingerprinting. The mother, child, and alleged father are all tested.

Therapeutic Phlebotomy

Therapeutic phlebotomy involves the withdrawal of a large volume of blood, usually measured by the unit (as in blood donation), or approximately 500 mL. It is performed by phlebotomists who have been specially trained in the procedure or in donor phlebotomy, in a manner similar to collecting blood from donors. It is used as a treatment for certain medical conditions such as polycythemia and hemochromatosis.

Polycythemia

Polycythemia is a disease characterized by an overproduction of red blood cells that is detrimental to the patient's health. The patient's red blood cell levels are monitored regularly, usually by means of the hematocrit test. Periodic removal of a unit of blood when the hematocrit exceeds a certain level helps to keep the patient's red blood cell levels within the normal range.

Hemochromatosis

Hemochromatosis is a disease characterized by excess iron deposits in the tissues. It can be caused by a defect in iron metabolism or as a result of multiple transfusions or excess iron intake. Periodic removal of single units of blood from the patient gradually causes depletion of excess iron stores because the body uses the iron to make new red blood cells to replace those removed.

Postprandial Glucose Testing

Postprandial (PP) means after a meal. Glucose levels in blood specimens obtained 2 hours after a meal are rarely elevated in normal people, but may be significantly increased in diabetic patients. Therefore, a glucose test collected 2 hours after a meal, a **2-hour PP,** is an excellent screening test for diabetes and other metabolism problems. The test is also used to monitor insulin therapy. Correct timing of specimen collection is very important. Glucose levels in specimens collected too early or too late may be falsely elevated or decreased, respectively, leading to misinterpretation of results.

Key Point ➤ The American Diabetes Association recommends a 2-hour glucose tolerance test for nongestational and pediatric patients. This tolerance consists of a fasting specimen and then a 2-hour specimen collected after administration of glucose. The nongestational adult is given 75 g of glucose and the pediatric patient is given 1.75 g/kg with a maximum of 75 g of glucose.

Test Procedure

1. Preparation for the test involves placing the patient on a high-carbohydrate diet for 2 to 3 days before the test.
2. It is important for the patient to be fasting before the test. This means no eating, smoking, or drinking other than water for at least 10 hours before the test.
3. The day of the test, the patient is instructed to eat a special breakfast containing the equivalent of 100 g of glucose.
4. A blood specimen for glucose determination is collected 2 hours after the patient finishes eating.

Glucose Tolerance Test

A **glucose tolerance test (GTT)** is performed to check for carbohydrate metabolism problems. The major carbohydrate in the blood is glucose. The two major types of disorders involving glucose metabolism are those in which the blood glucose level is increased (**hyperglycemia**), as in diabetes mellitus, and those in which the blood glucose levels are decreased (**hypoglycemia**). The enzyme insulin, produced by the pancreas, is primarily responsible for regulating blood glucose levels. The GTT evaluates insulin response to a measured dose of glucose by recording glucose levels collected at specific time intervals. Results are plotted on a graph creating what is referred to as a GTT curve (Fig. 11-10).

There are a number of variations of the GTT procedure, involving variations in doses of glucose and timing of collections. The standard procedure, on which most variations are based, follows.

Test Procedure

Patient preparation for a GTT is very important. A patient should receive verbal and written instructions.

1. The patient is instructed to eat balanced meals containing approximately 150 g of carbohydrate for 3 days before the test.
2. The patient must then fast at least 12 hours preceding the test, but not for more than 16 hours. The patient is allowed and encouraged to drink water during the fast because urine specimens are usually collected as part of the procedure. No other food or beverages are allowed. The patient is also not allowed to smoke or chew gum because these activities stimulate the digestive process and may cause erroneous test results.

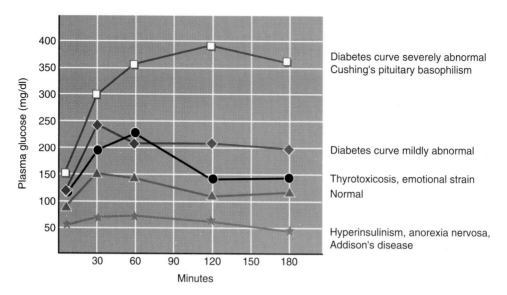

Diabetes curve severely abnormal
Cushing's pituitary basophilism

Diabetes curve mildly abnormal

Thyrotoxicosis, emotional strain
Normal

Hyperinsulinism, anorexia nervosa,
Addison's disease

■ FIGURE 11-10 ■

Glucose tolerance test (GTT) curves.

3. A fasting blood specimen is drawn and checked for glucose. (If the fasting blood glucose is higher than 200 mg/dL, the test is usually not performed.) A fasting urine specimen may also be collected.

4. An adult patient is given a commercial glucose beverage, containing between 50 and 100 g of glucose (Fig. 11-11). Children and small adults are given approximately 1 g/kg of weight. The patient must consume the drink within 5 minutes. If a patient vomits during the procedure, his or her physician should be consulted to determine if the test should be continued.

5. Timing for the test is started as soon as the patient finishes the glucose beverage. Blood is normally collected at 30 minutes, 1 hour, 2 hours, 3 hours, and so on, for the length of time specified by the physician; the test rarely exceeds 6 hours. Specimens should be labeled with both the exact time collected and the time interval of the test (e.g., ½ hour, 1 hour). Some physicians may request urine to be collected at the same time intervals.

6. No food, alcohol, smoking, or chewing gum is allowed throughout the test period. Water intake is allowed and encouraged.

In normal patients, blood glucose levels peak within 30 minutes to 1 hour after glucose ingestion. The peak in glucose levels triggers the release of insulin, which brings glucose levels back down to fasting levels within about 2 hours and no glucose spills over into the urine. Because diabetics have an inadequate or absent insulin response, glucose levels peak at higher levels and are slower to return to fasting levels. If blood is not drawn on time, it is important for the phlebotomist to note the discrepancy so that the physician will take this into consideration.

The method used to collect GTT specimens should be consistent for all specimens. That is, if the first specimen is collected by venipuncture, all succeeding specimens should be venipuncture specimens. If skin puncture is used to collect the first specimen, all succeeding specimens should also be skin puncture specimens.

Toxicology Specimens

Blood Alcohol (Ethanol) Specimens

Normally a **blood alcohol** (ethanol or ETOH) test is ordered by a patient's physician for medical reasons. Occasionally a blood alcohol test is requested by the police department for legal reasons. In such an event, special protocol, referred to as chain of custody, must be strictly followed (see the section on forensic specimens). Refer to state-specific law for legal regulations and requirements.

The 70% isopropyl alcohol used in skin preparation for routine venipuncture should not be used for blood alcohol determinations. Methanol can also affect results. In addition, tincture of iodine contains alcohol and likewise should not be used to clean the site. A nonalcohol-containing alternative antiseptic such as chlorhexidine gluconate or regular soap and water should be used instead.

A **gray top, sodium fluoride tube,** with or without an anticoagulant depending upon the need for serum or plasma in the test procedure, is generally required for specimen collection, although red stopper serum tubes or green stopper heparin tubes are sometimes used. Because alcohol is volatile (easily vaporized or evaporated), the tube should be filled until the vacuum is exhausted and the stopper should *not* be removed until absolutely necessary.

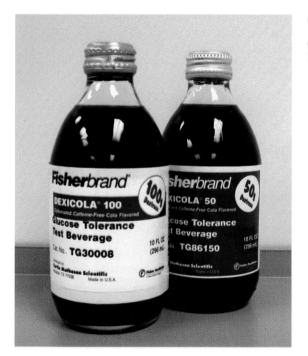

■ Figure 11-11 ■

Commercial Glucose Tolerance Test Beverage, 50 g and 100 g dosage.

Forensic Specimens

Occasionally a blood, urine, or other body fluid specimen is requested by law enforcement officials for forensic or legal reasons. Tests most frequently requested are blood alcohol levels, drug levels, and specimens for DNA analysis. In such an event, special protocol, referred to as **chain of custody,** must be strictly followed. Chain of custody requires detailed documentation that tracks the specimen from the time it is collected until the results are reported. The specimen *must* be accounted for at all times. If documentation is incomplete, any legal action may be impaired.

A special form (Fig. 11-12) is used to identify the specimen and the person or people who obtained and processed the specimen. Information on the form also includes the time, date, and place the specimen was obtained, along with the signature of the person from whom the specimen was obtained. Patient identification and specimen collection is performed in the presence of a witness, frequently a law enforcement officer. Special seals and containers may be required for the specimen. A phlebotomist involved in drawing a blood alcohol specimen for legal reasons can be summoned to appear in court.

Drug Screening

Many healthcare organizations, sports associations, and major companies require **drug screening** of employees, prospective employees, or athletes. Table 11-1 lists drugs commonly detectable by drug screening, along with the length of time after use that the drug is detectable in the body. Whether it is performed for legal reasons or not, there are legal implications to drug screening that require use of the chain of custody protocol described in the earlier section on Forensic Specimens. Screening is often performed without prior notice. Drug screening requires the following special patient preparation and collection procedures defined by the **National Institute on Drug Abuse (NIDA):**

Patient preparation requirements

- Explain the test purpose and procedure.
- Advise the patient of legal rights.
- Obtain a witnessed signed consent form.

Specimen collection requirements

- A special area must be maintained for urine collection.
- A proctor is required to be present during urine collection to verify that the specimen came from the correct person.
- A split sample may be required for confirmation or parallel testing.
- The specimen must be labeled appropriately to establish a chain of custody.
- To avoid tampering, a specimen must be sealed and placed in a clocked container during transport from the collection site to the testing site. Documentation must be carefully maintained from courier to receiver.

A Triage Urine Drug of Abuse Screen is manufactured by Biosite (Culver City, CA). This procedure uses a test device that simultaneously provides results for eight major classes of drugs of abuse (Fig. 11-13). These 8 drug classes are:

Amphetamines/methamphetamines

Barbiturates

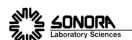

SONORA Laboratory Sciences
3401 E. Harbour Dr., Phoenix, Arizona 85034
602 431-5000
800 SONORA-1
800 766-6721

ORDERING PHYSICIAN/COMPANY OR FACILITY
2013AC
SOEHS-T'BIRD SAMARITAN MEDICAL
CENTER   2013A
5555 W THUNDERBIRD RD
GLENDALE, AZ 85306
602 588-5555   *RT14

CHAIN OF CUSTODY REQUISITION FORM

Failure to complete form properly could invalidate chain of custody.

DONOR INSTRUCTIONS (To be completed by donor)

**************************** IDENTIFICATION IS REQUIRED AT TIME OF COLLECTION ****************************
DONOR AFFIDAVIT
I certify that the specimen identified by the ID number on this form was provided by me on this date and is not adulterated. In my presence, the specimen was sealed with an evidence seal taken from this form. The ID Number on the seal and on this form are identical. I have initialed the seal. By my signature I consent to the release of laboratory test results to the doctor, facility, individual or company shown on this form.

| Donor Signature | Donor Name **(Print Clearly)** | Date |

| Birthdate | Social Security Number | Daytime Phone |

You have the right to list any drugs, prescription or non prescription, that you may have taken in the last two weeks or other relevant medical information. Please do so, if desired, in the space provided: _____

COLLECTOR INSTRUCTIONS (To be completed by collector)
1. Check donor identification **(preferably a picture I.D.)**
2. RECORD SPECIMEN TEMP: _____ (90° - 100°)
3. Specimen lid is tight, sealed properly with evidence seal, and initialed by donor.
4. I.D. number on specimen and form must match.
5. Place specimen in tamper-proof bag and seal in the presence of the donor.
6. Form is completed and signed by donor.
7. Collector signs this form, indicates date, time and collection site.

I certify that the specimen identified by this form was collected according to specified procedures, was properly identified and prepared for transport to the laboratory.

Check One Box
☐ Pre-Employment
☐ Post-accident
☐ Random
☐ Reasonable Cause
☐ Periodic
☐ Other_____

| Collector Signature | Printed Name | Date | Collection Time |

| Collection Site | Address | Phone |

COMMENTS: _____

LABORATORY USE ONLY
SPECIMEN RECEIVED BY:

SIGNATURE   PRINTED NAME   DATE
SPECIMEN SEAL CONDITION: ☐ INTACT ☐ NOT INTACT
COMMENTS: _____

TESTS

[X] 2406 (FORENSIC COM-
PREHENSIVE)

SOCIAL SECURITY NUMBER
_____ _____ _____

DEPT: _____

PHONE: _____

COLLECTION TIME/DATE
_____ / _____

************ SPECIMEN I.D. NUMBER 293012 ****************************

293012   293012
293012   293012
293012   293012

EVIDENCE SEAL

EVIDENCE SEAL

SPECIMEN I.D. NUMBER
293012
Donor Initials

_____
/ /
Date

EVIDENCE SEAL

EVIDENCE SEAL

ORIGINAL TO LABORATORY

■ FIGURE 11-12 ■

Chain of custody requisition form.   (Courtesy Sonora Laboratory Sciences, Phoenix, AZ.)

Table 11-1

Drugs Commonly Detectable at Drug Screening

Drug or Drug Families	Common Names	Detectable (time)	Comment
Alcohol		2-12 hours	
Amphetamines	Methamphetamine, speed, crystal, crank, ice	1-3 days 2-7 days	Single/light use Frequent/chronic use
Barbiturates	Downers, Seconal, Fiorinal, Tuinal, Phenobarbital	2 days to 4 weeks	Varies considerably with drugs in this class
Benzodiazepines	Valium, Librium, Xanax, Dalmane, Serax	1 week to >30 days	Varies considerably with drugs in this class
Cocaine (as metabolite)	Crack	1-3 days 3-14 days	Single/light use Frequent use/freebase
Cannabinoids	Marijuana, grass, hash	1-7 days >30 days	Single/light use Frequent/chronic use
Methadone	Dolophine	1-4 days	Single/light use
Opiates	Heroin, morphine, codeine, Dilaudid hydrocodone	2-4 days >7 days	Single/light use Frequent/chronic use
Phencyclidine	PCP, angel dust	2-7 days >30 days	Single/light use Frequent/chronic use
Propoxyphene	Darvon, Darvocet	1-2 days >7 days	Single/light use Frequent/chronic use

Courtesy Tox Talk, Sonora Laboratory Sciences, Phoenix, AZ (1996).

Benzodiazepines

Cocaine

Methadone

Phencyclidine (PCP)

Opiates (heroin)

Tetrahydrocannabinol (marijuana)

Tricyclic antidepressants

Therapeutic Drug Monitoring

Because the dosage of drug necessary to produce the desired effect varies widely among patients, **therapeutic drug monitoring (TDM)** is used by the physician to manage individual patient drug treatment. TDM helps the physician establish drug dosages, maintain dosages at beneficial levels, and avoid drug toxicity. Timing of specimen collection in regard to dosage administration is critical for safe and beneficial treatment and must therefore be consistent. A team effort is essential and requires co-

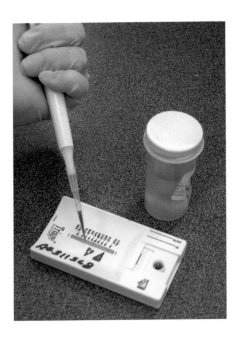

■ FIGURE 11-13 ■

Triage urine drug of abuse (DOA) screen. (Courtesy Biosite, San Diego, CA.)

ordination with pharmacy, nursing, and the lab. The phlebotomist is a key player in this team effort.

Some therapeutic drugs require the monitoring and evaluation of peak and trough drug levels for the physician to determine a safe and effective dosage for the patient (Fig. 11-14). Peak (or maximum) levels are collected when the highest serum concentration of the drug is anticipated, around 30 to 60 minutes after administration of the drug. Peak-level specimen collection requires careful coordination of sample collection with dosing. **Peak levels** screen for drug toxicity. Trough (or minimum) levels are easiest to collect because they are collected when the lowest serum concentration of the drug is expected, usually immediately before administration of the next scheduled dose. **Trough levels** are monitored to ensure that levels of the drug stay within the therapeutic (or effective) range.

Collection timing is most critical for aminoglycoside drugs, such as amikacin, gentamicin, and tobramycin, which have short half-lives. (A half-life is the time required for the body to metabolize half the amount of the drug.) The timing is less critical for drugs that have longer half-lives, such as phenobarbital and digoxin.

The FDA has approved some manufacturers of gel tubes for all analytes, including TDM; however, other gel tubes may affect TDM results. Refer to manufacture package inserts and test methodologies used in the laboratory for specific requirements.

Trace Elements

Trace elements or metals include aluminum, arsenic, copper, lead, iron, and zinc. These elements are measured in such small amounts that traces of these substances commonly found in the glass and stopper material of evacuated tubes may leach into the specimen, causing falsely elevated test values. For this reason, these tests must be collected in spe-

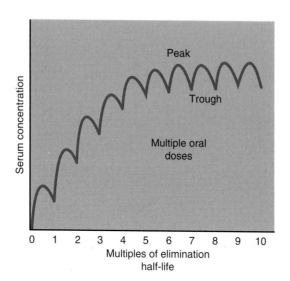

■ Figure 11-14 ■

Dose-response curve after multiple oral doses of a drug given each half-life.

cial trace element–free tubes made of materials that have been specially manufactured to be as free of trace elements as possible. An insert with each carton of tubes gives a detailed analysis of residual amounts of metals contained in the tubes. These tubes are usually royal blue in color and contain no additive, EDTA, or heparin. The type of additive is indicated on the label: red for no additive, lavender for EDTA, and green for heparin.

POINT-OF-CARE TESTING

Point-of-care testing (POCT), also known as alternate site testing (AST) or ancillary, bedside, or near-patient testing, brings laboratory testing to the location of the patient. Its benefits include convenience to the patient and a short results turnaround time (TAT) to the healthcare facility. A short TAT allows healthcare providers to address crucial patient needs, deliver prompt medical attention, and help expedite patient recovery.

POCT is possible owing to advances in laboratory instrumentation that have led to the development of small, portable, and often hand-held testing devices. These devices allow testing to occur in a variety of hospital settings including the bedside, emergency room, operating suite, and intensive care unit, and other direct patient care settings such as physician's offices, nursing homes, clinics, patient service centers, and even the patient's own home. Healthcare personnel trained to perform POCT include phlebotomists, nurses (RNs and LPNs), nursing assistants, medical assistants, home health aids, patient-care technicians, and respiratory therapy technicians.

In addition to being able to operate the analyzer according to manufacturer's instructions and perform the phlebotomy procedures required to collect the specimen, anyone performing POCT must understand quality assurance aspects of analyzer operation. Quality control and maintenance procedures are necessary to ensure that results obtained are accurate. At this time, no certification is required to perform POCT, however, anyone who performs POCT must meet the 1988 Clinical Laboratory Improvement Amendments qualifications and Occupational Safety and Health Administration guidelines for specimen handling. A number of POCT devices allow integration with a data networking system for transmission of test results into laboratory information systems or other computer systems.

Coagulation Monitoring

Coagulation point-of-care analyzers are used to monitor patient coumadin and heparin therapy. These devices include the Protime 3 and Hemochron Jr. (ITC, Edison, NJ), CoaguChek (Roche Diagnostics, Indianapolis, IN), a CLIA-waived PT and international normalization ratio (INR) performed on a whole blood fingerstick, and Rapidpoint Coag (Bayer Diagnostics, Tarrytown, NY). These analyzers perform a variety of tests:

- **prothrombin time (PT)** and INR
- **PTT or activated PTT (APTT)**
- **activated clotting time (ACT)**
- **heparin management test (HMT)**

Patients are able to perform protimes at home and transmit their results to the physicians' office. The physician can adjust medication over the phone and the patient does not need to make a physician's office visit. Many coumadin and anticoagulation clinics use point-of-care coagulation analyzers to provide timely laboratory results.

ACT

ACT, also called activated clotting time, has always been a bedside test. It analyzes activity of the intrinsic coagulation factors and is used to monitor heparin therapy. Heparin is given intravenously to patients who have blood clots, to patients whose blood is apt to clot too easily, or as a precaution after certain surgeries. Effects on intravenous heparin administration are immediate, but difficult to control. Too much heparin can cause the patient to bleed; therefore, heparin therapy is closely monitored. After a patient's condition is stabilized, the patient is placed on oral anticoagulant therapy such as coumadin, which can be monitored by the prothrombin test.

An automated variation of the ACT procedure, the Hemochron Jr. Signature (Fig. 11-15), is available from ITC (formerly called International Technidyne Corporation). With this system, the analyzer does the mixing and timing automatically. This system has the capability of performing the following tests:

- **ACT-LR:** monitors low to moderate levels of heparin useful in dialysis and cath lab procedures.
- **ACT+:** monitors moderate to high levels of heparin for use in cardiac bypass procedures.
- **APTT:** monitors low-dose heparin anticoagulation.
- **PT:** Provides the flexibility to utilize venous or fingerstick samples. Reports the result as a plasma equivalent value and an INR.
- **Citrate PT:** For PT testing of a whole blood sample collected in sodium citrate. Reports the result as a plasma equivalent value and an INR.

The Rapidpoint Coag from Bayer Diagnostics uses one drop of specimen on a credit card-sized test cartridge and is used for HMT (Fig. 11-16). HMT is a test for high-dose heparin monitoring for catheterization laboratories and surgery.

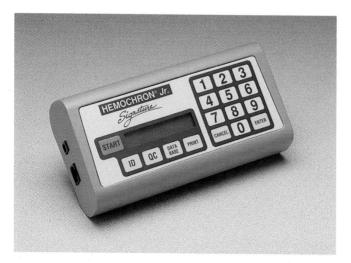

■ FIGURE 11-15 ■

The Hemochron Jr. Signature analyzer for ACT determinations. (ITC, Edison, NJ)

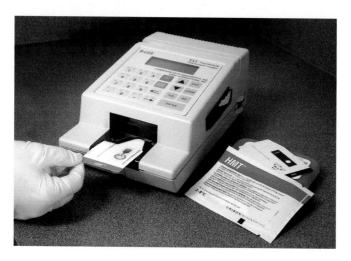

■ FIGURE 11-16 ■

Rapid Point Coag (Bayer, Tarrytown, NY) used for HMT.

Bleeding Time

The **bleeding time (BT)** test (Fig. 11-17) detects platelet function disorders by testing platelet plug formation in the capillaries. It is used in diagnosing problems with hemostasis and as a presurgical screening test.

BT is the time required for blood to stop flowing from a standardized puncture in the earlobe, finger, or the inner surface of the forearm. Prolonged bleeding can be caused by abnormal platelet function or the ingestion of aspirin or other salicylate-containing drugs within 2 weeks before the test. A number of other drugs such as ethanol, dextran, and streptokinase may also prolong bleeding time.

Bleeding time on the earlobe, originally described by Duke in 1910, is rarely ordered today. However, the test is still ordered by some facial surgeons who feel that the circulation of the ear more closely resembles that of the face. Ivy modified the Duke

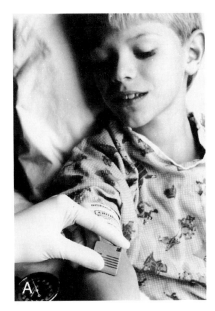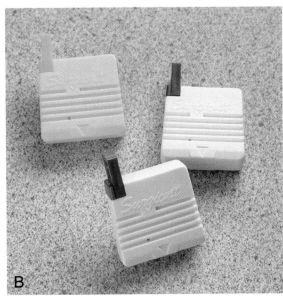

■ FIGURE 11-17 ■

(A) A bleeding time test being performed. (B) Closeup of automated bleeding time device.
(Courtesy ITC, Edison, NJ.)

bleeding time in 1941. The Ivy bleeding time is performed on the volar (inner) surface of the forearm using a blood pressure cuff to maintain constant pressure. The incision is made with a sterile lancet.

Most laboratories today use a modification of the Ivy procedure, controlling the width and depth of the incision by use of an automated incision device such as the Surgicutt (Fig. 11-18) (ITC) or Simplate (bioMerieux).

Materials needed for the modified Ivy are as follows:

1. Automated bleeding time device
2. Sphygmomanometer (blood pressure cuff)
3. Stopwatch, timer, or watch with sweep second hand
4. Filter paper (#1 Whatman or equivalent)
5. Alcohol prep pad
6. Butterfly bandage or Steri-Strip

TEST PROCEDURE

1. Determine whether the patient has taken aspirin or any other salicylate-containing drug within the last 2 weeks. Advise the patient of the potential for scarring.
2. Support the patient's arm on a steady surface.
3. Select an area on the inner (volar) surface of the forearm, distal to the antecubital area and devoid of surface veins, scars, or bruises. The lateral aspect is

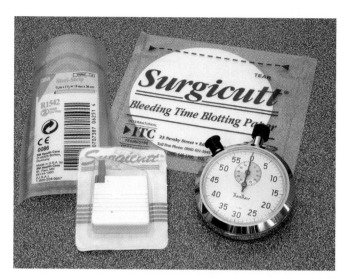

■ FIGURE 11-18 ■

Equipment for bleeding time test, including Surgicutt automated bleeding time device, blotting paper, stopwatch, and Steri-Strips. (ITC, Edison, NJ.)

preferred because using the medial aspect tends to cause more pain and has a higher incidence of scarring. It may be necessary to shave the test area lightly if it is covered with a large amount of hair.

4. Clean the selected area with alcohol and allow it to dry.
5. Place the blood pressure cuff around the arm.
6. Remove the puncture device from its package, being careful not to touch or rest the blade slot on any unsterile surface.
7. Inflate the blood pressure cuff to 40 mm Hg. (Time between inflation of the blood pressure cuff and making the incision should be between 30 and 60 seconds.) This pressure *must* be maintained throughout the entire procedure.
8. Remove the safety clip and place the puncture device firmly on the forearm without pressing. A horizontal incision parallel to the antecubital crease is recommended.
9. Depress the trigger while simultaneously starting the timer. Remove the device from the arm as soon as the blade has retracted (approximately 1 second after the device has been triggered).
10. Blot the blood flow at 30 seconds by bringing the filter paper close to the incision and absorbing or "wicking" the blood onto the filter paper without touching the wound. (Touching the wound will disturb platelet plug formation!)
11. Continue to blot every 30 seconds until blood no longer stains the filter paper. Stop the timer and record the time to the nearest 30 seconds. If bleeding persists beyond 30 minutes, the test is usually stopped and the time is recorded as 30 minutes or greater.
12. Remove blood pressure cuff, clean the arm, and apply a butterfly bandage. Cover with an adhesive bandage. The patient is instructed not to remove either bandage for 24 hours. *Normal:* Approximately 2 to 8 minutes depending on the method used.

1. Disturbing platelet plug formation will increase the bleeding time.
2. Failure to maintain 40 mm Hg will decrease the bleeding time.
3. Failure to start the timing as soon as the incision is made will decrease the bleeding time.

Arterial Blood Gas and Chemistry Panels

Several small, portable, and, in some cases, hand-held instruments are available that measure panels or groups of commonly ordered stat tests such as blood gases and electrolytes. The body normally maintains these analytes in specific proportions within narrow ranges, and any uncorrected imbalance can quickly lead to death. Consequently, these tests are often ordered in emergency and critical care situations where immediate response is vital to the patient's survival.

Common POCT Chemistry Panels

ARTERIAL BLOOD GASES

Arterial blood gases (ABGs) measured by POCT methods include **pH, partial pressure of carbon dioxide (pCO$_2$),** and **partial pressure of oxygen (PO$_2$).** The pH is a measure of the body's acid-base balance and is an indicator of a patient's metabolic and respiratory status. The normal range for arterial blood pH is 7.35 to 7.45. Below-normal pH is referred to as acidosis and above-normal pH is referred to as alkalosis. The pCO$_2$ is a measure of the pressure exerted by dissolved CO$_2$ in the blood and is proportional to the pCO$_2$ in the alveoli and, therefore, an indicator of how well air is being exchanged between the blood and the lungs. CO$_2$ levels are maintained within normal limits by the rate and depth of respiration. An abnormal increase in pCO$_2$ is associated with hypoventilation and a decrease with hyperventilation. The pO$_2$ is a measure of the pressure exerted by dissolved O$_2$ in the plasma and indicates the ability of the lungs to diffuse O$_2$ through the alveoli into the blood. It is used to evaluate the effectiveness of oxygen therapy.

ELECTROLYTES

The most common electrolytes measured by POCT are **sodium (Na$^+$), potassium (K$^+$), chloride (Cl$^-$), bicarbonate ion (HCO$_3^-$),** and **ionized calcium (iCa^{++}).**

* *Sodium* is the most plentiful electrolyte in the blood. It plays a major role in maintaining osmotic pressure and acid-base balance and in transmitting nerve impulses. Reduced sodium levels are referred to as **hyponatremia,** and elevated levels are referred to as **hypernatremia.**
* *Potassium* is primarily concentrated within the cells, with very little found in the bones and blood. It is released into the blood when cells are damaged. Potassium plays a major role in nerve conduction, muscle function, acid-base balance, and osmotic pressure. It influences cardiac output by helping to control the rate and force of heart contraction. Presence of a U wave on an electrocardiogram is indicative of potassium deficiency. Decreased blood potassium is called **hypokalemia;** increased blood potassium is called **hyperkalemia.**

- *Chloride* exists mainly in the extracellular spaces in the form of sodium chloride (NaCl) or hydrochloric acid. Chloride is responsible for maintaining cellular integrity by influencing osmotic pressure and acid-base and water balance. Chloride must be supplied along with potassium when correcting hypokalemia.
- *Bicarbonate ion* plays a role in transporting CO_2 to the lungs and in regulating blood pH. HCO_3^- is formed in the red blood cells and plasma from CO_2. Hydrogen ion (H^+) is released in the process, causing a decrease in pH, which means that the blood becomes more acid. HCO_3^- moves from the cells to the plasma and is carried to the lungs, where it re-enters the cells and releases CO_2 for removal through the walls of the alveoli. Removal of CO_2 by the lungs results in a decrease of H^+ ions and an increase in blood pH. Decreased ventilation (hypoventilation) results in higher CO_2 levels and production of more H^+ ions, which can lead to acidosis. Hyperventilation decreases CO_2 levels and can lead to alkalosis.
- *Ionized calcium* accounts for approximately 45% of the calcium in the blood; the rest is bound to protein and other substances. Only ionized calcium can be used by the body for such critical functions as muscular contraction, cardiac function, transmission of nerve impulses, and blood clotting.

POCT Chemistry Analyzers

The hand-held i-STAT (Fig. 11-19) (Abbott Diagnostics, Abbott Park, IL) measures blood gas values for pH, pCO_2, and O_2 and the electrolytes Na^+, K^+, Cl^-, and HCO_3^-. It can also measure blood urea nitrogen (BUN), glucose, hemoglobin (Hgb) and hematocrit (Hct), and ACT values. This system is based on small cartridges, with different cartridges having different test capabilities. Other instruments that measure blood gases

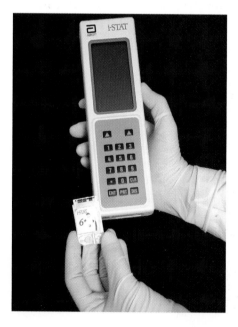

■ FIGURE 11-19 ■

i-STAT instrument   (Abbott Diagnostics, Abbott Park, IL.)

and electrolytes are the OPTI CCA (Critical Care Analyzer) (Roche Diagnostics, Indianapolis, IN), the Nova Stat Profile Analyzer (Nova Biomedical, Waltham, MA), and the Gem Premier (Instrumentation Laboratories, Lexington, MA).

The Careside (Fig. 11-20) (Careside, Inc., Culver City, CA) has more than 40 FDA-cleared tests covering chemistry and coagulation and is a dry film, unit-dose testing, closed cartridge-based system. This analyzer is often found in physician offices.

The small, portable IRMA (Fig. 11-21) (Phillips Medical) measures blood gas values for pH, pCO_2, and PO_2, and the electrolytes Na^+, K^+, and iCa^{++}. The IRMA system can also calculate other blood gas parameters such as HCO_3^- and O_2 saturation. A blood analysis is performed by a small cartridge that is inserted into the instrument. The cartridge automatically calibrates itself when it is inserted into the instrument. After calibration is complete, a small sample of blood is injected into the system's sensor cartridge. The test is performed in less than 2 minutes. The cartridge is then removed from the instrument and discarded in a biohazard container. Results are displayed on a screen and a hard copy printout is generated.

Cardiac Troponin T and I

Cardiac troponin T (TnT) and I (TnI) are proteins specific to heart muscle. Blood levels of cardiac TnT begin to rise within 3 to 4 hours of the onset of myocardial damage and may stay elevated for up to 14 days. Cardiac TnI levels rise within 3 to 6 hours and return to normal in 5 to 10 days. Measurement of these proteins is a valuable tool in the diagnosis of acute myocardial infarction or heart attack. TnT is also measured to monitor effectiveness of thrombolytic therapy in heart attack patients.

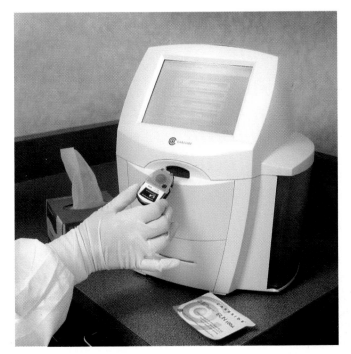

■ FIGURE 11-20 ■

Careside Point of Care Instrument. (Careside, Inc., Culver City, CA.)

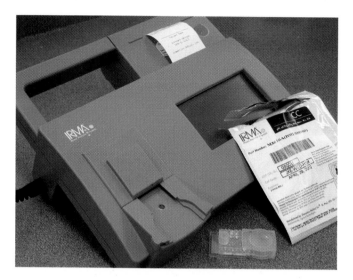

■ FIGURE 11-21 ■

Portable IRMA (Immediate Response Mobil Analysis) blood chemistry analyzer. (Phillips Medical, Inc., St. Paul, MN.)

A one-step, whole-blood bedside test for cardiac TnT, the CARDIAC T Rapid Assay (Roche Corp., Indianapolis, IN), uses disposable test kits to provide cardiac TnT results in minutes.

The Cardiac STATus from Spectral (Carepoint Cardiac Corporation, Toronto, CAN) and the Biosite Cardiac Triage (Fig. 11-22) (Biosite, San Diego, CA) provides results for three cardiac markers: Troponin I, CK-MB, and myoglobin.

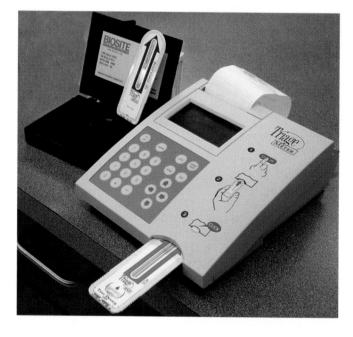

■ FIGURE 11-22 ■

Triage meter. (Biosite, San Diego, CA.)

Lipid Testing

The Cholestech LDX (Fig. 11-23) analyzer (Cholestech, Haywood, CA) can perform tests for cholesterol, triglyceride, low-density lipoprotein, and high-density lipoprotein. Blood can be obtained by fingerstick and collected in a lithium heparin coated capillary tube or by venipuncture. A quantitative result is obtained by visual evaluation of the intensity of a colored bar. A cartridge is also available which includes ALT, a liver enzyme that is monitored when patients are on some lipid reducing medications. Glucose testing is also available on some cartridges.

B-type Natriuretic Peptide

B-type natriuretic peptide (BNP) is a cardiac hormone produced by the heart in response to ventricular volume expansion and pressure overload. It is the first objective measurement for congestive heart failure (CHF). BNP levels help physicians differentiate chronic obstructive pulmonary disease and CHF. This facilitates early patient diagnosis and placement into the appropriate care plan. Circulation BNP concentrations increase with severity of CHF and have been shown to more accurately reflect final diagnosis than echocardiogram ejection fractions.

The BNP test uses a whole-blood EDTA specimen, which is placed in a cartridge and read on the Biosite Triage meter, where the BNP level is determined (Fig. 11-22).

Glucose

Whole blood glucose (WBG) testing or bedside glucose testing is one of the most common POCT procedures.

Glucose testing is most often performed to monitor glucose levels of patients with diabetes mellitus. Glucose levels are most commonly determined using small, portable,

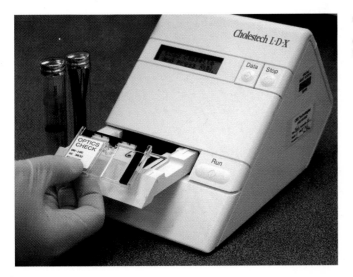

■ FIGURE 11-23 ■

Cholestech analyzer (Cholestech, Haywood, CA.)

relatively inexpensive glucose analyzers such as the Advantage (Roche Diagnostics, Indianapolis, IN), ONE TOUCH (LifeScan, Inc., Milpitas, CA), and the β-Glucose Analyzer (HemoCue, Inc., Mission Viejo, CA).

Most glucose analyzers use whole-blood specimens obtained by routine skin puncture. Some analyzers will also accept heparinized venous specimens.

The Advantage HQ (Roche) (Fig. 11-24) shows the meter connected to the nursing station computer. This allows data transfer of patient results to the lab, and in turn the laboratory can monitor results and quality control. The Advantage HQ, the newest model of the Advantage Inform (Fig. 11-25) (Roche), and ONE TOUCH (LifeScan) re-

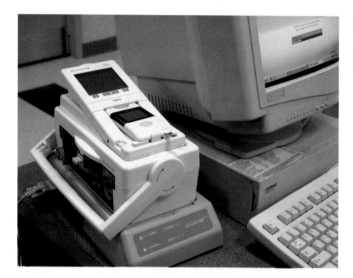

■ FIGURE 11-24 ■

Advantage HQ Blood Glucose Meter. (Roche Diagnostics, Indianapolis, IN.)

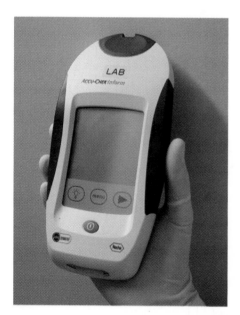

■ FIGURE 11-25 ■

Newest model of Advantage called Inform.
(Roche Diagnostics, Indianapolis, IN.)

quire use of a special reagent test strip. The test strips come in airtight containers that must not be left open for more than a few moments. It is also important to protect the test strips from heat. The test strip container has a code number. The code number in the analyzer must be set to match the code number of the test strip container. To perform the test, a drop of blood is applied to the test strip, which has been inserted into the analyzer. The analyzer determines the level of glucose in the blood and the result appears on a screen.

The HemoCue β-Glucose Analyzer (Fig. 11-26) accepts arterial specimens and skin puncture and venous specimens. The test is performed using a microcurette instead of a test strip. This unit is available with a data management system that allows operator and patient identification to be entered for record retention. The Glucose 201 (Fig. 11-27) is the latest hand-held glucose monitor from HemoCue.

NCCLS guidelines recommend that a phlebotomist receive institution authorization to perform WBG testing only after completing formal training in the facility-established procedures. Daily maintenance and quality control procedures must be performed and recorded before a WBG analyzer is used. These procedures should be repeated if the

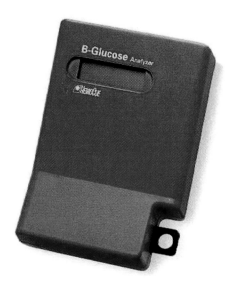

FIGURE 11-26

B-Glucose analyzer. (Courtesy HemoCue, Inc., Mission Viejo, CA.)

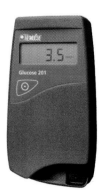

FIGURE 11-27

Glucose 201, the newest glucose system from HemoCue. (Courtesy HemoCue, Inc., Mission Viejo, CA.)

unit is dropped, the battery is replaced, patient results are questioned, or functioning of the unit is questioned.

Glycosylated Hemoglobin

Glycosylated hemoglobin, formed by the reaction of glucose with hemoglobin, is a diagnostic tool for monitoring diabetes therapy. Three hemoglobins, A_{1a}, A_{1b}, and A_{1c}, are types of Hgb A formed by glycosylation. Because glycosylation occurs at a constant rate during the 120-day life cycle of a red cell, glycosylated Hgb levels reflect the average blood glucose level during the preceding 4 to 6 weeks and therefore can be used to evaluate long-term effectiveness of diabetes therapy. Because this test measures glucose within a red blood cell, levels are more stable than with plasma or whole blood glucose.

Glycosylated hemoglobin values are reported as a percentage of the total hemoglobin within an erythrocyte. Because A_{1c} is present in larger quantity than the others, it is the one measured. Glycosylated Hgb can be measured using the FDA-waived A1cNOW from Metrika Inc. (Fig. 11-28). The device is a pager-sized monitor, needs only one drop of blood, and analyzes the result in 8 minutes.

Hematocrit

The Hct, also called packed cell volume, is a measure of the volume of red blood cells in a patient's blood. It is calculated by centrifuging a specific volume of anticoagulated blood and determining the proportion of red blood cells compared to plasma. Blood is collected in special microhematocrit tubes. The tubes are sealed at one end with clay and placed in a special centrifuge. The results can often be calculated while the tube is still in the centrifuge by lining the tube up with a special chart that is part of the machine and reading the results from the chart. The result is expressed as a percentage.

■ FIGURE 11-28 ■

A1c NOW meter. (Courtesy Metrika Inc. Sunnyvale CA.)

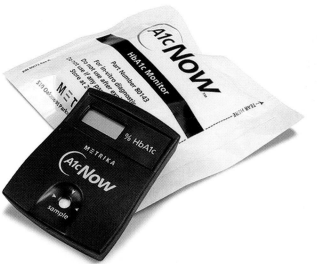

The hematocrit test is often performed in a physician's office labs, clinics, and blood donor stations to screen for anemia and to aid in the diagnosis and monitoring of patients with polycythemia.

Hemoglobin

Measurement of a patient's hemoglobin level is an important part of managing patients with anemia. A portable analyzer, the B-Hemoglobin System (Fig. 11-29) (HemoCue, Inc., Mission Viejo, CA) uses arterial, venous, or skin puncture specimens to determine hemoglobin levels. The sample is placed in a special microcuvette and inserted into the machine for a reading.

Occult Blood (Guaiac)

Detection of occult (hidden) blood in stool (feces) is an important tool in diagnosing and determining the location of a number of diseases of the digestive tract, including gastric ulcer and colon cancer. Most tests for detecting fecal blood use substances that depend upon peroxidase content as an indication of hemoglobin content to cause a color change in the specimen being tested. For this reason, a patient's diet should be free of meat and vegetable sources of peroxidase, which may lead to false-positive results. Other sources of false-positive results may be certain drugs, vitamin C, alcohol, and aspirin.

Testing for occult blood in POCT settings involves the use of special kits containing cards on which small amounts of feces are placed (Fig. 11-30). The specimen can be collected and tested onsite or the cards sent home with the patient to collect and mail

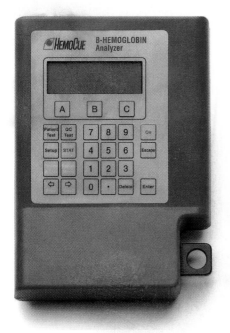

■ FIGURE 11-29 ■

Hemoglobin Data Management System. (Courtesy HemoCue, Inc., Mission Viejo, CA.)

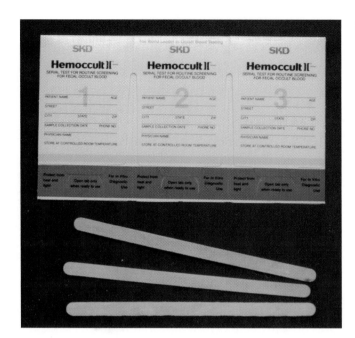

Hemoccult II occult blood collection cards. (Beckman Coulter, Fullerton, CA.)

back to the lab. Another type of occult blood test that can be done onsite or sent home with a patient involves a special reagent-impregnated pad that is dropped into the toilet after a bowel movement. A color change on the pad is compared with a result chart.

Pregnancy Testing

Most rapid pregnancy tests detect the presence of **human chorionic gonadotropin (HCG),** a hormone produced by the placenta that appears in both urine and serum beginning approximately 10 days after conception. Most rapid pregnancy testing is performed on urine. Peak urine levels of HCG occur at approximately 10 weeks of gestation.

A number of manufacturers supply urine pregnancy testing kits. Two examples are the Hybritech Icon II HCG urine assay (San Diego, CA) and the Quidel Quick Vue One Step (San Diego, CA) (Fig. 11-31). Each manufacturer's kit has unique reagents and timing and testing methods, and most test kits have a built-in control system. It is important to follow directions exactly.

Skin Tests

Although nurses most commonly perform skin testing, some laboratories do offer skin testing services, especially for outpatients. In addition, skin tests (especially for tuberculosis) are a part of employee screening programs. Skin tests do not involve the withdrawal of blood or body fluid; rather, they most often involve the intradermal (within the skin) injection of an allergenic substance (substance that causes an allergic reaction) to determine whether the patient has come in contact with a specific allergen (most commonly an antigen) and developed antibodies against it. Many disease-producing microorganisms will function as allergens and stimulate an antibody response in susceptible individuals. Intradermal skin testing can be performed to determine a patient's immune status associated with such microorganisms.

Types of Skin Tests

Common skin tests include the following:

- *Tuberculin (TB) test:* Also called PPD test because of the purified protein derivative used in testing; tests for tuberculosis. It is probably the most common skin test.
- *Schick test:* Tests for susceptibility to diphtheria.
- *Dick test:* Tests for susceptibility to scarlet fever caused by *Streptococcus pyogenes.*
- *Histoplasmosis (histo) test:* Tests for past or present infection by the fungus *Histoplasma capsulatum.*
- *Coccidioidomycosis (cocci) test:* Tests for an infectious fungus disease caused by *Coccidioides immitis.*

Skin Test Procedure

1. A site is selected on the volar surface of the forearm, below the antecubital crease. Areas with scars, bruises, burns, rashes, excessive hair, or superficial veins should be avoided.
2. The site is cleaned with 70% isopropyl alcohol and allowed to dry.
3. 0.1 mL of diluted antigen is drawn into a tuberculin syringe using a $\frac{1}{2}$-inch, 26- to 27-gauge needle.
4. The arm is held in the same manner as in venipuncture and the skin is stretched taut with the thumb.
5. The syringe is held at a very low angle (approximately 20 degrees) and the needle is slipped just under the skin.

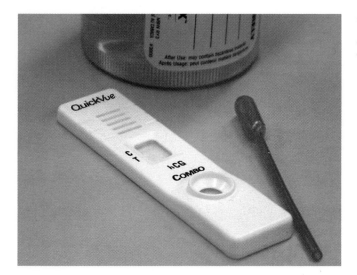

■ FIGURE 11-31 ■

QuickVue Pregnancy Test.
(Quidel Corp., San Diego, CA.)

6. The syringe plunger is pulled back slightly to make certain a vein has not been entered. (If blood appears in the syringe the procedure is discontinued and a new site chosen.)
7. The contents of the syringe are slowly expelled, creating a distinct, pale elevation of the skin 6 to 10 mm in diameter referred to as a bleb or wheal (Fig. 11-32).
8. The needle is removed and the arm remains extended until the site has time to close. Pressure is *not* applied to the site, nor is a bandage applied. (A bandage might absorb the fluid and also cause irritation, distorting test results.)
9. The reaction is read in 24 to 72 hours, depending upon the antigen tested.

Interpretation

Interpretation of the test is based upon the presence or absence of erythema (redness) or induration (hardness).

Negative: *Area (zone) of erythema and induration less than 5 mm in diameter (most tests).*

Doubtful: *Area of erythema and induration between 5 and 9 mm in diameter.*

Positive: *Area of erythema and induration 10 mm or greater in diameter.*

Strep Testing

Numerous kits are available for direct detection of group A streptococci on throat swab specimens. Examples are the Cards QS Strep A (Quidel Corp., San Diego, CA) (Fig. 11-33), the Strep A OIA (Optical Immuno Assay, BIOSTAR, Boulder, CO), and the Becton Dickinson Directigen 1-2-3 Group A Strep test (Franklin Lakes, NJ). Performance of the test normally requires two steps. The first involves nitrous acid or enzymatic extraction of the swab; the second involves a latex agglutination or enzyme immunoassay method of antigen detection. Results are available in minutes.

Urinalysis

A routine urinalysis consists of a physical and chemical analysis of the specimen and a microscopic analysis, if indicated. A medical laboratory technician or technologist must perform a microscopic analysis.

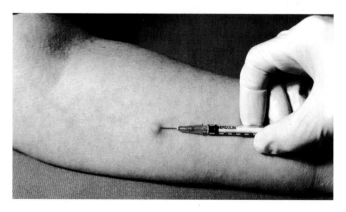

■ FIGURE 11-32 ■

Wheal (bleb) formed by intradermal injection of antigen during skin test procedure.

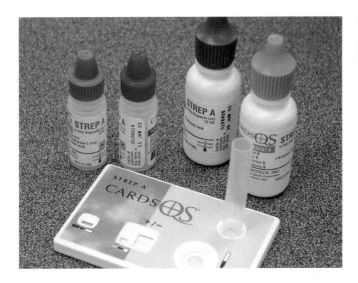

■ FIGURE 11-33 ■

Cards QS Strep A test kit.
(Quidel Corp., San Diego, CA.)

Chemical composition is most commonly determined by use of an inert plastic reagent strip containing pads impregnated with reagents that test for the presence of bacteria, blood, bilirubin, glucose, leukocytes, protein, and urobilinogen, and measure pH and specific gravity. (Specific gravity can also be measured separately using an instrument called a refractometer.) A chemical reaction resulting in color changes to the strip takes place when the strip is dipped in urine. The results can be determined by comparing the strip visually against a code on the container as shown in Fig. 11-34 or

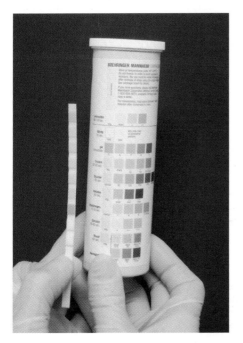

■ FIGURE 11-34 ■

Technician comparing urine reagent strip with chart on reagent strip container.

by inserting the strip into a machine called a reflectance photometer, which reads the strip and prints the results. Reflectance photometers include the Clinitek 200+ (Bayer, Bayer Diagnostics, Tarrytown, NY) and the Chemstrip 101 Urine Analyzer (Roche, Indianapolis, IN) that is a CLIA-waived analyzer. To ensure the integrity of the strips, they should remain tightly capped in their original containers when not in use to protect them from the deteriorating effects of light, moisture, and chemical contamination. The containers should be protected from heat.

Point-of-Care Analyzers: New Technologies

New POCT analyzers include invasive in vivo and ex vivo, noninvasive and chip-based systems.

Invasive systems include in vivo (inside the body) devices placed inside the patient's body that monitor changes in the patient's condition. Examples are the Phillips Medical Trendcare (Andover, MA) (formerly Agilent Technologies), which uses a fiber optic chemical measurement principle to monitor pH, PO_2, PCO_2, and temperature, and the MiniMed (Northridge, CA), which is a subcutaneous electrochemical continuous glucose monitoring system.

Invasive ex vivo systems test blood samples by drawing blood out of the body through a catheter placed inside the patient. The blood is tested externally (ex vivo). After the testing is complete some devices reinfuse the blood back into the patient. In vivo and ex vivo systems are beneficial to the patient because monitoring is continuous and eliminates the need for excess blood being withdrawn.

Noninvasive technology evaluates patient chemistries without the need for phlebotomy or fingerstick. An example of this technology is the Gluco Watch Biographer (Cygnus, Redwood City, CA). This device is worn like a wrist watch and measures glucose extracted through the skin, monitoring results every 20 minutes. The Bili Chek system (SpecRx, Norcross, GA) is a hand-held device that measures bilirubin levels from the skin of newborns, thereby eliminating heel stick serum bilirubin measurements.

Chip-based technology is in the research and development stage and has the potential to allow hundreds of tests to be performed on microchips. Currently this technology is used for analysis in research laboratories and has future applications for determining tumor markers, gene mutations and genetically inherited diseases.

STUDY & REVIEW QUESTIONS

1. When drawing a blood alcohol, it is acceptable to clean the arm with

   a. isopropanol.
   b. methanol.
   c. soap and water.
   d. tincture of iodine.

2. The most important part of blood culture collection is

   a. adequately filling two media vials.
   b. preparing the collection site.
   c. selecting the collection site.
   d. timing of the second set of cultures.

3. TDM peak concentration may be defined as the

   a. highest concentration of the drug during a dosing interval.
   b. lowest concentration of the drug during a dosing interval.
   c. maximum effectiveness of the drug.
   d. time when the amount of drug entering the body is equal to the amount
      leaving the body.

4. When performing a glucose tolerance test, the fasting specimen is drawn
   at 8:15 AM and the patient finishes the glucose beverage at 8:20. When
   should the 1-hour specimen be collected?

   a. 9:15
   b. 9:20
   c. 9:45
   d. 9:50

5. A bleeding time test detects

   a. abnormalities in drug metabolism.
   b. diabetes mellitus.
   c. platelet function disorders.
   d. septicemia

6. Removing a unit of blood from a patient and not replacing it is used as a
   treatment for

   a. autologous donation.
   b. ABO Rh incompatibility.
   c. leukemia.
   d. polycythemia.

Continued

STUDY & REVIEW QUESTIONS *(CONTINUED)*

7. Which of the following tests may require special chain-of-custody documentation when collected?

   a. Blood culture
   b. Cross match
   c. Drug screen
   d. TDM

8. What type of specimen is needed for a Guaiac test?

   a. Amniotic fluid
   b. Blood
   c. Feces
   d. Urine

9. The phlebotomist collects a blood specimen and wraps it in foil. Which of the following specimens could it have been?

   a. Bilirubin
   b. Cryoglobulin
   c. Glucose
   d. Protime

10. Which of the following specimens is collected in a trace-element–free tube?

    a. ABGs
    b. BUN
    c. Lead
    d. Occult blood

11. Common chemistry tests performed by POCT instruments include

    a. Hgb and Hct.
    b. Na and K.
    c. PT and PTT.
    d. T_4 and TSH.

12. A test that measures packed cell volume is

    a. ECG.
    b. hematocrit.
    c. hemoglobin.
    d. troponin T (TnT).

■ CASE STUDY: PERFORMANCE OF A GLUCOSE TOLERANCE TEST

Nancy, a phlebotomist, helped Mr. Smith prepare for a glucose tolerance test over the telephone last week. Today Mr. Smith comes in to have his tolerance performed. Nancy asks Mr. Smith if he ate regular, balanced meals for 3 days before today and did not eat, smoke, drink coffee or alcohol, or exercise strenuously for 12 hours before coming in. Mr. Smith answered that he had followed all the directions exactly. Nancy drew the fasting blood at 5:15 AM. Mr. Smith was given the drink at 5:25.

QUESTIONS:
1. How quickly must Mr. Smith completely finish the drink?
2. At what time would Nancy collect the 1-hour specimen?
3. If Mr. Smith's glucose was 300 at 30 minutes, is this normal?
4. If Mr. Smith vomits after 45 minutes, what should Nancy do?

Bibliography and Suggested Readings

Bishop, M. L., Duben-Engelkirk, J. L., & Fody, E. P. (1996). *Clinical chemistry: Principles, procedures, correlations* (3rd ed.). Philadelphia: Lippincott-Raven Publishers.

Dunne, W. M., Nolte, E., Wilson, M. (1997). *Cumitech 1B-blood cultures III.* American Society for Microbiology Press, Washington, DC.

Fischbach, F. (1996). *A manual of laboratory & diagnostic tests* (5th ed.). Philadelphia: Lippincott-Raven Publishers.

Joint Commission on the Accreditation of Healthcare Organizations. *2002-2003 Comprehensive accreditation manual for pathology and clinical laboratory services.* Joint Commission Resources, 2002. Oakbrook Terrace, IL: JCAHO.

Lotspeich-Steininger, C. A., Stiene-Martin, E. A., & Koepke, J. A. (1992). *Clinical hematology: Principles, procedures, correlations.* Philadelphia: J. B. Lippincott.

Louie, R., Kost, G. (September 2001). *Emerging technologies for point of care testing,* Advance for Administrators of the Laboratory. Vol 10, No 9, page 64-68, Merion Publications, Inc., King of Prussia, PA.

Morris, L. D., Pont, A., & Lewis, S. M. (2001). Use of a new HemoCue system for measuring haemoglobin at low concentrations. *Clinical and Laboratory Haematology* 91–96.

National Committee for Clinical Laboratory Standards, AST2-A. (1999). *Point-of-care in vitro diagnostic (IVD) testing: Approved guideline.* Villanova, PA: NCCLS.

National Committee for Clinical Laboratory Standards, C30-A. (1994). *Ancillary blood glucose testing in acute and chronic care facilities.* Villanova, PA: NCCLS.

Quality point of care testing: A Joint Commission handbook. (1999). Oakbrook Terrace, IL: Joint Commission.

National Committee for Clinical Laboratory Standards, H18-A2. (1999). *Procedures for the handling and processing of blood specimens: Approved guideline.* Villanova, PA: NCCLS.

National Committee for Clinical Laboratory Standards, H7-A3. (2000). *Procedures for determining packed cell volume by the microhematocrit method. Third edition: Approved standard.* Villanova, PA: NCCLS.

National Committee for Clinical Laboratory Standards, H21-A3, 18, No. 20. (1998). *Collection, transport and processing of blood specimens for coagulation testing and performance of coagulation assays: Approved guideline, 3rd edition.* Villanova, PA: NCCLS.

12

ARTERIAL PUNCTURE PROCEDURES

KEY TERMS

ABGs

Allen test

arteriospasm

brachial artery

collateral circulation

femoral artery

radial artery

steady state

thrombus

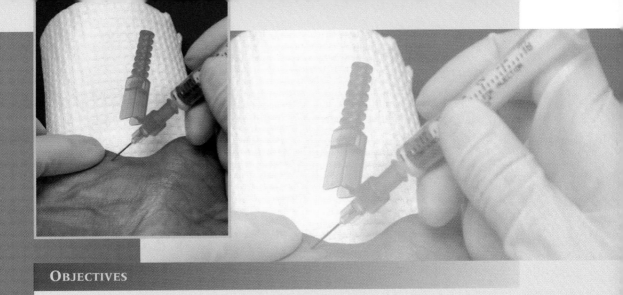

Upon successful completion of this chapter, the reader will be able to:

1 Define the key terms and abbreviations listed at the beginning of this chapter.

2 State the primary reason for performing arterial punctures and identify the personnel who may be required to perform them.

3 Identify the sites that can be used for arterial puncture, the criteria used for selection of the site, and the advantages and disadvantages of each site.

4 List equipment and supplies needed for arterial puncture.

5 Describe patient assessment and preparation procedures, including the administering of local anesthetic, before performing arterial blood gases.

6 Explain the purpose of the Allen test, describe how it is performed, define what constitutes a positive or negative result, and give the procedure to follow for either result.

7 Describe the procedure for collecting radial arterial blood gases, and the role of the phlebotomist in other site collections.

8 List complications associated with arterial puncture, identify factors that may affect the integrity of the blood gas sample, and describe the criteria for sample rejection.

INTRODUCTION

An arterial blood specimen is collected anaerobically by directly puncturing an artery with a sharp short-beveled hypodermic needle or winged infusion set attached to a syringe or other collection device. Arterial blood is the ideal specimen for many analyses because its composition is consistent throughout the body, whereas the composition of venous blood varies relative to the metabolic needs of the areas of the body it serves. However, because arterial puncture is technically more difficult to perform and potentially more painful and hazardous to the patient than venipuncture, arterial specimens are not used for routine blood tests. The primary reason for performing arterial puncture is to obtain blood for evaluation of **arterial blood gases (ABGs).**

ABGS

ABG evaluation is used in the diagnosis and management of respiratory disease to provide valuable information about a patient's oxygenation, ventilation, and acid-base balance, and in the management of electrolyte and acid-base balance in patients with other disorders such as diabetes. Because arterial blood is one of the most sensitive specimens analyzed, accurate patient assessment and proper specimen collection and handling are necessary to ensure accurate diagnostic results. Most instruments used to process ABG specimens directly measure pH, partial pressure of carbon dioxide (PCO_2), oxygen pressure (PO_2), calculate bicarbonate (HCO_3), base excess (or deficit), and oxygen (O_2) saturation. See Table 12-1 for an explanation of commonly measured ABG parameters. Many instruments now also measure other critical care analytes such as sodium, potassium, chloride, ionized calcium, glucose, and hemoglobin.

PERSONNEL WHO PERFORM ARTERIAL PUNCTURE

Paramedical personnel (healthcare workers other than physicians) who may be required to perform arterial puncture include nurses, medical technologists and technicians, respiratory therapists, emergency medical technicians, and level II phlebotomists. Personnel who perform ABG procedures are normally certified by their healthcare institutions after successfully completing training involving theory, demonstration of technique, observation of the actual procedure, and performance of arterial puncture under the supervision of qualified personnel. Skills are typically reverified annually.

ARTERIAL PUNCTURE SITES

Several different sites can be used for arterial puncture. The criteria for site selection include the presence of collateral circulation, how large and accessible the artery is, and the type of tissue surrounding the puncture site. The site chosen should not be inflamed, irritated, edematous, or in close proximity to a wound or hematoma. Sites recently used for arterial puncture should be avoided, if possible. In addition, *never* select a site in a limb with an arteriovenous shunt or fistula. The following are sites commonly chosen for arterial puncture.

Table 12-1

Commonly Measured Arterial Blood Gas (ABG) Parameters

Parameter	Normal Range	Description
pH	7.35-7.45	A measure of the acidity or alkalinity of the blood; used to identify a condition as acidosis or alkalosis.
PO_2	80-100 mm Hg	Partial pressure of oxygen. A measure of how much oxygen is dissolved in the blood. Indicates if ventilation is adequate. Decreased oxygen levels in the blood increase the respiration rate and vice versa.
PCO_2	35-45 mm Hg	Partial pressure of carbon dioxide. A measure of how much carbon dioxide is dissolved in the blood. Evaluates lung function. Increased CO_2 levels in the blood increase the respiratory rate and vice versa. *Respiratory* disturbances alter PCO_2 levels.
HCO_3	22-26 mEq/L	Bicarbonate. A measure of the amount of bicarbonate in the blood. Evaluates the bicarbonate buffer system of the kidneys. *Metabolic* disturbances alter HCO_3 levels.
O_2 saturation	97-100%	Oxygen saturation. The percent of oxygen bound to hemoglobin. Determines if hemoglobin is carrying the amount of oxygen it is capable of carrying.
Base excess (or deficit)	(-2) - $(+2)$ mEq/L	A calculation of the nonrespiratory part of acid-base balance based on the PCO_2, HCO_3, and hematocrit.

The Radial Artery

The first choice and most common site used for arterial puncture is the **radial artery,** located in the thumb side of the wrist (Fig. 12-1). Although smaller than arteries in other sites, the radial artery is readily accessible in most patients.

Advantages

The biggest advantage of using the radial artery is the presence of **collateral circulation.** Having collateral circulation means that the area is supplied with blood from more than one artery. Under normal circumstances, both the radial and the ulnar artery supply the hand with blood. If the radial artery were to be inadvertently damaged as a consequence of arterial puncture, the ulnar artery could supply blood to the hand. For this reason, the ulnar artery is never used for arterial puncture. Collateral circulation can be evaluated by an instrument called the Doppler ultrasonic flow indi-

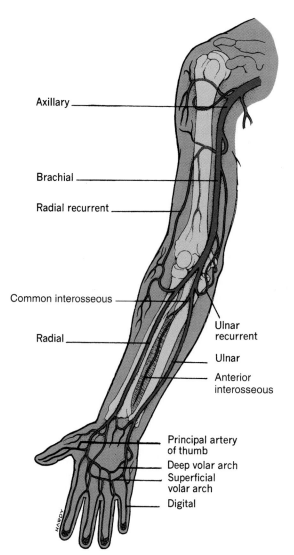

Axillary

Brachial

Radial recurrent

Common interosseous

Radial

Ulnar recurrent

Ulnar

Anterior interosseous

Principal artery of thumb

Deep volar arch

Superficial volar arch

Digital

cator or by performing the modified Allen test. If collateral circulation is absent, the radial artery should not be punctured.

Another advantage of using the radial artery is that there is less chance of hematoma formation after the procedure, because the radial artery can be easily compressed over the ligaments and bones of the wrist.

Disadvantages

Disadvantages of using the radial artery include the fact that considerable skill is required to puncture it successfully owing to its small size, and that it may be difficult or impossible to locate on patients with low cardiac output.

The Brachial Artery

The **brachial artery** (Fig. 12-1) is the second choice for arterial puncture. It is located in the medial anterior aspect of the antecubital fossa near the insertion of the biceps muscle.

Advantages

Advantages of the brachial artery are that it is large and easy to palpate and puncture. The brachial artery has adequate collateral circulation, though not as much as the radial artery.

Disadvantages

There are a number of disadvantages to puncturing the brachial artery:

- It is deeper than the radial artery.
- It lies close to a large vein (the basilic) and the median nerve, both of which may be inadvertently punctured.
- Unlike the radial artery, there are no underlying ligaments or bone to support compression of the brachial artery, resulting in an increased risk of hematoma formation after the procedure.

The Femoral Artery

The **femoral artery** (Fig. 12-2) is the largest artery used for arterial puncture. It is located superficially in the groin, lateral to the pubis bone. Femoral puncture is performed primarily by physicians and specially trained emergency room personnel.

Advantages

The femoral artery is large and easily palpated and punctured. It is sometimes the only site where arterial sampling is possible, especially on patients with low cardiac output.

Disadvantages

Disadvantages of femoral arterial puncture include poor collateral circulation, increased risk of infection because of the location of the site, difficulty in achieving aseptic technique because of the presence of pubic hair, and the possibility of dislodging plaque buildup from the inner artery walls of older patients. In addition, the femoral artery lies close to the femoral vein, which may be inadvertently punctured.

Because of the numerous disadvantages associated with femoral puncture, it is generally used only in emergency situations or when other sites are not available.

Other Sites

Other sites where arterial specimens may be obtained include the scalp and umbilical arteries in infants and the dorsalis pedis arteries of the adult. The phlebotomist is not trained to perform arterial punctures at these locations or to obtain specimens from cannulae, catheters, or other indwelling devices at these or any other locations.

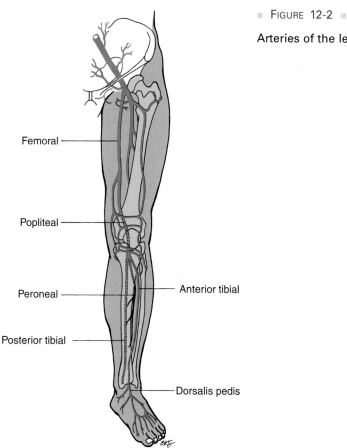

■ FIGURE 12-2 ■

Arteries of the leg.

Femoral

Popliteal

Peroneal

Anterior tibial

Posterior tibial

Dorsalis pedis

ABG SPECIMEN COLLECTION

Test Requisition

As with any other test, a physician's order is needed before collecting ABGs. In addition to normal patient identification information, specific information such as current body temperature, respiratory rate, and ventilation status must be recorded at the time of specimen collection.

Required information may vary according to regulatory requirements. Typical ABG requisition information is listed in Box 12-1.

Equipment and Supplies

Personal Protective Equipment

Personal protective equipment needed by the blood drawer when collecting arterial specimens includes a fluid-resistant lab coat, gown, or apron, gloves, and face protection because of the possibility of blood spray during arterial puncture.

Box 12-1

TYPICAL ARTERIAL BLOOD GAS REQUISITION INFORMATION

Required information:
1. Patient's full name
2. Medical record or identification number
3. Age or birth date
4. Room number or other patient location
5. Date and time of test collection
6. Fraction of inspired oxygen (FiO_2)
7. Body temperature
8. Respiration rate
9. Clinical indication for specimen collection
10. Blood drawer's initials
11. Requesting physician

Supplemental information as required by institutional policy or regulatory agencies:
12. Ventilation status
13. Method of ventilation
14. Sampling site and type of procedure
15. Patient activity and position
16. Working diagnosis or ICD-9 codes

Specimen Collection Equipment and Supplies

ABG specimen collection equipment (Fig. 12-3) includes special heparinized syringes for specimen collection and special caps or other devices to plug or cover the syringe after specimen collection to maintain anaerobic conditions. ABG specimens are collected in syringes rather than tubes because evacuated tube pressure can change results. Many ABG syringes contain special filters that vent residual air, then seal upon contact with blood. ABG equipment is commonly available in sterile prepackaged kits that contain the heparinized syringe, special capping device, and safety needle or needle removal device. ABG collection equipment and supplies are listed in Box 12-2.

Patient Assessment and Preparation Procedures

Identification and Assessment

The blood drawer must properly identify the patient, explain the procedure, and obtain his or her consent. Collection conditions must be verified and documented. In addition it should be determined whether or not the patient is on anticoagulant therapy.

Box 12-2

ARTERIAL BLOOD GAS COLLECTION EQUIPMENT AND SUPPLIES

1. Antiseptic pads such as isopropanol, povidone-iodine, or chlorhexidine for site cleaning.
2. (Optional) Local anesthetic to numb the site; 1% lidocaine without epinephrine is recommended.
3. Sharp short bevel hypodermic needle in 20 g to 23 g or 25 g and $\frac{5}{8}$ to 1-$\frac{1}{2}$ inches in length, depending on the collection site, the size of the artery, and the amount of blood needed. Typically, a 22 g, 1-inch needle is used for radial and brachial puncture and a 22 g 1-$\frac{1}{2}$-inch needle is used for femoral puncture. The needle should have a safety feature to prevent accidental needlesticks or be used with an approved safety needle-removal device or safety syringe.
4. Special glass or plastic 1 to 5 mL self-filling syringe or other collection device (prefilled with the appropriate amount and type of lyophilized heparin salt) selected according to the type of tests ordered, the method of analysis, and the amount of blood required. The syringe should contain a safety device to prevent accidental needlesticks or be used with a safety needle or approved safety needle-removal device.
5. (Optional) 1- or 2-mL plastic syringe with a 25 g or 26 g $\frac{1}{2}$- to $\frac{5}{8}$-inch long needle for administration of anesthetic solution. Either the syringe or the needle should contain a safety device to prevent accidental needlesticks.
6. A safety needle removal device or small block of rubber or latex in which to insert the needle unless the needle or syringe has a safety feature to prevent accidental needlesticks.
7. Luer tip cap or other suitable device to cover the end of the syringe after needle removal to maintain anaerobic conditions within the specimen.
8. (As required) Coolant capable of maintaining the specimen at a temperature between 1°C and 5°C to slow the metabolism of white blood cells, which consume oxygen. A container of crushed ice and water big enough to completely submerge the syringe barrel is typically used.
9. 2 × 2-inch gauze squares to hold pressure over the site until bleeding has stopped.
10. Self-adhering gauze bandage to wrap the site after collection.
11. Identification and labeling materials such as waterproof labels and indelible ink pens or makers.
12. A puncture-resistant sharps container to dispose of used needles and syringes.

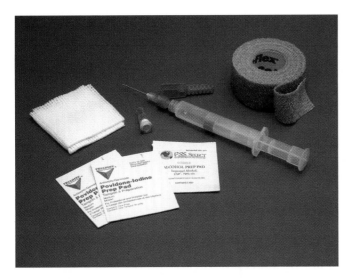

Arterial blood gas equipment.

If an anesthetic is to be used, it should also be determined if the patient is allergic to any anesthetics.

Steady State

Current body temperature, breathing pattern, and the concentration of oxygen inhaled, affect the amount of oxygen and carbon dioxide in the blood. Consequently a patient should have been in a stable or **steady state** (i.e., no exercise, suctioning, or respirator changes) for at least 20 to 30 minutes before obtaining blood gases. This is especially important for patients with abnormal respiratory function such as patients with chronic lung disease. With the exception of certain emergency situations, ABG collection should not be performed until a steady state that meets required collection conditions has been achieved.

Modified Allen Test

It must be determined that the patient has collateral circulation before performing arterial puncture. The modified **Allen test** (Fig. 12-4) is an easy way to assess collateral circulation before collecting a blood specimen from the radial artery. It is performed without the use of special equipment. If the test is positive, arterial puncture can be performed on the radial artery. If the test is negative, arterial puncture should not be performed on that arm and the patient's nurse or physician should be notified of the problem. The procedure for the modified Allen test is described in Box 12-3.

Administration of Local Anesthetic

The advent of improved thin-wall needles has made the routine administration of anesthetic before arterial puncture unnecessary. However, it may be a reassuring option for some patients, especially children, who are fearful of the procedure. A fearful patient may respond by breath-holding, crying, or hyperventilation, all of which may

Box 12-3

MODIFIED ALLEN TEST

1. Have the patient make a tight fist.
2. Using the middle and index fingers of both hands, apply pressure to the patient's wrist, compressing both the radial and ulnar arteries at the same time.
3. While maintaining pressure, have the patient open the hand slowly. The hand should appear blanched or drained of color.
4. Lower the patient's hand and release pressure on the ulnar artery only.

   Positive Allen test: The hand flushes pink or returns to normal color within 15 seconds, indicating the return of blood to the hand via the ulnar artery and the presence of collateral circulation. If the Allen test is positive, proceed with arterial blood gas collection.

   Negative Allen test: The hand *does not* flush pink or return to normal color within 15 seconds, indicating the inability of the ulnar artery to adequately supply blood to the hand and therefore the absence of collateral circulation. If the Allen test is negative, the radial artery should not be used and another site must be selected.
6. Record the results on the request slip.

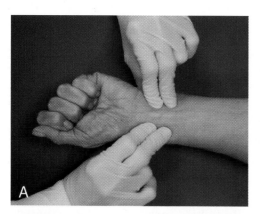
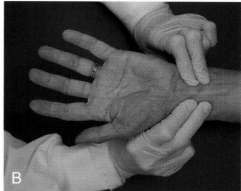
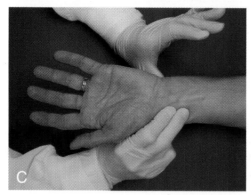

■ FIGURE 12-4 ■

Allen test. (*A*) The fingers are used to compress the radial and ulnar arteries while the patient makes a fist. (*B*) A blanched appearance to the open hand is observed while both arteries are being pressed. (*C*) The patient's hand flushes with color when the ulnar artery is released, signifying a positive Allen test.

affect blood gas results. In addition to minimizing or preventing such patient reactions, local anesthesia may prevent vasoconstriction. The recommended local anesthetic for ABG collection is 1% lidocaine without epinephrine; however, it may cause prolonged bleeding in patients on anticoagulant therapy. The procedure for preparing and administering local anesthetic is described in Box 12-4.

Box 12-4

PREPARING AND ADMINISTERING LOCAL ANESTHETIC

Prepare the anesthetic syringe:
Attach a 25 g needle to a 1-mL syringe.
Clean the stopper of the anesthetic (i.e., lidocaine) bottle with alcohol.
Insert the needle through the stopper of the anesthetic bottle and withdraw 0.5 mL anesthetic.
Carefully replace the needle cap and leave the syringe in a horizontal position.
Administer anesthetic:
Insert the needle of the anesthetic syringe into the skin over the arterial puncture site at an angle of approximately 10 degrees.
Pull back slightly on the plunger to be certain a vein was not inadvertently penetrated.
If blood appears in the syringe, withdraw the syringe, prepare a fresh syringe and needle, and repeat the procedure in a slightly different spot.
If no blood appears in the syringe, slowly expel the contents into the skin, forming a raised wheal.
Wait 1 to 2 minutes for the anesthetic to take effect before proceeding with arterial puncture. Note anesthetic application on the request form.

Radial ABG Procedure

Puncture of the radial artery can be performed if it is determined that there is collateral circulation provided by the ulnar artery and the site meets other selection criteria previously described. Individual steps for collecting ABGs from the radial artery are listed in Box 12-5. Major points of radial ABG procedure are explained as follows.

Position the Arm

Position the patient's arm out to the side (abducted) with the palm facing up and the wrist supported. (A rolled towel placed under the wrist is typically used to provide support.) Ask the patient to extend the wrist at an approximate 30-degree angle to stretch and fix the tissue over the firm ligaments and bone of the wrist.

Box 12-5

RADIAL ARTERIAL BLOOD GAS (ABG) PROCEDURE

1. Receive the physician's order and note the requested collection time.
2. Assemble and transport equipment to the patient's bedside.
3. Identify the patient and explain the procedure.
4. Record the patient's temperature, respiratory rate, and breathing mixture (e.g., room air) and other required information on the laboratory slip.
5. Wash hands and put on gloves.
6. Position the patient's arm with the palm facing up and a rolled towel underneath for support and assess collateral circulation using the modified Allen test (see Fig. 12-4), a Doppler ultrasonic flow indicator, or both. If collateral circulation is present, continue with ABG collection. If collateral circulation is absent, choose another site.
7. With the arm abducted (out to the side) the palm facing up and the wrist supported, have the patient extend the wrist at an approximate 30-degree angle.
8. Use an index finger to locate the radial artery proximal to the crease on the thumb side of the wrist and palpate it to determine its size, direction, and depth.
9. Prepare the site by cleaning first with alcohol and then with povidone-iodine or other suitable antiseptic. Prep the nondominant index finger in the same manner. Allow the site to dry, being careful not to touch it with any unsterile object.
10. (Optional) Administer local anesthetic according to the procedure in Box 12-4.
11. Pick up and hold the ABG syringe or collection device in the dominant hand as if holding a dart and relocate the artery by placing the index finger of the opposite hand directly over the pulse.
12. Warn the patient of the imminent puncture and ask him or her to relax the wrist as much as possible.
13. Direct the needle away from the hand, facing into the arterial blood flow and insert it bevel up into the skin at a 30- to 45-degree angle approximately 5 to 10 mm distal to the index finger that is locating the pulse (Fig. 12-5).
14. Slowly direct the needle toward the artery. Stop advancing the needle when a "flash" of blood appears in the needle hub. Allow the blood to pump into the syringe until the desired amount of blood is collected.
15. If the artery is missed, slowly withdraw the needle until just the bevel is under the skin and redirect the needle into the artery. Do not probe.

continued

continued

16. After obtaining the specimen, withdraw the needle and immediately place clean dry gauze over the site with one hand and activate the needle safety device with the other.

17. Apply firm pressure to the puncture site for a minimum of 3 to 5 minutes, longer for patients on anticoagulant therapy.

18. While applying pressure to the site, use your free hand to eject any air bubbles from the specimen, remove the needle, discard it in a sharps container, and cap the syringe (Fig. 12-6) or use an appropriate needle removal safety device and air bubble removal cap.

19. Gently mix the specimen by inversion or rotation to prevent clot formation.

20. Label the specimen.

21. Check the site for swelling or bruising. If none is noted, clean the povidone-iodine from the site with an alcohol prep pad, wait 2 minutes, and check the site again. Check the pulse distal to the site. If the pulse is absent or faint, alert the patient's nurse or physician immediately. If the site appears normal, apply a pressure bandage and make a notation when the bandage may be removed.

22. Thank the patient.

23. Dispose of used equipment properly. Remove gloves and mask and wash hands.

24. Transport the specimen according to laboratory policy and deliver to the lab as soon as possible or place the specimen on ice if a delay greater than 30 minutes is anticipated.

Locate the Artery

Using the index finger of the nondominant hand, locate the radial artery pulse proximal to the skin crease on the thumb side of the wrist. Palpate the artery to determine its size, direction, and depth.

Key Point ➤ Never use the thumb to palpate. It has a pulse that can be misleading.

Clean the Site

Prepare the site by cleaning first with alcohol and then with povidone-iodine or other suitable antiseptic. Prep the nondominant index finger that will be used to palpate in the same manner. Allow the site to dry, being careful not to touch it with any unsterile object.

Insert the Needle

Pick up and hold the syringe or collection device in the dominant hand as if holding a dart. Relocate the artery by placing the index finger of the opposite hand directly over the pulse. Warn the patient of the imminent puncture and ask him or her to relax the wrist as much as possible while maintaining its extended position. Direct the needle away from the hand, facing into the arterial blood flow and insert it bevel up into the skin at a 30- to 45-degree angle (femoral puncture requires a 90-degree angle) approximately 5 to 10 mm distal to the index finger that is locating the pulse (Fig. 12-5).

Advance the Needle into the Artery

Slowly advance the needle, directing it toward the artery just under the finger. When the artery is pierced, a "flash" of blood will appear in the hub of the needle. When the flash appears, stop advancing the needle. Do not pull back on the syringe plunger. The blood will continue to pump into the syringe unless a needle smaller than 23g is used, in which case a gentle pull on the plunger may be required. Hold the syringe very steady until the desired amount of blood is collected.

Key Point ➤ If the artery is missed, slowly withdraw the needle until the bevel is just under the skin before redirecting it into the artery. Do not probe. Probing is painful and can cause hematoma or thrombus formation or damage the artery.

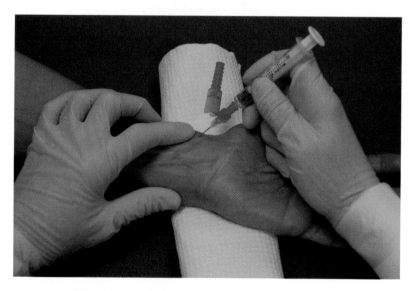

■ Figure 12-5 ■

Performing an arterial puncture.

Withdraw the Needle and Apply Pressure

When the desired amount of blood has been obtained, withdraw the needle, immediately place a folded clean dry gauze square over the site with one hand and simultaneously activate the needle safety device with the other hand or place the needle in an approved needle removal safety device. Apply firm pressure to the puncture site for a minimum of 3 to 5 minutes. Longer application of pressure is required for patients on anticoagulant therapy.

 Key Point ➤ *Never* allow the patient to apply the pressure. A patient may not apply pressure firmly enough. In addition *do not* replace manually holding the site for the required time with the application of a pressure bandage.

Remove Air, Cap Syringe, and Mix Specimen

While applying pressure to the site, use your free hand to immediately eject any air bubbles from the specimen. Remove the safety needle, being careful not to introduce air bubbles into the specimen. Discard the needle in a sharps container and cap the syringe (Fig. 12-6), preferably using an air bubble removal cap. Gently but thoroughly mix the specimen by inversion or rotation to prevent clot formation.

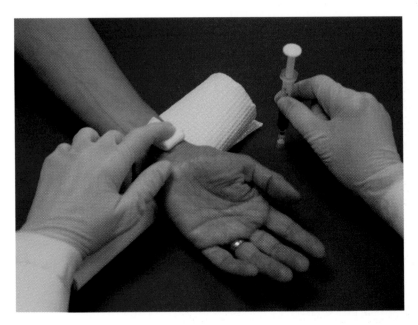

■ FIGURE 12-6 ■

Capping the arterial blood gas syringe while holding pressure over the patient's artery.

Check the Site

After applying pressure for 3 to 5 minutes, check the site. If bleeding, swelling, or bruising is noted, reapply pressure for an additional 2 minutes.

 Key Point ➤ Never leave a patient if the site is still bleeding. Notify the patient's nurse or physician of the problem.

If the site appears normal, clean the povidone-iodine from the site with an alcohol prep pad, wait 2 minutes, and check it again. Next check the pulse distal to the site. If the pulse is absent or faint, alert the patient's nurse or physician immediately as a thrombus may be blocking blood flow. If the site appears normal and the pulse is normal, apply a pressure bandage and make a notation when the bandage may be removed.

Wrap-up Procedures

Label the specimen before leaving the patient's bedside. Dispose of used equipment properly. Remove gloves and mask and wash hands. Thank the patient.

Transportation and Handling

Transport the specimen according to laboratory protocol and deliver to the laboratory as soon as possible. Typically, ABG specimens collected in plastic syringes are transported at room temperature provided the specimen will be analyzed within 30 minutes. If the patient has an elevated leukocyte or platelet count the specimen should be analyzed within 5 minutes of collection. If a delay in analysis is expected, specimens should be collected in glass syringes and placed on ice as soon as possible. Specimens for electrolyte testing in addition to ABG evaluation should not be cooled because cooling affects potassium levels. Such specimens should be transported and tested as soon as possible.

ABG Collection from Other Sites

Collection of ABGs from other sites is similar to the procedure for radial ABGs. Because phlebotomists are not normally trained to collect specimens from these sites, specific procedures are not given in this text. Phlebotomists may, however, be asked to provide the equipment and assist in labeling and transporting specimens collected from these sites by others (e.g., an emergency room physician).

HAZARDS AND COMPLICATIONS ASSOCIATED WITH ARTERIAL PUNCTURE

Arteriospasm. Pain or irritation caused by needle penetration of the artery muscle, and even patient anxiety, can cause a reflex constriction of the artery referred to as an **arteriospasm.** The condition is transitory but may make it difficult to obtain a specimen. To help minimize the chance of arteriospasm reassure the patient by fully explaining the procedure and its purpose and answer questions to help relieve patient anxiety.

Discomfort. Some discomfort is generally associated with arterial puncture, even with use of a local anesthetic. Extreme pain during arterial puncture may indicate nerve involvement and the procedure should be terminated.

Infection. Infection can result from improper site preparation or contamination of the site before specimen collection. Proper antiseptic preparation of the site and avoiding activities that recontaminate the site before specimen collection minimizes the chance of infection.

Hematoma. Blood is under considerable pressure in the arteries and is initially more likely to leak from an arterial puncture site than from a venipuncture site. However, arterial puncture sites tend to close more rapidly because of the elastic nature of the arterial wall. Elasticity tends to decrease with age, increasing the probability of hematoma formation in older patients. The probability of hematoma formation is also greater in patients receiving anticoagulant therapy.

Numbness. Numbness of the hand or wrist can result from nerve irritation or damage as a result of error in technique such as improper redirection of the needle when the artery is missed.

Thrombus formation. Injury to the intima or inner wall of the artery can lead to thrombus or clot formation. A thrombus may grow until it blocks the entire lumen of the artery, obstructing blood flow and impairing circulation. A thrombus can also be the source of an embolus and result in an embolism in another area of the body.

Vasovagal syncope. Sudden fainting related to hypotension caused by a nervous system response to abrupt pain or trauma can occur during arterial puncture. If a patient faints during arterial puncture remove the needle immediately, activate the safety device, hold pressure over the site, and follow syncope procedures discussed in Chapter 9.

SAMPLING ERRORS

Errors in sample collection that can affect the integrity of a blood gas sample and lead to erroneous results include the following:

Air bubbles. If air bubbles are not immediately or completely expelled from the sample, oxygen from the air bubbles can diffuse into the sample and carbon dioxide can escape from the sample, changing test results.

Delay in analysis. Blood cells continue to metabolize or consume oxygen and nutrients and produce acids and carbon dioxide at room temperature. If the specimen remains at room temperature for more than 30 minutes, the pH, blood gas, and glucose values will not accurately reflect the patient's status. Processing the specimen as soon as possible after it is obtained helps ensure the most accurate results.

Improper mixing. Inadequate or delayed mixing of the sample can lead to clotting, making the sample unacceptable for testing. Undetected microclots can lead to erroneous results.

Improper syringe. Use only syringes especially designed for ABG procedures. The use of regular plastic syringes will lead to erroneous values. Use of commercially available ABG kits can eliminate this source of error.

Obtaining a venous sample by mistake. Markedly inaccurate ABG values will result if a venous sample is obtained by mistake. Normal arterial blood is bright cherry red in color. Venous blood is a darker bluish-red color. However, it is sometimes difficult to distinguish between arterial and venous blood in poorly ventilated patients because their arterial blood may appear as dark as venous blood. The best way to be certain that a specimen is arterial is if the blood pulses into the syringe. In some instances, such as low cardiac output, a specimen may need to be aspirated. In these cases it is hard to be certain that the specimen is truly arterial.

Use of improper anticoagulant. Heparin is the acceptable anticoagulant for blood gas specimens. Oxalates, EDTA, and citrates may alter results, especially pH.

Use of too much or too little heparin. Too much heparin in the syringe can cause erroneous results owing to acidosis. Too little heparin can result in clotting of the specimen. Use of commercially available kits containing preheparinized syringes can eliminate this source of error.

CRITERIA FOR ABG SPECIMEN REJECTION

- Air bubbles in specimen
- Clotted specimen
- Improper or absent labeling
- Inadequate volume of specimen for the test
- Prolonged delay in delivery to the lab
- Use of wrong type of syringe

STUDY & REVIEW QUESTIONS

1. The primary reason for performing arterial puncture is to

   a. determine hemoglobin levels.
   b. evaluate blood gases.
   c. measure potassium levels.
   d. obtain calcium values.

2. Locations to obtain arterial blood gases are all of the following *except* the

   a. brachial artery.
   b. ulnar artery.
   c. femoral artery.
   d. radial artery.

3. One of the following items is not ABG equipment. Which is it?

   a. Povidone-iodine prep pad
   b. Heparinized syringe
   c. Syringe cap
   d. Tourniquet

4. A phlebotomist has a request to collect an ABG specimen while the patient is breathing room air. When the phlebotomist arrives to collect the specimen the patient is still on a ventilator. What should the phlebotomist do?

   a. Call the phlebotomy supervisor and ask what to do
   b. Collect the specimen and write the ventilator setting on the requisition
   c. Consult with the patient's nurse
   d. Take the patient off of the ventilator and draw the specimen

5. The purpose of the modified Allen test is to determine

   a. blood pressure in the radial artery.
   b. the presence of collateral circulation.
   c. the coagulation time of the arteries.
   d. whether the patient is absorbing oxygen.

6. Which of the following is an acceptable angle of needle insertion for radial ABGs?

   a. 10 degrees
   b. 20 degrees
   c. 45 degrees
   d. 90 degrees

Continued

STUDY & REVIEW QUESTIONS *(CONTINUED)*

7. Which of the following complications are associated with arterial puncture?
   a. Arteriospasm
   b. Hematoma
   c. Infection
   d. All of the above

8. Which of the following will *not* produce erroneous ABG values?
   a. Air bubbles in the sample
   b. Cooling a specimen with a high white blood count
   c. Delay in analysis exceeding 30 minutes
   d. Improper mixing

9. Which statement is *not* true? An arteriospasm
   a. is a reflex constriction of the artery.
   b. can be caused by irritation of the artery muscle by the needle.
   c. makes it difficult to obtain a specimen.
   d. results in permanent damage to the artery.

10. What would cause you to suspect that a thrombus formed in the radial artery while you were collecting an ABG specimen from it?
    a. A hematoma forms at the site
    b. The patient complains of extreme pain
    c. The pulse distal to the site is weak or absent
    d. There is no way to tell

■ CASE STUDY: ABG COMPLICATIONS

A phlebotomist has a requisition to collect an ABG specimen from a patient in the cardiac care unit. The phlebotomist identifies the patient and records required requisition information. The patient has an intravenous line in the left arm in the area of the wrist so the phlebotomist chooses the right arm. The patient is having a hard time breathing and appears quite restless and agitated. The phlebotomist performs the modified Allen test. The result is positive. The phlebotomist attempts puncture of the radial artery. The patient moves his arm as the needle is inserted and it misses the artery. The phlebotomist redirects the needle several times and finally hits the artery. The blood pulses into the syringe but is dark reddish blue in color. The phlebotomist completes the draw, removes the needle, holds pressure over the site, and at same time activates the needle safety device, removes the needle, and caps the syringe, being careful not to introduce air bubbles into it.

After holding pressure for 5 minutes and cleaning the povidone-iodine from the site, the phlebotomist checks the pulse distal to the site. The pulse is barely discernible.

QUESTIONS:
1. What should the phlebotomist do now?
2. What might be affecting the pulse?
3. How might the patient have contributed to the problem?
4. How might the phlebotomist's technique have contributed to the problem?
5. Can the phlebotomist be certain that the specimen is arterial?

Bibliography and Suggested Readings

Bishop, M., Duben-Engelkirk, J., & Fody, E. (2000). *Clinical chemistry, principles, procedures, correlations* (4th ed.). Philadelphia: Lippincott Williams & Wilkins.

Burtis, C., & Ashwood, E. (2001). *Tietz fundamentals of clinical chemistry* (3rd ed.). Philadelphia: W.B. Saunders.

National Committee for Clinical Laboratory Standards, H11-A3. (May 1999). *Procedures for the collection of arterial blood specimens: Approved standard* (3rd ed.). Wayne, PA: NAACLS.

University of Iowa Web site. Introduction to interpreting arterial blood gases for medical students. Available at: http://www.int-med.uiowa.edu/education/abg.htm.

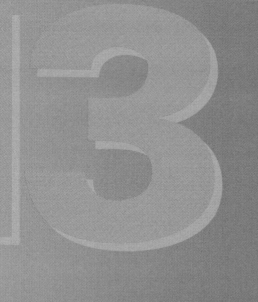

NONBLOOD SPECIMENS AND TESTS

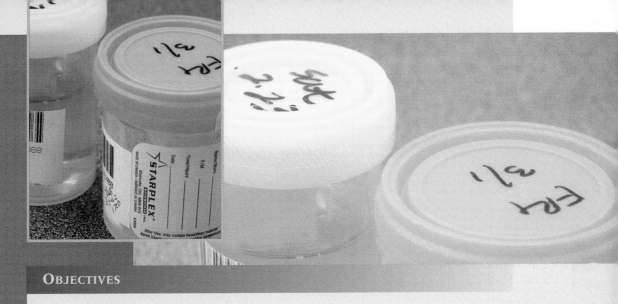

OBJECTIVES

Upon successful completion of this chapter, the reader will be able to:

1 Define the key terms and abbreviations listed at the beginning of the chapter.
2 Describe nonblood specimen labeling and handling.
3 Name and describe the various urine tests, specimen types, and collection methods.
4 Identify and describe the types of nonblood specimens and explain why these specimens are tested.
5 Describe collection and handling procedures indicated for nonblood specimens.
6 Identify tests performed on various nonblood specimens.

INTRODUCTION

Although blood is the type of specimen most frequently analyzed in the medical laboratory, other body fluids are also analyzed. The phlebotomist may be involved in obtaining the specimen (as in throat swab collection); test administration (as in sweat chloride collection); instruction (as in urine collection); processing (accessioning and preparing the specimen for testing); or merely labeling or transporting specimens to the lab.

NONBLOOD SPECIMEN LABELING AND HANDLING

As a minimum, nonblood specimens should be labeled with the same identifying information as blood specimens. Most institutions also require information on the type or source of the specimen. Before accepting specimens collected by other hospital personnel, the phlebotomist must check that the specimen is properly labeled. Standard precautions should be observed when handling nonblood specimens because body fluids are potentially infectious.

BODY FLUID SPECIMENS

Urine

Urine is the most frequently analyzed nonblood body fluid. Analysis of urine can aid in the diagnosis and treatment of urinary tract infections and the detection of metabolic disease. Accuracy of results depends on the method of collection, type of container used, transportation and handling of the specimen, and timeliness of testing to prevent multiplication of bacteria and breakdown of components such as cellular elements and bilirubin. Collection of urine specimens on inpatients is usually handled by nursing personnel. Phlebotomists, however, often handle outpatient urine specimen collection.

The phlebotomist must be able to explain urine collection procedures to a patient without causing him or her embarrassment. Verbal instructions must be followed by written instructions, preferably with illustrations. In outpatient areas, written instructions are often posted on the wall in the restroom designated for patient urine collections. The type of specimen preferred for many urine studies is the first urine voided (passed naturally from the bladder or urinated) in the morning because it is the most concentrated. However, the type of specimen and the method of urine collection vary depending on the type of test ordered. The most common urine tests, types of urine specimens requested, and various collection methods follow.

Common Urine Tests

ROUTINE URINALYSIS

A routine **urinalysis (UA)** includes a physical, chemical, and microscopic analysis of the specimen. Physical characteristics noted include color, odor, transparency, and specific gravity or concentration. Chemical composition is most commonly determined by use of a plastic strip containing areas impregnated with reagents that test for the presence of bacteria, blood, white blood cells, protein, glucose, and other substances. The strip is dipped into the urine and compared to a color chart, usually found on the label of the reagent strip container. Special timing is involved in reading the results. The manner in which the results are to be reported is indicated on the reagent label. Most results are reported using the terms **trace, 1+, 2+,** and so on to indicate the degree of a positive result, and **negative (neg) or (−)** symbol when no reaction is noted. Machines are available that read the strips automatically (see the discussion of point-of-care testing in Chapter 11). The strip is used once and discarded.

Urine components such as cells, crystals, and microorganisms can be seen by microscopic examination of a sample of urine sediment obtained through centrifugation. A measured portion of urine is centrifuged in a special plastic tube. After centrifugation, the supernatant, or top portion of the specimen, is discarded and a drop of the remaining sediment is placed on a glass slide and covered with a small square of glass called a coverslip, or placed in a special chamber, and examined under the microscope by either a laboratory technician or technologist. There are UA machines in the laboratory that also perform this function.

Specimens for routine UA should be collected in clear, dry, chemically clean containers with tight-fitting lids. If a culture and sensitivity (C&S) is also ordered on the specimen, the container should be sterile. Urine specimens should be transported to the lab promptly. Specimens for routine UA that cannot be transported or analyzed promptly can be held at room temperature and protected from light for up to 2 hours. Specimens held longer should be refrigerated. Specimens for which both a C&S and a UA are requested should be refrigerated if immediate processing is not possible.

A regular voided specimen is acceptable for routine urinalysis. However, to avoid contamination of the specimen by genital secretions, pubic hair, and bacteria surrounding the urinary opening, the ideal procedure for collecting a specimen for routine urinalysis is referred to as **midstream collection.** (See section on Urine Collection Methods in this chapter for regular voided and midstream collection methods).

URINE CULTURE AND SENSITIVITY

A urine **culture and sensitivity (C&S)** may be requested on a patient with symptoms of **urinary tract infection (UTI).** When performing a urine culture, a measured portion of urine is transferred onto a special nutrient medium. The medium is incubated for 18 to 24 hours and then checked for bacterial growth. If an organism is identified, a sensitivity or **antibiotic susceptibility** test is performed to determine which antibiotics will be effective against the organism.

Urine for C&S must be collected in a sterile container (Fig. 13-1) after midstream **clean-catch** (see Collection Methods) procedures to ensure that the specimen is free of contaminating matter from the external genital areas.

Key Point ➤ Specimens for C&S and other microbiologic studies should be transported to the lab and processed immediately. If a delay in transportation or processing is unavoidable the specimen should be refrigerated.

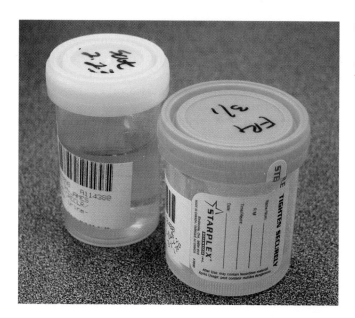

Urine specimens collected in sterile containers for C & S testing.

URINE CYTOLOGY STUDIES

Cytology studies are performed on urine to detect cancer, cytomegalovirus, and other viral and inflammatory diseases of the bladder and other structures of the urinary system. Because cells from the lining of the urinary tract are readily shed into the urine, a smear can be easily prepared from urinary sediment or filtrate. The smear is stained by the Papanicolaou (PAP) method and examined under a microscope for the presence of abnormal cells. A fresh, clean-catch specimen is required for the test. Ideally, the specimen should be examined as soon after collection as possible. If a delay is unavoidable, the specimen may be preserved by the addition of an equal volume of 50% alcohol.

URINE DRUG SCREENING

Urine drug screening is performed to detect illicit recreational drug use, use of anabolic steroids to enhance performance in sports, and unwarranted use of prescription drugs; to monitor therapeutic drug use to minimize withdrawal symptoms; and to confirm a diagnosis of drug overdose. With the exception of alcohol, urine is preferred for drug screening because many drugs can be detected in urine but not blood.

Screening tests are typically performed in groups based on drug families (see Chapter 11, Table 11-1). A random sample in a chemically clean, covered container is required for the test. Specimens containing blood cells or having a high or low urine pH (highly acid or alkaline) or a low specific gravity will yield erroneous results and will require recollection of the specimen. (For additional information see Forensic Specimens in Chapter 11.)

URINE PREGNANCY TESTING

Pregnancy can be confirmed by testing urine for the presence of human chorionic gonadotropin (HCG), a hormone produced by cells within the developing placenta that appears in serum and urine approximately 8 to 10 days after conception or fertilization.

Although a random urine specimen can be used for testing, the first morning specimen is preferred because it is more concentrated and therefore would have the highest HCG concentration. HCG also appears in the urine of patients with melanoma, tumors of the ovaries or testes, and certain types of cancer including breast, lung, and renal.

OTHER URINE TESTS

Numerous chemistry tests, including electrophoresis, tests for heavy metals (e.g., copper, lead), myoglobin clearance, creatinine clearance, and porphyrins, can be performed on urine specimens. Many of these tests require a pooled timed specimen such as a 24-hour collection.

Types of Urine Specimens

RANDOM

Random urine specimens are collected at any time. They are used primarily for routine UA and screening tests. Random refers only to the timing of the specimen and not the method of collection.

TIMED

Some tests require individual urine specimens collected at specific times. Others require the collection and pooling of urine throughout a specific time period. Some of the most frequently encountered timed urine tests are as follows.

First morning (8-hour)

A **first morning** or **8-hour** urine specimen is usually collected immediately upon awakening in the morning after approximately 8 hours of sleep. This type of specimen normally has a higher specific gravity, which means that it is more concentrated than a random specimen. For this reason, 8-hour specimens are often requested to confirm results of random specimens and specimens with low specific gravity.

Tolerance tests

Tolerance tests typically require the collection of urine at specific times. The standard glucose tolerance test requires individual urine specimens collected serially at specific times that correspond with the timing of blood collection, such as fasting, $\frac{1}{2}$ hour, 1 hour, and so on. Timing of the specimens is important in the interpretation of test results. For this reason, the specimens must be collected as close to the requested time as possible, and the label of the specimen should include the time of collection and the type of specimen (e.g., fasting, $\frac{1}{2}$ hour).

Twenty-four hour

A **24 hour** urine specimen is collected to allow quantitative analysis of a urine analyte. Collection of all urine voided in the 24-hour period is critical. The best time to begin a 24-hour collection is when the patient wakes in the morning, typically between 6 and 8 AM. Collection of the specimen requires a large, clean, preferably wide-mouth container capable of holding several liters (Fig. 13-2). A special collection device that fits

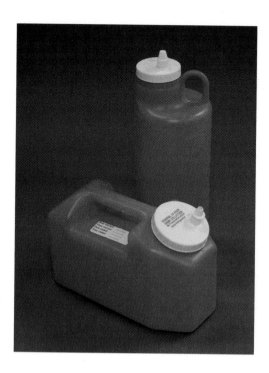

■ FIGURE 13-2 ■

Two styles of 24-hour urine specimen collection containers.

over the toilet and looks somewhat like an upside down hat is sometimes provided to the patient to make collection of the specimen easier. Some 24-hour specimens require the addition of a preservative before collection. Others must be kept refrigerated throughout collection. Information on proper handling of the specimen can be obtained by consulting the laboratory procedure manual. The label of the specimen, in addition to standard patient identification, must state that the specimen is a 24-hour specimen and, if applicable, the type of preservative added to the container and any precautions associated with it. The procedure for 24-hour urine collection is shown in Box 13-1.

Box 13-1

24-HOUR URINE COLLECTION PROCEDURE

1. Void into toilet as usual after awakening; note the time and date on the specimen container label and begin the timing.
2. Collect all urine voided for the next 24-hour period. Refrigerate the specimen throughout the collection period (except for urate testing). This can be accomplished by placing the specimen container in an ice chest placed in the bathtub, for example.

continued

3. To prevent contamination of the specimen by fecal material, it is best to urinate *before* having a bowel movement rather than after.
4. At the end of the 24-hour period, void one last time and add this specimen to the collection container.
5. Put the container in a portable cooler and transport the specimen to the lab as soon as possible.

Fractional (double-voided)

A **fractional** or **double-voided** specimen is collected to compare the urine concentrations of an analyte to its concentration in the blood. It is most commonly used to test urine for glucose and ketones. The procedure requires the patient to collect a urine specimen, emptying the bladder in the process. The time is recorded and the specimen is tested for the analyte. In the meantime, the patient drinks approximately 200 mL of water. Urine is given time to accumulate in the bladder for a specified time, commonly 30 minutes. At the end of the time period, another urine specimen is collected and tested for the analyte. Tolerance test urine specimens are also considered fractional specimens.

Urine Collection Methods

REGULAR VOIDED

A **regular voided** urine collection requires no special patient preparation and is collected by having the patient void (urinate) into a clean urine container.

MIDSTREAM

A **midstream** urine collection is performed to obtain a specimen that is free of genital secretions, pubic hair, and bacteria surrounding the urinary opening. To collect a midstream specimen, the patient voids the initial urine flow into the toilet. The urine flow is interrupted momentarily and then restarted, at which time a sufficient amount of urine is collected into a specimen container. The last of the urine flow is voided into the toilet.

MIDSTREAM CLEAN-CATCH

A **midstream clean-catch** urine is collected in a sterile container and yields a specimen that is suitable for microbial analysis or culture and sensitivity testing. Clean-catch procedures are necessary to ensure that the specimen is free of contaminating matter from the external genital areas. Special cleaning of the genital area is required before the specimen is collected. The cleaning methods vary somewhat depending upon whether the patient is male or female. A phlebotomist must be able to explain the proper procedure to both male and female patients. Clean-catch procedures are described in Box 13-2 for females and in Box 13-3 for males.

Box 13-2

CLEAN-CATCH PROCEDURES FOR FEMALE PATIENTS

1. Stand in a squatting position over the toilet.
2. Separate the folds of skin around the urinary opening. Cleanse the area around the opening with special towelettes (or sterile soapy cotton balls).
3. Cleanse the area again with clean towelettes (or water-soaked sterile cotton balls), wiping from front to back.
4. Void the first portion of urine into the toilet. Stop the urine flow momentarily, then resume the flow, and collect a portion of urine into the container, being careful not to touch the inside or lip of the container with the hands or any other part of the body.
5. Void the remainder of urine into the toilet.
6. Cover the specimen with the lid provided, touching only the *outside* surfaces of the lid and container.

Box 13-3

CLEAN-CATCH PROCEDURES FOR MALE PATIENTS

1. Wash hands thoroughly.
2. Cleanse the end of the penis with sterile, soapy cotton balls (or special towelettes) beginning at the urethral opening and working away from it (the foreskin of an uncircumcised male must first be retracted).
3. Repeat the above procedure using two successive sterile, water-soaked cotton balls (or clean towelettes).
4. Void the first portion of urine into the toilet. Stop the urine flow momentarily, then resume the flow and collect a portion of urine into the container. Be careful not to touch the inside or lip of the container with the hands or any other part of the body.
5. Void the remainder of urine into the toilet.
6. Cover the container with the sterile lid, touching only the *outside* surfaces of the lid and container.

CATHETERIZED

A **catheterized** urine specimen is collected from a sterile catheter inserted through the urethra into the bladder. A catheterized specimen is collected when a patient is having trouble voiding or is already catheterized for other reasons. Catheterized specimens are sometimes collected on babies to obtain a specimen for C&S, on female patients to prevent vaginal contamination of the specimen, and on bedridden patients when serial specimen collections are needed.

SUPRAPUBIC

A **suprapubic** urine specimen is collected in a sterile syringe by inserting a needle through the abdominal wall directly into the urinary bladder and aspirating the urine directly from it. The specimen is then transferred into a sterile urine container or tube. The procedure normally requires use of local anesthetic and is performed by a physician. If the patient has a catheter, the specimen can be collected from the catheter by a nurse using a sterile needle and syringe. Suprapubic collection is used for samples for microbial analysis or cytology studies. It is sometimes used to obtain uncontaminated samples from infants and young children.

PEDIATRIC URINE COLLECTION

A plastic urine collection bag with hypoallergenic skin adhesive is used to collect a urine specimen from an infant or small child that is not yet potty trained. The patient's genital area is cleaned and dried before the bag is taped to the skin. The bag is placed around the vagina of a female and over the penis of a male. A diaper is placed over the collection bag. The patient is checked every 15 minutes until an adequate specimen is obtained. The bag is then removed, sealed, labeled, and sent to the lab as soon as possible. A 24-hour specimen can be obtained by using a special collection bag with a tube attached that allows the bag to be emptied periodically.

Amniotic Fluid

Amniotic fluid is the clear almost colorless to pale yellow fluid that fills the membrane (amnion or amniotic sac) that contains a fetus within the uterus. It is preferably collected after 15 weeks of gestation and is obtained by transabdominal amniocentesis, a procedure that involves inserting a needle through the mother's abdominal wall into the uterus and aspirating approximately 10 mL of fluid from the amniotic sac.

Amniotic fluid can be analyzed to detect genetic disorders such as Down syndrome, hemolytic disease resulting from blood incompatibility between the mother and fetus, and to determine gestational age. However, the most common reasons for testing amniotic fluid are to detect problems in fetal development, particularly neural tube defects such as spina bifida, and to assess fetal lung maturity.

Genetic disorders can be detected by chromosome studies done on fetal cells removed from the fluid, although the procedure has for the most part been replaced by studies on chorionic villi or placental tissue because it can be obtained earlier in the gestational period than amniotic fluid. Hemolytic disease can be detected by measuring bilirubin levels.

Although ultrasonography has become the accepted means of estimating gestational age, amniotic fluid creatinine levels have been used to estimate gestational age because levels are related to fetal muscle mass.

Problems in fetal development can be detected by measuring **alpha-fetoprotein (AFP),** an antigen normally present in the human fetus that is also found in amniotic fluid and maternal serum. (AFP is also present in certain pathologic conditions in males and nonpregnant females.) Abnormal AFP levels may indicate problems in fetal development such as neural tube defects. AFP testing is initially performed on maternal serum and abnormal results are confirmed by amniotic fluid AFP testing. Because normal AFP levels are different in each week of gestation, it is important that the gestational age of the fetus be included on the specimen label. Fetal lung maturity can be assessed by measuring the levels of substances called phospholipids that act as surfactants to keep the alveoli of the lungs inflated. Amniotic fluid testing to assess fetal lung maturity may be ordered on or near the patient's due date and is often ordered STAT when the fetus is in distress.

Amniotic fluid is normally sterile and must be collected in a sterile container. The specimen should be protected from light to prevent breakdown of bilirubin, and delivered to the laboratory as soon as possible. Specimens for chromosome analysis must be kept at room temperature. However, specimens for some chemistry tests must be kept on ice. Follow laboratory protocol.

Cerebrospinal Fluid

Cerebrospinal fluid (CSF) is a clear, colorless liquid that circulates within the cavities surrounding the brain and spinal cord. CSF has many of the same constituents as blood plasma. Specimens are obtained by a physician; most often through lumbar (spinal) puncture. The primary reason for collecting CSF is to diagnose meningitis. Routine tests performed on spinal fluid include cell counts, chloride, glucose, and total protein. Other tests are performed if indicated. CSF is generally collected in three special sterile tubes numbered in order of collection. Laboratory protocol dictates which tests are to be performed on each particular tube, unless indicated by the physician. Normally, the first tube is used for chemistry and immunology tests, the second tube for microbiology studies, and the third tube for cell counts. CSF should be kept at room temperature, delivered to the lab stat and analyzed immediately.

Gastric Secretions/Gastric Analysis

Gastric secretions are obtained by aspiration via a tube passed through the mouth or nose, down the throat, and into the stomach. Gastric specimens are collected in sterile containers.

A **gastric analysis test** examines gastric acid secretions to determine gastric function in terms of stomach acid production. A basal tube gastric analysis involves aspirating a sample of gastric secretions by means of a tube passed through the mouth and throat (oropharynx) or nose and throat (nasopharynx) into the stomach after a period of fasting. This sample is tested to determine acidity before stimulation. After the basal sample has been collected, a gastric stimulant, most commonly histamine or pentagastrin, is administered intravenously and several more samples are collected at timed intervals. The role of the phlebotomist in gastric analysis testing is to assist in labeling specimens and to draw blood specimens for serum gastrin determinations.

Nasopharyngeal Secretions

Nasopharyngeal (NP) secretions are cultured to detect the presence of the microorganisms that cause diphtheria, meningitis, pertussis (whooping cough), and pneumonia. NP specimens are collected using a sterile Dacron or cotton-tipped flexible wire swab. The swab is inserted gently into the nose and passed into the nasopharynx. After it is in the nasopharynx, the swab is gently rotated, then carefully removed, placed into transport media, labeled, and transported to the lab.

Saliva

Saliva specimens are increasingly being used to monitor hormone levels and detect alcohol and drug abuse because they can be collected quickly and easily in a noninvasive manner. Numerous kits are available for collecting and testing specimens. Detection of drugs in saliva is a sign of recent drug use. Many saliva tests are point-of-care tests. However, saliva specimens for hormone tests are typically frozen to ensure stability and sent to a laboratory for testing.

Semen

Semen is analyzed to assess fertility and also to determine the effectiveness of sterilization after vasectomy. Semen specimens are collected in sterile containers similar to sterile urine containers. Semen specimens must be kept warm and delivered to the lab immediately.

Key Point ➤ A semen specimen should *never* be collected in a condom. Condoms often contain **spermicides** (substances that kill sperm) that invalidate test results.

Serous Fluids

Serous fluid is a pale yellow watery fluid found between the double-layered membranes that enclose the **pleural, pericardial,** and **peritoneal** cavities. It lubricates the membranes and allows them to slide past one another with minimal friction. The fluid is normally present in small amounts but volumes increase when inflammation or infection is present or when serum protein levels decrease.

Key Point ➤ Accumulation of excess serous fluid in the peritoneal cavity is called ascites (a-si' tez).

The fluid can be aspirated (withdrawn by syringe) if increased amounts are interfering with normal function of associated organs, or for testing purposes. A physician performs the procedure. Fluid withdrawn for testing is typically collected in EDTA tubes if cell counts or smears are ordered, oxalate or fluoride tubes for chemistry tests, and sterile containers for cultures. The type of fluid should be indicated on the specimen label. Serous fluids are identified according to the body cavity of origin as follows:

- Pleural fluid: aspirated from the pleural cavity surrounding the lungs
- Peritoneal fluid: aspirated from the abdominal cavity
- Pericardial fluid: aspirated from the pericardial cavity surrounding the heart

Sputum

Sputum specimens are sometimes collected in the diagnosis or monitoring of lower respiratory tract infections such as tuberculosis (TB). Sputum is mucus or phlegm that is ejected from the trachea, bronchi, and lungs through deep coughing. First-morning specimens are preferred because secretions tend to collect in the lungs overnight and a larger volume of specimen can be produced. The patient must first remove dentures if applicable, then rinse the mouth and gargle with water to minimize contamination with mouth flora and saliva. The patient then brings up the sputum through deep coughing into a special sterile container.

Key Point ➤ The patient must cough up material from deep in the respiratory tract and not simply spit into the container.

Specimens are transported at room temperature and require immediate processing upon arrival in the laboratory to maintain specimen quality.

Sweat

Sweat is analyzed for chloride content in the diagnosis of **cystic fibrosis,** primarily in children and adolescents younger than the age of 20 years. Cystic fibrosis is caused by a disorder of the exocrine glands, affecting primarily the lungs, liver, and pancreas. Patients with cystic fibrosis have abnormally high levels (2 to 5 times normal) of chloride in their sweat.

Chloride levels in sweat are measured by means of the **sweat chloride test.** The test involves transporting **pilocarpine** (a sweat-stimulating drug) into the skin by means of electrical stimulation **(iontophoresis)** from electrodes placed on the skin. Sweat is collected, weighed to determine the volume, and analyzed for chloride content.

Sweat specimens can also be used to detect illicit drug use. Sweat is collected on patches placed on the skin for extended periods, then tested for drugs.

Synovial Fluid

Synovial fluid is a clear, pale yellow viscous fluid that lubricates and decreases friction in moveable joints. It is normally present in small amounts but increases when inflammation is present. It can be tested to identify or differentiate arthritis, gout and other inflammatory conditions. It is typically collected in three tubes: EDTA or heparin for cell counts, identification of crystals, and smear preparation; a sterile tube for culture and sensitivity; and a nonadditive tube for macroscopic appearance, chemistry, and immunology tests, and to observe clot formation.

OTHER NONBLOOD SPECIMENS

Bone Marrow

Because it is the site of blood cell production, **bone marrow** may be aspirated or withdrawn and examined to detect and identify blood diseases. A bone marrow biopsy may be performed at the same time. To obtain bone marrow, a physician inserts a special large-gauge needle into the bone marrow in the iliac crest (hip bone) or sternum (breast bone). When the bone marrow is penetrated, a 10 mL or larger syringe is attached to the needle to aspirate 1.0 to 1.5 mL of specimen. A laboratory hematology technologist is typically present and makes special slides from part of the first marrow aspirated. Additional syringes may be attached to collect marrow for other tests such as chromosome studies or bacterial cultures. Part of the first sample may be placed in an EDTA tube for other laboratory studies. Remaining aspirate is sometimes allowed to clot and placed in formalin or other suitable preservative and sent to histology for processing and examination. In an alternate method, blood and particles from the EDTA tube are filtered through a special paper. The filtered particles are then folded in the paper and placed in formalin. If a bone marrow biopsy is also collected the cylindrical core of material obtained is touched lightly to the surface of several clean slides before being placed in a special preservative solution. The slides are air dried and later fixed with methanol and stained with Wright's stain in the hematology department. The biopsy specimen and several slides are sent to the histology department for processing and evaluation. The remaining slides including biopsy touch slides are sent to the hematology department for staining and evaluation under the microscope.

Breath Samples

Breath specimens are collected and analyzed in the detection of **Helicobacter pylori (H. pylori)**, a type of bacteria that secretes substances that damage the lining of the stomach, causing chronic gastritis and leading to peptic ulcer disease. One common breath test used to detect H pylori is the **C-urea breath test.** The test is based on the fact that H. pylori bacteria produce urease, an enzyme that breaks down urea. This enzyme is not normally present in the stomach. To perform the test, a baseline breath sample is collected, after which the patient drinks a special substance that contains synthetic urea. The urea contains a nonradioactive form of carbon called carbon-13. If H. pylori organisms are present, urease will be present and the urea will be broken down, releasing carbon dioxide (CO_2) that contains carbon-13, in the process. The CO_2 will be absorbed into the blood stream and exhaled in the patient's breath. The patient breathes into a special Mylar balloon or other collection device at specified intervals. The breath specimens are analyzed for carbon-13 content. If carbon-13 is found in amounts higher than those in the baseline sample, the bacteria are present in the stomach.

Feces (Stool)

Examination of **feces (stool)** is helpful in the evaluation of gastrointestinal disorders. Stool specimens can be evaluated for the presence of intestinal parasites and their eggs (ova and parasites [O & P]); checked for fat and urobilinogen content; cultured to detect the presence of pathogenic bacteria; and tested for the presence of **occult** (hidden) **blood** by means of the **guaiac** test.

Stool specimens are normally collected in clean, dry containers. They should be covered and sent to the laboratory immediately after collection. Special O & P specimen containers are available (Fig. 13-3). Most specimens, especially those for detection of parasites, should be kept at body temperature (37°C). Gallon containers, similar to paint cans, are used for 24-, 48-, and 72-hour stool collections for fat and urobilinogen; these specimens are refrigerated throughout the collection period.

Special test cards, such as Hematest (Miles Inc., Elkhart, IN) and Hemoccult (Smith-Kline Diagnostics, San Jose, CA), are often used by outpatients to collect stool specimens for occult blood. The patient is usually instructed to have a meat-free diet for 3 days before the test. Patients are then instructed to collect separate specimens for 3 successive days. Cards can be mailed or brought to the lab after collection.

Hair

Samples of hair are sometimes collected for trace and heavy metal analysis and the detection of drugs of abuse. Use of hair samples for drug testing is advantageous because hair cannot be easily altered or tampered with and is easy to obtain. Hair can show evidence of chronic drug use rather than recent use. Although use of hair for drug testing is on the rise, lack of standardization in this area has held up widespread acceptance.

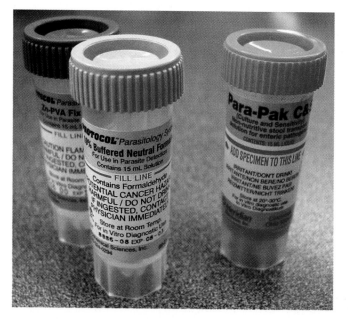

▓ FIGURE 13-3 ▓

Ova and parasite specimen containers.

Throat Swabs

Throat swab specimens are most often collected to aid in the diagnosis of streptococcal (strep) infections. Nursing staff typically collect throat swab specimens on inpatients. However, it is not unusual for phlebotomists to collect throat culture specimens on outpatients. A throat culture is collected in the following manner using a culture kit containing a sterile polyester-tipped swab and covered transport tube containing transport media (Fig. 13-4). The procedure for throat swab collection is shown in Box 13-4.

Box 13-4

THROAT CULTURE COLLECTION PROCEDURE

1. The patient is instructed to open his or her mouth wide while tilting the head back.
2. A small flashlight or other light source can be directed at the back of the throat to illuminate areas of inflammation. A tongue blade may be used to depress the tongue.
3. Both tonsils, the back of the throat, and any areas of ulceration, exudation, or inflammation should be brushed with the sterile swab, being careful not to touch the swab to the lips or tongue.
4. Because proper collection will often cause the patient to have a gag reflex or cough, the phlebotomist may wish to wear a mask or stand to the side of the patient.
5. After the specimen is collected, the swab is placed back into the collector tube. The ampule containing transport media is then crushed between the fingers and the swab embedded in the released media. The cover is secured and the specimen is properly labeled and sent to the lab immediately.

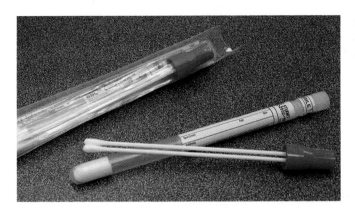

■ FIGURE 13-4 ■

Throat swab and transport tube.

Tissue Specimens

Tissue specimens from biopsies may also be sent to the laboratory for processing. Most tissue specimens arrive at the laboratory in formalin or suitable solution and need only to be accessioned and sent to the proper department. However, with more biopsies being performed in outpatient situations, a phlebotomist in specimen processing may encounter specimens that have not yet been put into the proper solution. It is important for the phlebotomist to check the procedure manual to determine the proper handling for any unfamiliar specimen. (For example, tissues for genetic analysis should *not* be put in formalin.) Improper handling may ruin a specimen from a procedure that is, in all probability, expensive, uncomfortable for the patient, and not easily repeated.

STUDY & REVIEW QUESTIONS

1. Additional information necessary on a nonblood specimen label includes the

   a. party to be charged.
   b. patient's diagnosis.
   c. physician.
   d. type of sample.

2. Which type of urine specimen is used to detect the presence of infection?

   a. 2-hour
   b. 24-hour
   c. Clean catch
   d. Midstream

3. Which of the following statements describes proper 24-hour urine collection?

   a. Collect the first morning specimen, start the timing, and collect all urine for the next 24-hour period, except the first specimen voided the following morning
   b. Collect the first morning specimen, start the timing, and collect all urine for the next 24-hour period, including the first specimen voided the following morning
   c. Discard the first morning specimen, start the timing and collect all urine for the next 24 hours except the first specimen voided the following morning
   d. Discard the first morning specimen, start the timing and collect all urine for the next 24 hours including the first specimen voided the following morning

4. Which nonblood specimen is most frequently analyzed in the lab?

   a. CSF
   b. Pleural fluid
   c. Synovial fluid
   d. Urine

5. Which of the following fluids comes from the lung area?

   a. Gastric
   b. Peritoneal
   c. Pleural
   d. Synovial

Continued

STUDY & REVIEW QUESTIONS *(CONTINUED)*

6. A procedure called iontophoresis is used in the collection of this specimen:
   a. Amniotic fluid
   b. CSF
   c. Saliva
   d. Sweat

7. Saliva specimens can be used to detect
   a. alcohol.
   b. drugs.
   c. hormones.
   d. all the above.

8. Which test typically requires a refrigerated stool specimen?
   a. Guaiac
   b. Occult blood
   c. Ova and parasites
   d. 72-hour fecal fat

9. A breath test can be used to detect organisms that cause
   a. meningitis.
   b. peptic ulcers.
   c. TB.
   d. whooping cough

10. Serous fluids come from the
    a. amnion.
    b. joints.
    c. spinal cavity.
    d. ventral body cavities.

■ CASE STUDY: 24-HOUR URINE SPECIMEN COLLECTION

A patient arrives at an outpatient lab with a 24-hour urine specimen. The specimen container is properly labeled and appears to hold a normal volume of urine. In speaking with the patient, however, the phlebotomist learns that the patient did not include the final morning specimen because he woke up several hours past the 24-hour collection deadline.

QUESTIONS:

1. Should the phlebotomist accept the specimen? Why or why not?
2. Should the specimen have been accepted if the patient had included the specimen that was several hours late? Why or why not?
3. What can be done to ensure that future 24-hour collections are handled properly?

Bibliography and Suggested Readings

Bishop, M., Duben-Engelkirk, J., & Fody, E. (2000). *Bishops clinical chemistry.* (4th ed.). Philadelphia: Lippincott Williams & Wilkins.

Burtis, C., & Ashwood, E. (2001). *Tietz, Fundamentals of clinical chemistry.* (5th ed.). Philadelphia: W. B. Saunders.

Fischbach, F. (2000). *A manual of laboratory & diagnostic tests* (6th ed.). Philadelphia: Lippincott Williams & Wilkins.

Harmening, D. (2002) *Clinical hematology and fundamentals of hemostasis* (4th ed.). Philadelphia: F. A. Davis.

Linne, J., & Ringsrud, K. (1999). *Clinical laboratory science, the basics and routine techniques* (4th ed.). St. Louis: Mosby, Inc.

National Committee for Clinical Laboratory Standards, GP16-A2. (2001). *Urinalysis and collection, transportation, and preservation of urine specimens, approved guideline* (2nd ed.). Wayne, PA: NCCLS.

14

COMPUTERS AND SPECIMEN HANDLING AND PROCESSING

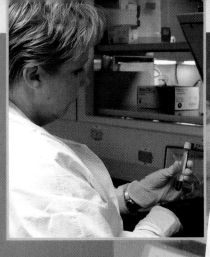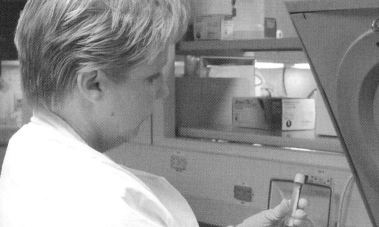

Upon successful completion of this chapter, the reader will be able to:

1 Define the key terms and abbreviations listed at the beginning of this chapter.

2 Describe components and elements of a computer, identify general computer skills, and define associated computer terminology.

3 Trace the flow of specimens through the laboratory with an information management system.

4 List information found on a computer label.

5 Define how barcodes are used in healthcare.

6 Describe specimen-handling procedures for routine specimens, and special handling procedures for specimens that are light or temperature sensitive.

7 Identify time constraints and exceptions for delivery of specimens.

8 Identify Occupational Safety and Health Administration (OSHA)–required protective equipment worn when processing specimens.

9 Describe the various steps involved in processing the different types of specimens and identify the criteria for specimen rejection.

COMPUTERIZATION IN HEALTHCARE

Introduction

Computers are very common in the United States and are an essential tool in healthcare today. The computer can now be found throughout all departments of a hospital, group practice, or health maintenance organization. Various types of computer hardware and software are being used to manage **data** (information collected for analysis or computation), monitor patients' vital signs, and, most recently, aid in diagnosis. With the sophisticated support that computers provide in the healthcare context, we see healthcare and computer technology becoming increasingly interrelated. There is no doubt that today's healthcare providers encounter computers on the job, making computer literacy a required skill in all areas of healthcare. To be considered "computer literate" an individual must be able to do the following:

1. Understand the computer and the functions it performs.
2. Perform basic operations to complete required tasks.
3. Demonstrate willingness to adapt to the changes that computers are making on the quality of life.

Computer technology comes with its own vocabulary. The terms listed in Table 14-1 represent a few of the more common ones used in a computer-oriented healthcare environment.

Computers range in size from large supercomputers that fill entire rooms to small, very convenient, hand-held models. A hand-held model is ideal for patient identification using barcode systems and paperless collection of data because it can go anywhere the patient may be.

Computer Networks

A computer network is a group of computers that are all linked for the purpose of sharing resources. In a computer network, individual computer stations are called *nodes*. The network interconnection allows all the computers to have access to each other's information or to a large database of information at a remote site through a special node called a server. The computers can be connected by coaxial cables, optical fibers, or standard telephone lines. These systems are also known as local area networks.

Networking can take the form of simple interoffice connections or complex systems between several organizations in different cities or across continents. A good example of a large and complex system is the Internet, in which computers all over the world (through the use of telephone lines, fiber optics, and satellite connections) can access multiple sites and unlimited information (Fig. 14-1). The advantage of networking for businesses, such as healthcare institutions, is its efficiency. The immediate access it provides speeds up processing, increases productivity and reduces costs.

The Internet has greatly expanded access and sharing of information. Most major manufacturers of laboratory analyzers have the capability to connect their computer via the Internet with an analyzer in their customer's laboratory, thus improving inventory management, quality control programs, and instrument maintenance by monitoring indicators through the Internet. This Web connection provides real-time inter-

Table 14-1

Common Computer Terminology

Term	Defintion
Accession number	A unique number generated when the test request is entered into the computer
CPU	Central processing unit
Cursor	Flashing indicator on the monitor
Data	Information collected for analysis or computation
Hardware	Equipment used to process data
Icon	Image that signifies a computer application (program or document)
ID code	A unique code used to identify a person for purposes of tracking
Input	Data entered into the computer
LIS	Laboratory information system
Logging on	Entering as a user on the system via a password
Mnemonic	Memory-aiding code or abbreviation
On-line	The computer is connected to the system and is operational
Output	Processed information generated by the computer
Password	Secret word or phrase used to enter the system
Peripherals	All additional equipment attached to the CPU
RAM	Random access memory; temporary storage of data in the memory of the CPU
ROM	Read-only memory; contains instructions for operation of the computer installed by the manufacturer
Software	Coded instructions required to control the hardware in the processing of data
Storage	A place for keeping data; outside the computer it is called secondary storage
Verify	To confirm or check for correctness of input

vention for times that an analyzer malfunctions by decreasing down time and increasing efficiency.

Computer Components

When operating any type of computer, the user will employ the three basic components of any system. These components provide a means to **input** information, a way to **process** information, and a method to **output** information.

Input

There are several ways to input or move information into a computer. The most common way is to use a keyboard, much like a typewriter keyboard with additional keys for computer functions. Other methods of input include a light pen designed to read information on the computer screen and scanners programmed to read barcodes.

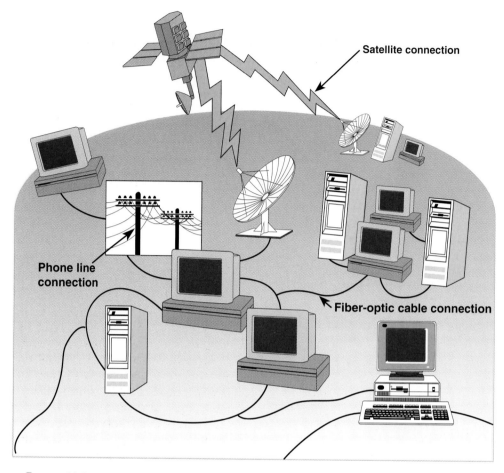

■ FIGURE 14-1 ■

Structure of the Internet. (Adapted from Carey, P., & Ambrosia, A. (1995). *The Internet*. Cambridge, MA: Course Technology)

Process

After information has been input, it is processed through a component called the **central processing unit (CPU).** The CPU, made up of many electrical components and microchips, has three elements as shown in Figure 14-2. The communications and control unit manages or oversees the processing and completion of each task required by the operator. The arithmetic and logic unit performs mathematical processes and makes decisions based on logical comparisons of input data. The third element, memory, may be of two types: **random-access memory (RAM)** and **read-only memory (ROM).** RAM serves as temporary storage for data that will be lost when the computer is shut off. If the information needs to be kept for a later date, the operator must transfer it to a hard drive, diskette, or compact disks (CDs). ROM storage, installed by the manufacturer, instructs the computer to carryout operations requested by the user.

Key Point ➤ ROM has characteristics of both hardware and software, so the term "firmware" has been applied to it to lessen confusion.

Output

Output describes the return of processed information or data to the user or to someone in another location. Just as there are several ways to input information, there are several means by which processed data can be received. One of the most common ways is through a printer. When data are printed on paper, they are said to be "hard copy." Another output device is the monitor, which looks like a television screen and displays data as they are entered and during the processing.

Elements of the Computer

There are three elements that make up computer systems. These elements are called hardware, software, and storage.

Hardware is the equipment that is used to process data and includes the CPU and peripherals (all additional equipment attached to the CPU) used for the input or output of information. Examples of hardware peripherals are keyboards, monitors, barcode readers, scanners, tablets, facsimile machines, printers, and modems (devices that transfer data to other computers over telephone lines). A monitor and keyboard combination is called a "terminal" (Fig. 14-3); these are necessary peripherals for most computers. With portable computers (laptops and hand-helds), the display and keypad are built into the device.

Software is the programming (coded instructions) required to control the hardware in processing of data. Two basic types exist: systems software and applications software. Systems software controls the normal operation of the computer. Applications software refers to programs prepared by software companies or in-house programmers to per-

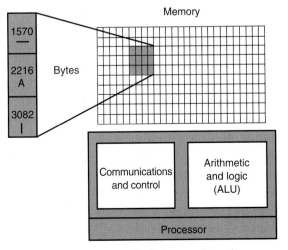

■ FIGURE 14-2 ■

The three elements of the central processing unit, showing memory bytes (characters of data) represented by blocks that have been assigned a unique location in RAM (random access memory). (Adapted from Trainor, D., & Krasnewich, D. (1994). *Computers!* New York: McGraw-Hill)

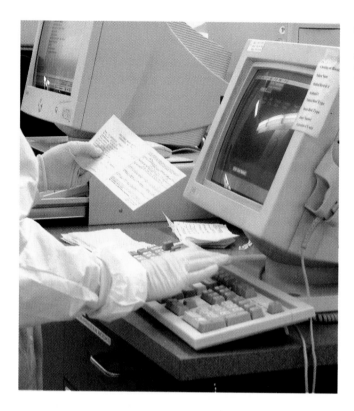

A computer terminal in the specimen-processing area of the laboratory.

form specific tasks required by users. Software applications come in five basic types: spreadsheets, communication systems, database systems, word processing, and graphics. Packages that perform more than one application, such as word processing, spreadsheet, and database, are called integrated software. The advantage of integrating applications is that it allows the different functions to be merged easily in one document.

Storage of information outside the CPU is necessary because RAM, as mentioned previously, is limited temporary storage, which will be lost when the computer is turned off. Storage outside the CPU is called secondary storage. Examples of permanent secondary storage devices for documents and programs are diskettes, external hard drives, magnetic tapes, cartridges, and CDs.

Computers and the Laboratory

As previously discussed, computers are accurate processors of information at incredible speeds. For this reason, computer systems in healthcare are considered more efficient and cost-effective than relying on manual methods. Today most analyzers in the laboratory have a sophisticated computer system that has been designed to manage patient data and **interface** (connect for the purpose of interaction) with the main hospital information system.

In the laboratory multiple computers can connect to each other and share data. There are two types of interfaces used in laboratory information systems (LIS). One is a unidirectional interface, which means information only goes one way, from the analyzer to the LIS computer. The second interface is bidirectional, meaning data can go back and forth between two systems. Competition between companies that sell laboratory information systems is based on the ease of input, the format of output, and the availability of customized software. Extensive research goes into selecting the right computer system for specific laboratory needs. After selecting a vendor, it will take several months to bring a system **online** (make it operational). Usually one or two people are put in charge of the system's daily operation; they are called "system managers." These individuals have the responsibility to train other personnel in the laboratory and keep them updated as changes are made to the software. They must readily develop troubleshooting skills as they solve day-to-day problems that develop after the system is installed.

Today's healthcare facility may be totally integrated (connected) through networking of computers and a common software system. Some point-of-care analyzers used outside of the main laboratory can be interfaced with data management systems, which in turn connect to the LIS.

This means that patient information can be accumulated in a central database and shared with ancillary services and any outside agency involved in that particular patient's care. A totally integrated system will have an "electronic chart" and will make a paperless facility possible.

Key Point ➤ Intranets (networks within companies) connect multiple LIS systems, and the Internet (network outside companies) connects them to the world.

General Computer Skills

General skills that the phlebotomist must learn, regardless of what LIS is used, involve the following.

Logging on. A person who is allowed to access a computer system is given a password. The password uniquely identifies that person and allows him or her to become a system user. The process of entering a password and gaining access to the system is called "logging on." Most systems require a username to be entered before the password. When the log-on sequence is completed, a **menu** is displayed listing the options from which the user may choose. For security and authorization purposes, most systems are designed to allow users unique access to different menus or programs.

Cursor movement. After logging on, a flashing indicator on the screen, called the **cursor,** indicates the starting point for input. When entering patient information in a LIS, the cursor will automatically reset itself at the correct point for data input after the **Enter** key has been pressed.

Using icons. Access to documents and software programs can be initiated by using the mouse to click on a small, representative image called an icon that opens a document or launches a software program.

Entering data. After necessary information has been input, the Enter key must be pressed for information to be processed. If an error in spelling or selection is made, it can easily be deleted by back spacing before pressing the Enter key. If the wrong information is entered, however, it is still possible to correct errors.

Correcting errors. This procedure is necessary to correct mistakes that are detected after the Enter key has been pressed. The procedure to delete errors is program-dependent and must be learned with each system. Some LIS programs use order verification, an additional step in the process, to allow a review of the information before it is accepted.

Verifying orders. After all patient information has been entered, it will appear on the monitor screen as a complete order. At this point, the user can review the information again and can choose to modify, delete, or accept it. When all orders have been entered, the user can request an inquiry of the orders as another check.

Making order inquiries. Selecting "order inquiry" allows the user to retrieve any or all the test orders associated with a patient.

Deleting orders. If, after entering an order, a user finds that it is incorrect, he or she can request the computer delete or reject it. The command "delete" can also be used when an order is canceled.

Laboratory Information Systems

The objectives of LIS are to file results, accumulate statistics to determine workload, generate report forms, and monitor quality assurance and quality control in the laboratory.

 Key Point ➤ There are multiple vendors and types of laboratory information systems on the market at this time. Those with more than 1,000 installation sites include Cerner Corporation/Cerner Citation/Cerner DHT, Medical Information Technology, INC (Meditech), and Misys, formerly Sunquest.

Each type of information system allows users to define their own parameters for terms and conditions that make the system unique to that facility. Several programs within the system allow the users to do specific tasks, seemingly at the same time, such as (1) admit patients, (2) request test orders, (3) print labels, (4) enter results, (5) inquire about results, and (6) generate reports.

ID Code

In laboratory settings, users are given an identification **(ID) code** and a password. Passwords are used for each individual to gain access to the system. Passwords must be kept strictly confidential because the security associated with each password determines what system functions can be accessed. Passwords are also logged with every transaction on the system, allowing the system manager to identify the person performing each transaction. Tech codes, on the other hand, are used to further identify each person entering data into the system, mainly for the purpose of accruing workload. ID codes are not always confidential because it is not always possible for phlebotomists to verify their own collections. A data entry clerk may verify all collections and must have access to the list of ID codes so that he or she can associate the proper phlebotomist with each draw.

Icons

The Cerner Millenium LIS uses icons (as in Windows MS) to request the appropriate program or function necessary to enter data. Other laboratory information systems may use a menu of **mnemonic** (memory-aiding) codes or a numeric system for selecting a function.

For example, in the Cerner Millenium Laboratory Information System a phlebotomist would select the "dept order entry" icon. This requisition entry program can be called by many different names, but it is basically the same procedure for any of the systems. During this data entry phase, an **accession number** is given to each requested order. This number is generated by the LIS when the specimen request is entered into the computer and will be identified with the specimen as long as it is in the laboratory.

To create labels and collection lists for the phlebotomist to use in collecting the appropriate samples, it is necessary to select another icon to either "label reprint" individual labels if not done at time of order entry or to generate or regenerate "order result viewer," which is a collection list by using the "collection list" icon. After collection has been accomplished, the phlebotomist returns to the laboratory and verifies the collection through another application, "specimen log-in." Other programs in the lab system that the phlebotomist might use are "order result viewer" to search for lab orders or results and "request a chart" to print or send a patient's report via fax.

A mnemonic code to identify the type and volume of tube required is always printed whenever a label is generated. For example, if the phlebotomist knows that a complete blood count is ordered and the code on the label reads 5.0 mL LAV, he or she knows what tube type to choose and the amount to draw. This demonstrates one of the benefits of computerized label generation; the label aids the phlebotomist in acquiring the proper specimen in a timely fashion (Fig. 14-4).

The steps an LIS uses for processing a typical specimen, from arrival in the lab through reporting of results, are shown in Figure 14-5.

Barcode

A barcode is a parallel array of alternately spaced black bars and white spaces representing a code. The code may represent numbers or letters. Some of the uses of barcodes in healthcare include identification of patients (barcoded ID bands), supply inventory, specimen identification, and pharmaceutical drug name, dose, and route. Many laboratory analyzers use barcode technology for specimen identification. A barcoded label, produced by the LIS on a bar code label printer as seen in (Fig. 14-6), is applied to the collected specimens, making specimen processing in the laboratory more efficient. Hand-held systems are being used to read barcoded patient identification bands and generate the labels used for specimen collection at the patient's bedside. One system that performs this function is the BD DX System from Becton Dickinson (Franklin Lakes, NJ).

 Key Point ➤ Computer technology makes sharing of information so easy that patient confidentiality can be violated. Congress took steps to eliminate confidentiality violation by enacting the Health Insurance Portability and Accountability Act (see

Chapter 1), which is designed to protect the privacy and security of patient information by standardizing the electronic transfer of data. This Act affects everyone involved in healthcare: patients, physicians and other healthcare personnel, healthcare organizations, vendors, and insurance companies.

Interfacing

Computers and the ability of computers to be able to talk to each other are important components in effective communication in healthcare. The Connectivity Industry Consortium (CIC) was recently established to ensure that any point-of-care (POC) analyzer could talk to any LIS, thereby standardizing all data management tools. This will make it possible for healthcare workers to ensure all POC testing they perform will be transferred to the computer and become part of the patient's chart. A guideline was developed by POC analyzer manufacturers, LIS vendors, and healthcare providers that resulted in the National Committee for Clinical Laboratory Standards (NCCLS) *Point-of-Care Connectivity, Approved Standard.*

■ FIGURE 14-4 ■

A computerized label generated when the requisition order is entered. (Cerner Corp., Kansas City, MO.)

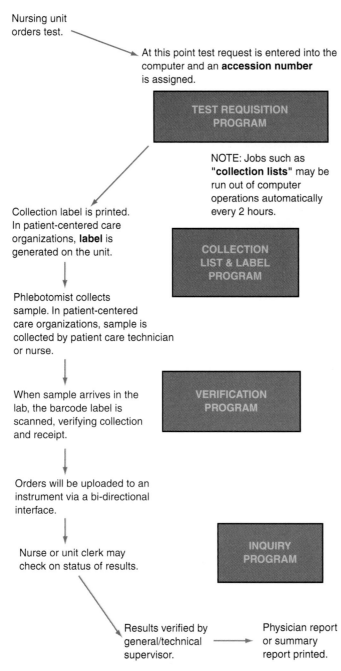

Nursing unit orders test.

At this point test request is entered into the computer and an **accession number** is assigned.

TEST REQUISITION PROGRAM

NOTE: Jobs such as **"collection lists"** may be run out of computer operations automatically every 2 hours.

Collection label is printed. In patient-centered care organizations, **label** is generated on the unit.

COLLECTION LIST & LABEL PROGRAM

Phlebotomist collects sample. In patient-centered care organizations, sample is collected by patient care technician or nurse.

When sample arrives in the lab, the barcode label is scanned, verifying collection and receipt.

VERIFICATION PROGRAM

Orders will be uploaded to an instrument via a bi-directional interface.

Nurse or unit clerk may check on status of results.

INQUIRY PROGRAM

Results verified by general/technical supervisor.

Physician report or summary report printed.

■ FIGURE 14-5 ■

Example of a workflow chart.

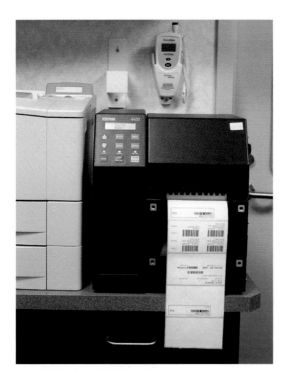

■ FIGURE 14-6 ■

Bar code label printer at the nursing station.

Computerization Trends

Current trends in healthcare indicate that clinical laboratory operations will continue to decentralize and that POC testing will increase. The need for complete networking becomes even more apparent as remote laboratory testing facilities increase in numbers. Large reference laboratories, totally separate from the hospital, will need to download results from automated instruments into patient charts or centralized databases. Barcode label systems for the identification of patients and their samples, medications, and supplies will decrease the risk of human error.

With the further development of microchip technology in POC analyzers, testing of patient specimens is being moved from the traditional laboratory to anywhere the patient might be. This new technology is referred to as a "lab-on-a-chip." Additionally, researchers are using the computer's ability to aggregate and analyze massive amounts of medical data. The outcome of this "artificial intelligence" will continue to revolutionize medicine.

SPECIMEN HANDLING

Introduction

As part of the computerization network that connects many aspects of patient care, the laboratory network tracks patient specimens from the time they are collected until the results are reported. The quality of those results, however, is dependent upon proper handling of the specimen in the preanalytical (before analysis) phase, which includes all the steps taken before the actual testing of the sample. Improper handling can render the most skillfully obtained specimen useless or cause erroneous test results, which in turn cause delays or incorrect care for the patient.

Unfortunately, it is not always easy to tell when a specimen has been handled improperly. Therefore, to assure delivery of a quality specimen for analysis, it is imperative that all phlebotomists be adequately instructed in this area so that established policies and procedures are followed. In addition, to protect the phlebotomist and others from accidental exposure to potentially infectious substances, all specimens should be handled according to the standard precautions guidelines outlined in Chapter 3.

Key Point ➤ Of interest is the fact that CLIA, the federal regulation governing all laboratories, does not address specimen handling even though it is estimated that 46% to 68% of all laboratory errors occur in the preanalytical phase.

General Guidelines

Preanalytical errors are those factors that are introduced into the specimen before and during collection, transport, processing, or storage that alter patient test results (Table 14-2). Because the scope in methodologies for the variety of tests performed is extensive, a phlebotomist must follow the specific procedures and policies defined by his or her laboratory to avoid errors and ensure that a quality specimen is made available for patient testing. These policies and procedures are found in the laboratory **user manual.** When a laboratory sends specimens to another laboratory (i.e., reference laboratory) for testing, the reference laboratory's user manual must be consulted for instructions on collection, handling, and transportation of those specimens.

Proper handling of specimens begins with the initiation of the test request and includes patient identification, preparation, equipment selection, and "order of draw," all covered elsewhere in this text. This chapter deals with proper handling after the specimen is collected until it is delivered to the proper lab area for testing.

Handling of Routine Specimens

Additive Tube Mixing

Additive tubes should be gently inverted three to eight times as soon as they are drawn. The required number of inversions depends upon the type of additive. Gentle inversion as in Figure 14-7 helps to evenly distribute the additive while minimizing the chance of hemolysis. Vigorous mixing may cause hemolysis and should be avoided. Examples of tests that cannot be performed on hemolyzed specimens include potassium, magnesium, and most enzyme tests. Inadequate mixing of anticoagulant tubes leads to microclot formation, which may cause erroneous test results, especially for hematology studies. Inadequate mixing of gel separation tubes may prevent the additive from functioning properly and clotting may be incomplete. Nonadditive tubes do not require mixing.

Table 14-2

Possible Sources of Preanalytical Errors

Prior to Collection	At Time of Collection	Specimen Transport	Specimen Processing	Specimen Storage
Patient treatments (i.e., intravenous medications, radioisotopes)	Misidentification of patient	Inappropriate temperature requirements	Failure to centrifuge specimens according to test requirements	Temperature change outside defined limits
Dehydration of patient	Wrong collection time	Delay preventing appropriate processing	Multiple centrifugations	
Wrong test ordered	Incorrect collection tube	Exposure to light	Rimming of clots	
Duplicate test	Expired tubes	Agitation causing hemolysis	Delay in separating cells from plasma/serum	
Incomplete requisition	Tourniquet tied more than 1 minute	Method of transport (i.e., hand delivery vs. pneumatic tube)	Aliquot mislabeled	
Fasting too long/too short	Nonsterile site preparation		Evaporation	
Strenuous exercise	Incorrect position of needle causing hemolysis		Contamination: dust or powder from gloves	
Altitude	Patient position		Incomplete centrifugation	
Age of patient	Incorrect order of draw			
Sex of patient	Inadequate volume of blood			
Pregnancy	Failure to mix tubes with additives			
Patient stress	Use of plasma separator tube or serum separator tube inappropriate			
Smoking	Mislabeling of tube			
Medications				

Transporting Specimens

Blood specimen tubes must be transported carefully. Rough handling can hemolyze specimens and can even lead to tube breakage. Tubes should be transported with the stopper up, which aids in clot formation of serum tubes, reduces agitation (which can cause hemolysis), and prevents contact of the contents of the tube with the tube stopper. Blood in contact with tube stoppers can be a source of specimen contamination and contributes to **aerosol** (a fine mist of the specimen) formation during stopper removal.

Nonblood specimens should be transported in leak-proof containers with adequately secured lids. Specimens transported through pneumatic tube systems as shown in Figure 14-8, should be protected from shock and sealed in zipper-type plastic bags to contain

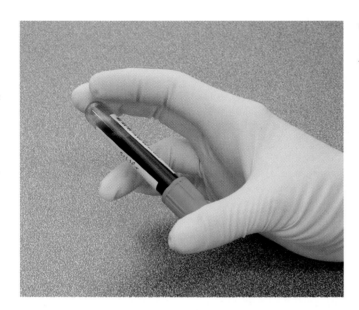

■ FIGURE 14-7 ■

Mixing of anticoagulated tube.

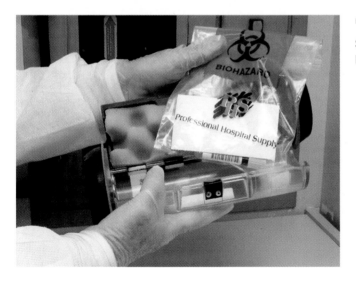

■ FIGURE 14-8 ■

Specimen received in pneumatic tube.

spills. NCCLS and Occupational Safety and Health Administration (OSHA) guidelines require specimen transport bags to have a biohazard logo, a liquid-tight closure, and a slip pocket for paperwork.

Specimens arriving in the lab from off-site locations by courier or mail systems need to be transported as defined by the Department of Transportation (DOT) and the Federal Aviation Administration (FAA) regarding packaging and transport. In addition, special care should be taken to protect specimens from the effects of extreme heat or cold.

Specimens Requiring Special Handling

Specimens Requiring Protection from Light

Some analytes (**analyte** is a general term for a substance undergoing analysis) are broken down in the presence of light, causing falsely decreased values. The most common of these is bilirubin. Other light sensitive analytes include vitamin C, B_{12}, B_2, B_6, carotene, serum, red cell folate, and urine porphyrins and porphobilinogen. Specimens can be easily protected from light by wrapping them in aluminum foil as shown in Figure 14-9. Light-inhibiting, amber-colored microcollection containers are available for collection of bilirubin specimens from infants.

Specimens that Need to be Chilled

Chilling slows down certain metabolic processes that continue even after a specimen is drawn. Specimens that require chilling should be completely immersed in a slurry of crushed ice and water (Fig. 14-10). The use of large cubes of ice without water added prevents adequate cooling of the entire specimen. Placing the specimen in contact with a solid piece of ice can cause parts of the specimen to freeze, resulting in hemolysis and possible breakdown of analytes. Table 14-3 lists examples of specimens that require chilling after collection.

Some tests require the specimen to be refrigerated or frozen for analyte stability. Remember to be aware of specimen processing instructions regarding centrifugation and separation of serum or plasma from the cells before refrigeration or freezing.

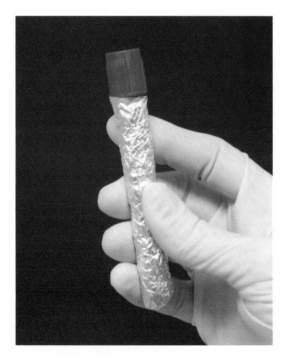

▩ FIGURE 14-9 ▩

Specimen wrapped in aluminum foil.

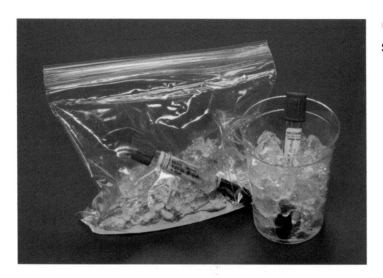

■ FIGURE 14-10 ■

Specimen in ice slurry.

Table 14-3

Examples of Specimens Requiring Chilling

Blood gases
Ammonia
Lactic acid
Plasma rennin activity
Glucagon

Key Point ➤ Some specimens such as potassium should not be chilled. When a potassium test is ordered with other analytes that require chilling, it should be collected in a separate tube.

Specimens that Need to be Kept Warm

Some specimens will precipitate or agglutinate if allowed to cool below body temperature after collection. These specimens need to be transported at or near the normal body temperature (37°C). In addition, some of these tests require the collection tube to be prewarmed to 37°C before collection of the specimen. Small, portable heat blocks that are kept in a 37°C incubator until needed and that hold this temperature for approximately 15 minutes after removal from the incubator are available for transporting temperature-sensitive specimens. Temperature-sensitive specimens that can withstand temperatures higher than 37°C can be wrapped in an activated heel warmer for transport (Fig. 14-11).

Some of the specimens that require body temperature transport are as follows:

• **Cryoglobulins,** abnormal serum proteins (globulins) that precipitate when cooled and dissolve when brought back to body temperature. Their presence is usually associated with immunologic diseases such as myeloma, chronic lymphocytic leukemia, chronic active hepatitis, and viral infections.

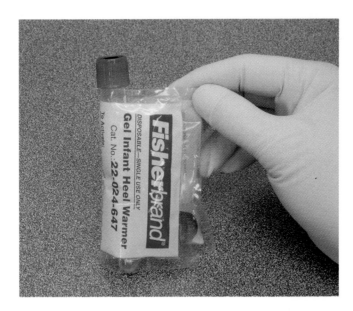

■ FIGURE 14-11 ■

Specimen wrapped in a heel warmer.

- **Cold agglutinin,** an antibody that attaches to red blood cells and causes them to clump together or agglutinate at temperatures below body temperature. Cold agglutinin antibodies are present in the serum of persons with *Mycoplasma pneumonia* (atypical pneumonia) and certain blood diseases such as hemolytic anemia. To prevent the antibody from attaching to the red blood cells, a cold agglutinin specimen must be collected in a tube prewarmed to 37°C and kept at this temperature until the serum is separated from the cells.
- **Cryofibrinogen,** an abnormal fibrinogen that precipitates when cooled and dissolves when brought back to body temperature. It is present in diseases associated with coagulation disorders and patients with cold intolerance.

Key Point ➤ It is important to familiarize yourself with the following temperatures related to specimen handling:

- Body temperature 37°C
- Room temperature 15°C-30°C
- Refrigerated temperature 2°C-10°C
- Frozen temperature −20°C or lower; some specimens require −70°C or lower.

Time Constraints for Specimen Delivery

All specimens should be transported to the lab promptly. Ideally, routine blood specimens should arrive at the lab within 45 minutes of collection and be centrifuged within 1 hour.

Guidelines recommended by NCCLS document H18-A set the maximum time limit for separating serum and plasma from the cells at 2 hours from time of collection. Less time is recommended for certain specimens, particularly potassium and cortisol specimens.

Prompt processing of specimens is easily achieved with an onsite lab, as in a hospital setting, but it is not always possible when specimens come to the lab from off-site locations, such as doctors' offices. Specimens that cannot reach their destination within the allotted time period should be allowed to clot (if applicable), then centrifuged, and the serum or plasma separated and transferred to a suitable container for transport.

If the specimens are drawn in serum separator tubes or plasma separator tubes (PSTs), they need only be centrifuged after they have clotted, if applicable (Fig. 14-12). After the tubes have been centrifuged, the separator gel prevents glycolysis for up to 24 hours. Applicable temperature requirements should be maintained until the specimens reach the laboratory.

Exceptions to the Preceding Guidelines

Specimens for glucose determination drawn in sodium fluoride tubes are stable for 24 hours at room temperature and up to 48 hours when refrigerated at 2°C to 8°C. Hematology tests drawn in lavender stopper (EDTA) tubes are performed on whole blood specimens and should never be centrifuged. EDTA specimens are stable for 24 hours. However, it is important to make smears from EDTA blood within 1 hour of collection to preserve the integrity of the blood cells and prevent artifact formation because of prolonged contact with the anticoagulant. "Stat" or "medical emergency" specimens take priority over all other specimens and should be transported and processed immediately.

 Key Point ➤ Prothrombin time results are reliable unrefrigerated and uncentrifuged for up to 24 hours after collection. Partial thromboplastin time requires analysis within 4 hours of collection regardless of storage conditions.

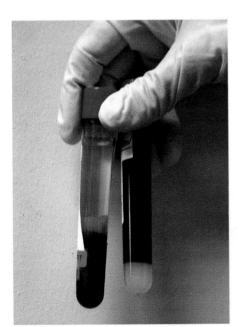

■ FIGURE 14-12 ■

Hemogard SSTs. (Becton Dickinson, Franklin Lakes, NJ.) *Right,* before being centrifuged. *Left,* after being centrifuged.

SPECIMEN PROCESSING

Protective Equipment

OSHA regulations require the wearing of protective equipment when processing specimens. Protective equipment includes gloves, fully closed lab coats or aprons, and protective face gear such as mask and goggles with side shields or chin-length face shields.

Central Processing

Most laboratories have a specific area commonly called **central processing** or triage (screening and prioritizing area) where specimens are received and prepared for testing. Here, the specimens are identified, logged and accessioned, and sorted by department and type of processing required. It is in this area that the specimens are accepted or rejected for analysis. The possible reasons for rejection of specimens are varied; Box 14-1 lists these criteria. Specimens not requiring centrifugation, such as urine and hematology specimens, are then distributed to the proper department. Specimens for tests requiring serum or plasma must be centrifuged as shown in Figure 14-13 and labels generated for the **aliquot** tube that will receive the serum or plasma obtained through centrifugation. (Aliquot is defined as a portion of the specimen used for testing.) Great care must be taken to match each specimen with the corresponding aliquot tube.

Plasma Specimens

Specimens for tests performed on plasma are collected in tubes containing anticoagulants and may be centrifuged without delay. For example, (Fig. 14-14) shows a specimen collected for prothrombin time that was immediately spun down using a StatSpin Express. PSTs are available to maintain specimen stability after centrifugation. Some laboratories use plasma in place of serum specimens for chemistry testing to reduce turnaround time

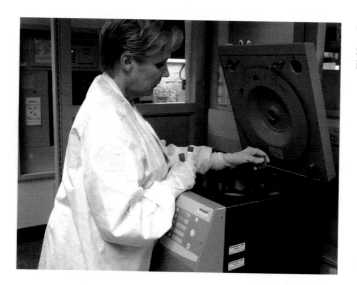

■ FIGURE 14-13 ■

Specimen processor loading a centrifuge.

Box 14-1

CRITERIA FOR SPECIMEN REJECTION

Specimens received by the lab may be rejected for analysis for the following reasons:

1. Inadequate, inaccurate, or missing specimen identification (e.g., a urine specimen that is not labeled).
2. Additive tubes containing an inadequate volume of blood (e.g., a partially filled coagulation tube).
3. Hemolysis (e.g., a hemolyzed specimen intended for potassium determination).
4. Wrong tube (e.g., a complete blood count [CBC] collected in a red top tube).
5. Outdated tube (e.g., a CBC collected in an expired tube.
6. Improper handling (e.g., a lavender top drawn for a CBC that has clots in it because of improper mixing).
7. Contaminated specimen (e.g., a urine for culture and sensitivity in an unsterile container).
8. Insufficient specimen, referred to as "quantity not sufficient" (QNS) for the test ordered (e.g., a specimen for an erythrocyte sedimentation rate submitted in a microtainer).
9. Collected at the wrong time (e.g., a specimen for therapeutic drug monitoring (TDM) collected before the drug was given).
10. Bilirubin specimens exposed to light. Bilirubin results can be 50% lower after 1 hour of exposure to light.
11. Delay in testing. For sedimentation rates an EDTA tube is only stable for 12 hours refrigerated and 4 hours at room temperature. Partial thromboplastin time older than 4 hours will give incorrect results.
12. Delay or error in processing. Serum tubes that have not been spun within 2 hours or refrigeration of serum tubes before centrifugation will increase some analytes such as potassium, creatinine, phosphorus, and LDH and decrease analytes such as glucose, ionized calcium, and carbon dioxide.

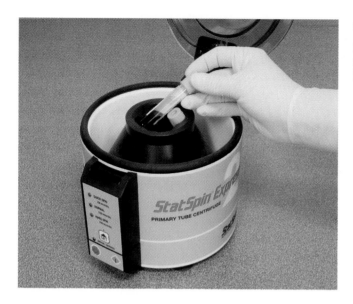

Prothrombin specimen after centrifugation in a StatSpin Express.

(TAT) because no time has to be spent waiting for the specimen to clot. Not all chemistry tests can be performed on plasma; therefore, follow established procedures.

Key Point ➤ Be aware of the type of anticoagulant in the PST and other heparin-containing tubes. For example, lithium heparin cannot be used for lithium levels, ammonium heparin cannot be used for ammonia levels, and sodium heparin cannot be used for sodium levels.

Serum Specimens

Specimens for tests performed on serum must be completely clotted before centrifugation. If clotting is not complete when the specimen is centrifuged, the resultant serum may clot and interfere with the performance of the test. Complete clotting normally takes approximately 30 to 45 minutes at room temperature. Specimens from patients on anticoagulant medication, such as heparin or dicumarol, and specimens from patients with high white blood counts, may take longer to clot. Chilled specimens may also take longer to clot. Serum separator tubes and other tubes containing clot-activating glass particles usually clot within 15 minutes. Thrombin tubes normally clot in 5 minutes. There are also several commercially available clot activators, which can be added to the tube after the specimen is drawn. Proper mixing of clot activator tubes will help ensure proper clotting.

Special Precautions for Handling Specimens

Stoppers should remain on tubes awaiting **centrifugation.** Removing the stopper from a specimen can cause a loss of carbon dioxide (CO_2) and an increase of pH, leading to inaccurate results for tests such as pH, CO_2, and acid phosphatase. In addition, leaving the stopper off exposes the specimen to possible contamination and evaporation. Sources of contamination can be as simple as a drop of sweat, which interferes with electrolyte results, or powder from gloves, which may interfere with calcium determinations (some powders contain calcium). Evaporation leads to inaccurate results because of concentration of analytes.

Centrifugation

Specimen preparation. After blood specimens have fully clotted, they may be centrifuged. A centrifuge is a device that spins the blood at a high number of revolutions per minute. The centrifugal force created causes the cells and plasma or serum to separate (Fig. 14-15). Tubes should remain capped during centrifugation to prevent contamination, evaporation, **aerosol** formation, and changes to pH.

If stoppers are removed for aliquoting, the tubes should be recapped or covered with suitable closure devices after completion. Use of applicator sticks to "rim" or release a clot is a potential source of contamination as well as hemolysis and is no longer recommended.

Centrifuge operation. It is imperative that equal-size tubes with equal volumes of specimen be placed opposite one another or "balanced" in the centrifuge. An unbalanced centrifuge may break specimen tubes, ruining specimens and causing the contents to form aerosols. The lid to the centrifuge should remain closed

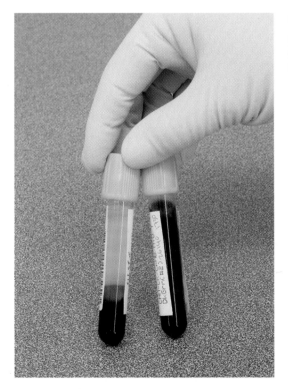

■ FIGURE 14-15 ■

Sodium citrate tubes. *Left,* after being centrifuged. *Right,* before being centrifuged.

during operation and should not be opened until the rotor has come to a complete stop. Newer centrifuges do not allow the user the capability of opening the centrifuge until the rotor has completely stopped.

Centrifuge each specimen only once. Repeated centrifugation can cause hemolysis and analyte deterioration and alter test results. In addition, after the serum or plasma has been removed, the volume ratio of plasma to cells changes. Because a centrifuge generates heat during operation, specimens requiring chilling should be processed in a temperature-controlled refrigerated centrifuge.

Stopper Removal

Some testing instruments sample the specimen directly from the collection tube through the stopper. For those that do not, the stopper has to be removed to obtain the serum or plasma needed for testing. Stoppers can be removed using commercially available stopper removal devices or by use of robotics. When not using such a device, the stoppers should first be covered with a 4 × 4-inch gauze or tissue to catch any aerosol that may be released or the tube should be held behind a "splash shield" safety device. The stopper should be pulled straight up and off and not "popped." Becton Dickinson manufactures a different type of stopper for evacuated tubes that does not require gauze or other devices to contain the spray. This tube stopper system is called Hemogard (Becton Dickinson, Franklin Lakes, NJ) (Fig. 14-16) and is designed to protect personnel from splatters and aerosols caused by blood that remains on the stopper or around the outer rim of the tube.

Aliquot Preparation

Serum or plasma should be transferred into aliquot tubes using disposable transfer pipets as shown in Figure 14-17. Pouring specimens into aliquot tubes increases the

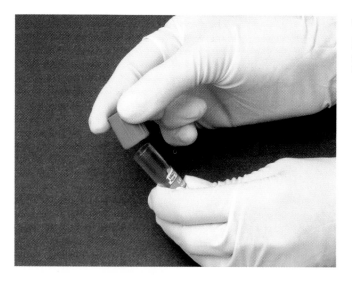

■ FIGURE 14-16 ■

Examples of a Hemogard closure tube. (Becton Dickinson, Franklin Lakes, NJ)

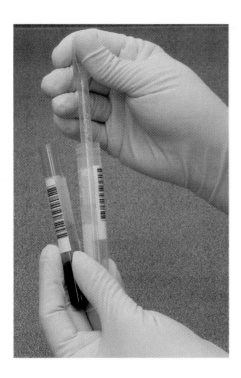

■ FIGURE 14-17 ■

Aliquoting a sample.

possibility of aerosol formation or splashing and is not recommended. OSHA's *Occupational Exposure to Bloodborne Pathogens: Final rule,* published in December 1991, states "All procedures involving blood or potentially infectious materials shall be performed in such a manner as to minimize splashing, spraying, splattering, and generation of droplets of these substances." After the serum or plasma is transferred into the aliquot tube, the tube is covered or capped.

 Key Point ➤ Serum or plasma from specimens with different additives should never be placed in the same aliquot tube.

STUDY & REVIEW QUESTIONS

1. Peripherals on a computer include all of the following *except* a
   a. barcode reader.
   b. scanner.
   c. modem.
   d. CPU.

2. Logging on to most computer systems requires the use of a/an:
   a. accession number.
   b. barcode reader.
   c. modem.
   d. password.

3. After arriving in the laboratory, all specimens are immediately
   a. centrifuged to stop glycolysis.
   b. logged or accessioned.
   c. refrigerated until delivered to the appropriate department.
   d. uploaded to an instrument for analysis.

4. All of the following are found on a lab generated computer label except
   a. accession number.
   b. patient identification.
   c. department for testing.
   d. ordering physician.

5. Barcoding in healthcare is used for all of the following except
   a. bidirectional interfacing.
   b. drug administration.
   c. labeling and supply inventory.
   d. physical location of the patient.

6. Which of the following specimens should be protected from light?
   a. BUN
   b. Complete blood count (CBC)
   c. Bilirubin
   d. Glucose

7. The machine used to separate the serum or plasma from blood samples is called a/an
   a. Autolet.
   b. centrifuge.
   c. glucometer.
   d. hemostat.

8. After obtaining a plasma renin activity level, the blood must be transported
   a. as "stat."
   b. away from light.
   c. in ice.
   d. at body temperature.

Continued

STUDY & REVIEW QUESTIONS *(CONTINUED)*

9. Contamination with perspiration could falsely elevate which blood levels?

    a. Amylase
    b. Calcium
    c. Chloride
    d. Magnesium

10. Which of the following instances would *not* be a reason for a specimen to be rejected for analysis?

    a. A CBC collected in a lavender top tube
    b. A specimen for potassium determination that is hemolyzed
    c. A protime specimen in a partially filled tube
    d. A specimen lacking an identification label

11. According to NCCLS guidelines, serum for analysis should not be in contact with cells for longer than

    a. 30 minutes.
    b. 60 minutes.
    c. 90 minutes.
    d. 120 minutes.

12. All of the following are required personal protective equipment when processing specimens except

    a. a chin-length face shield.
    b. a fully closed impervious lab coat.
    c. impervious shoe covers.
    d. gloves.

■ CASE STUDY: MISSING RESULTS

Nurse Susan collected blood for blood urea nitrogen (BUN) and creatinine tests on patient Mr. Jones in bed 201 at 9:30 AM, and sent the specimen to the lab. At 10:30, Susan calls the lab and states she is not able to find Mr. Jones' results in the computer. The technologist, Frank, tells Susan he does not have a specimen with that name on it; however, he did run a BUN and creatinine on patient Betty Smith in bed 202 drawn at 9:30 AM by Susan. Susan says there could not have been an error because she labeled the specimen with the only label she found on the barcoded label printer at the time.

QUESTIONS:
1. What do you think has happened to Mr. Jones' specimen?
2. Why does the lab have results on Mrs. Smith?
3. What steps should Susan take to get the results on Mr. Jones?
4. What is to be done with the results on Mrs. Smith?

Bibliography and Suggested Readings

Advance Laboratory. (February 2002). *10th Annual Information Systems Buyers Guide.* King of Prussia, PA.

Biosite Diagnostics. (July 1996). *Triage panel for drugs of abuse assay manual.* San Diego, CA.

Bishop, M. L., Duben-Engelkirk, J. L., & Fody, E. P. (1992). *Clinical chemistry: Principles, procedures, correlations* (2nd ed.). Philadelphia: J. B. Lippincott.

CAP TODAY. (January 1999). Intranet technology seeping into laboratories.

Carraro, P. M. (1997). Mistakes in a stat laboratory: Types and frequency. *Clinical Chemistry 43*(8), 1348–1351.

Clinical Lab Products. (1999). Medical World Communications. *Clinical Lab Products 28*(9).

Department of Transportation. Hazardous Materials Regulations; Title 49, Code of Federal Regulations, Parts 100-185. 2001.

Henry, J. B. (1996). *Clinical diagnostic and management of laboratory methods* (19th ed.). Philadelphia: W. B. Saunders.

HIPPA, Health Insurance Portability and Accountability Act. (August 17, 2000). *Federal Register.*

Jacobs, D., DeMott, W., Oxley, D. (1994). *Laboratory test handbook* (3rd ed.). Hudson, OH: Lexi-Comp Inc.

Joint Commission on the Accreditation of Healthcare Organizations (JCAHO). (2001). *2001 Accreditation manual for hospitals.* Oakbrook Terrace, IL: JCAHO.

National Committee for Clinical Laboratory Standards, H18-A. (December 1999). *Procedures for the handling and processing of blood specimens.* Wayne, PA: NCCLS.

National Committee for Clinical Laboratory Standards, H21-A3. (December 1999). *Collection, transport and preparation of blood specimens for coagulation testing and general performance of coagulation assays.* Wayne, PA: NCCLS.

National Committee for Clinical Laboratory Standards, POCT1. (2001). *Point of care connectivity, approved standard.* Wayne, PA: NCCLS.

Occupational Safety and Health Administration. (1991). *Occupational exposure to bloodborne pathogens; Final Rule.* 29 CFR 1910.1030. *Federal Register* (December 6), 6404–6418.

Occupational Safety and Health Administration. (2001). *Occupational exposure to bloodborne pathogens: Needlestick and other sharps injuries; Final Rule.* 29 CFR 1910. *Federal Register* (January 18), 5318–5325.

Quest Diagnostics Nichols Institute. (April 2001). *Reference manual.*

Wilson, D. D. (1999). *Nurses' guide to understanding laboratory and diagnostic tests.* Philadelphia, PA: Lippincott Williams & Wilkins.

GLOSSARY

ABGs: arterial blood gases

ABGT: ancillary blood glucose testing

ABO blood group system: a genetically determined blood group system that recognizes four blood types: A, B, AB, and O, based on the presence or absence of the A and B antigens on the red blood cells

accepting assignment: when a provider agrees to accept a fixed amount from an insurer as payment in full for a given service

accession number: a unique number given to each test request

accreditation: the process by which a professional or governmental agency evaluates an educational institution according to accepted criteria or standards to assure that graduates are qualified for professional employment

ACD: acid citrate dextrose

acid citrate dextrose (ACD): an additive that is used for certain immunohematology tests such as DNA testing and HLA phenotyping used in paternity evaluation and to determine transplant compatibility. It acts as both a red blood cell nutrient and a preservative by maintaining red cell viability

ACT: activated coagulation time

activated coagulation time (ACT): also referred to as activated clotting time, this procedure tests the activity of the intrinsic coagulation factors and is used to monitor heparin therapy

additive: any substance such as an anticoagulant, antiglycolytic agent, separator gel, cell preservative, or clot activator added to a blood collection tube. Additives do not include tube or closure coatings

aerobic: with oxygen

aerosol: a substance released in the form of a fine mist

agglutinate: clump together

agglutination: an antigen–antibody reaction that causes clumping (such as seen when antibodies attach to antigens on the surface of the RBCs of a different blood type)

agglutinins: antibodies present in the plasma of a person's blood that will react against and agglutinate RBCs carrying antigens of a different blood type

agranulocytes: WBCs lacking easily visible granules

AHCCCS: Arizona Health Care Cost Containment System

airborne precautions: precautions to follow in addition to standard precautions for patients known or suspected to be infected with microorganisms transmitted by airborne droplet nuclei. Anyone entering the room of a patient with airborne precautions must wear an N95 respirator

albumin: a plasma protein manufactured by the liver that functions to help regulate osmotic pressure of the blood

aliquot: a portion of a sample used for testing

Allen test: a test performed to ascertain collateral blood flow to the hand prior to performing radial ABCs

alveoli: thin-walled, sac-like chambers in the lungs where the exchange of O_2 and CO_2 takes place between the air and blood

ambulatory care: care provided outside of inpatient institutions, or "care for the walking client"

Ambulatory Patient Classification (APC): a new classification system for determining payment to hospitals for outpatient services

American Medical Technologists (AMT): an organization that approves phlebotomy programs, certifies phlebotomy personnel, and provides continuing education in phlebotomy

American Society for Clinical Laboratory Sciences (ASCLS): Organization that provides continuing education in phlebotomy

American Society of Clinical Pathologists (ASCP): Certifying agency and professional organization for laboratory personnel

American Society for Medical Technology (ASMT): Professional organization for laboratory personnel

American Society for Phlebotomy Technicians (ASPT): Certifying agency and professional organization for phlebotomists

amniotic fluid: the liquid in the amniotic sac that surrounds and cushions the fetus

AMT: American Medical Technologists

anabolism: The process by which the body converts simple compounds into complex substances needed for the cellular activities of the body.

anaerobic: without oxygen

analyte: a general term for a substance undergoing analysis

anatomic position: a way of referring to the body or body parts when the patient is standing erect, arms at the side, with palms and eyes facing forward

anatomy: study of the structural components of the body

anchor: to grasp an area of the body 1 to 2 inches below the intended venipuncture site with the nondominant hand, using your thumb to pull the skin taut

ancillary blood glucose testing: instant or "rapid" glucose testing commonly performed using small, portable glucose analyzers. Also called bedside glucose testing

anemia: an abnormal reduction in the number of RBCs in the circulating blood

aneurysm: a localized dilation or bulging in the wall of a blood vessel, usually an artery

antecubital fossa: the area of the arm located anterior to and below the bend of the elbow, where the major veins for venipuncture are located

antecubital veins: major superficial arm veins located in the antecubital fossa

anterior: also called ventral, refers to the front

antibody: protein substance manufactured by the body as a response to a foreign protein or antigen and directed against it

antibiotic susceptibility: procedure to determine the ability of an antibiotic to slow or stop the growth of a specific microorganism

anticoagulant: a substance that prevents blood from clotting

antigen: a substance that causes the formation of antibodies that are directed against it

antiglycolytic agent: a substance that inhibits the metabolism of glucose by the cells of the blood. The most common antiglycolytic agents are sodium fluoride and lithium iodoacetate

antimicrobial removal device (ARD): a blood culture bottle containing a resin that removes antimicrobials (antibiotics) from the specimen

antimicrobial therapy: use of chemical substances to kill or stop the growth of microorganisms

antiseptics: bacteriostatic solutions that are used to clean the skin before venipuncture or skin puncture

anuclear: without a nucleus

aorta: the largest artery in the body, arising from the left ventricle of the heart and approximately 1 inch (2.5 cm) in diameter

APC: Ambulatory Patient Classification

approval: a process similar to accreditation

ARD: antimicrobial removal device

arm/wrist band: the patient's identification bracelet which normally lists the patient's name and hospital identification number or medical record

Arizona Health Care Cost Containment System (AHCCCS): a unique form of public welfare offered by the state of Arizona to replace Medicaid

arrhythmia: an irregularity in the heart rate, rhythm, or beat

arterial blood gases (ABGs): an evaluation of arterial blood to provide valuable information about a patient's oxygenation, ventilation, and acid-base balance, which is needed for the diagnosis and management of respiratory disease

arteries: thick-walled vessels that carry blood away from the heart

arterioles: the smallest branches of arteries

arteriosclerosis: a disease that involves thickening, hardening, and the loss of elasticity of artery walls

arteriospasm: involuntary contraction of an artery

ASAP: as soon as possible

ASCLS: The American Society for Clinical Laboratory Sciences

ASCP: American Society for Clinical Pathology

ASMT: American Society for Medical Technology

ASPT: American Society for Phlebotomy Technicians

assault: an intentional threat or movement that could make a person feel in danger of harmful physical contact

atherosclerosis: a form of arteriosclerosis involving changes in the intima of the artery due to an accumulation of lipid material

atria: The upper chambers on each side of the heart which receive blood before it enters the ventricles.

atrioventricular (AV) node: a structure located in the lower right atrium of the heart that slows conduction of the electrical pulse generated by the sinoatrial node, creating a slight delay before electrical impulses are carried to the ventricles

atrioventricular valves: valves at the entrance of the ventricles

autologous donation: the process by which a person donates blood for his or her own use

AV bundle (bundle of His): a group of cardiac muscle fibers that form part of the electrical impulse-conducting system of the heart

A-V shunt: Arteriovenous passage artificially constructed to divert blood flow

avascular: containing no blood vessels

avulsion: forcibly tearing away of a part or structure

bacteremia: bacteria in the blood

bactericidal: an agent that destroys bacterial microorganisms

bacteriostatic: prevents or inhibits the growth of bacteria

barcode: a series of black and white stripes of varying widths corresponding to letters and numbers; the stripes can be grouped together to represent patient names, identification numbers, or laboratory tests

barriers: things that impede, block, obstruct, or separate; as in communication barriers that interfere with messages between senders and receivers, chemical and physical barriers that prevent glycolysis, and protective barriers that reduce the likelihood of exposure to bloodborne pathogens

basal state: metabolic state early in the morning, while the body is still at rest, and approximately 12 hours after the last intake of food, exercise, or activity

basilic vein: the large vein on the inner side of the arm in the antecubital fossa; the third-choice vein for venipuncture

basophils: the least numerous of the WBCs, comprising less than 1% of the WBC population. The granules of basophils are large, stain dark blue, and often obscure the nucleus

battery: intentional, unconsented-to physical contact with one person by another person

BBP: bloodborne pathogen

bedside manner: the behavior of a healthcare provider as perceived by a patient. Positive bedside manner puts a patient at ease.

bevel: the point of the needle that has been cut on a slant for ease of entry

biconcave: indented from both sides

biohazard: anything that is potentially harmful to the environment and man

bleeding time (BT): the time required for blood to stop flowing from a standardized incision. The BT is dependent on platelet plug formation in the capillaries, and is measured to determine platelet and vascular function

bloodborne pathogen (BBP): a term applied to any infectious microorganism present in the blood and other body fluids and tissues

bloodborne pathogen standard: OSHA's regulations for all employees with occupational exposure to pathogens found in the blood

blood pressure: a measure of the force exerted by the blood on the walls of blood vessels

blood smear: a drop of blood spread into a thin film on a microscope slide; also called a blood slide

blood volume: an individual's calculated amount of blood based on his or her body weight. In adults it is calculated on 70 mL of blood per kilogram of body weight, and in infants, on 100-110 mL per kilogram of body weight

B-lymphocytes: WBCs that give rise to plasma cells, which produce antibodies

body cavities: large hollow spaces that house various organs of the body

body fluids: fluids in the body that are found within the cell, outside of the cell, and some around and across the cell. Examples of body fluids other than blood are urine and cerebrospinal, amniotic, and serous fluids. The chemical composition of these fluids in the various areas is carefully regulated

body plane: a flat surface determined by making a real or imaginary cut through a body in the normal anatomic position

body substance isolation (BSI): a type of infection control precautions that preceded standard precautions. BSI differed from universal precautions by requiring glove use when contacting *any* moist body substance.

brachial artery: main artery of the arm, which is located in the medial anterior aspect of the antecubital fossa near the insertion of the biceps muscle

bradycardia: a slow heart rate, less than 60 beats per minute

breach of confidentiality: an unauthorized release of information concerning a patient

BSI: body substance isolation

BT: bleeding time

bundle of His: part of the electrical conduction system of the heart. It is located between the ventricles, and conducts impulses from the AV junction to the right and left bundle branches

butterfly needle: also called a winged-infusion needle system; made up of a small needle attached to a thin tubing with an adapter at one end that can used with a syringe or evacuated tube system for venipuncture

calcaneus: heel bone

calcium (Ca): a mineral that is essential to the clotting process and also needed for proper bone and teeth formation, nerve conduction, and muscle contraction

CAP: College for American Pathologists

capillaries: tiny vessels, one cell layer thick, that connect the arterioles and venules and allow the exchange of oxygen and nutrients between the cells and the blood

capillary action: process by which blood is drawn up, by contact only, into a small tube

capillary blood gases: blood gas determinations performed on arterialized capillary (skin puncture) specimens

capitation: a method of reimbursement in which the provider is paid an established fee for each patient in a panel or group of assigned patients

carbaminohemoglobin (HbCO$_2$): hemoglobin combined with CO_2

cardiac cycle: one complete contraction and subsequent relaxation of the heart, with each cycle lasting approximately 0.8 seconds

cardiac output: the volume of blood pumped by the heart in 1 minute: approximately 5 liters per minute

cardiopulmonary resuscitation (CPR): revival of heart and lung activity after they have stopped functioning

catabolism: the process by which complex substances are broken down into simple substances

catheter: a tube passed through the body for injecting or withdrawing fluids from body cavities or blood vessels

catheterized: a term that describes a urine specimen collected from a sterile catheter inserted through the urethra into the bladder

cathode ray tube (CRT): monitor or screen for displaying computer output

causative agent: the pathogen responsible for causing an infection; also referred to as an infectious agent

CDC: Centers for Disease Control and Prevention

Celsius: a temperature scale on which melting point is 0 degrees and boiling point is 100 degrees. Normal body temperature expressed in Celsius (or Centigrade) is 37 degrees. Also known as the Centigrade scale

Centers for Disease Control and Prevention (CDC): a division of the U.S. Public Health Service that investigates diseases that have epidemic potential

Center for Medicare and Medicaid Services (CMS): an agency of the U.S. Department of Health and Human Services that manages the federal Medicare and Medicaid programs; formerly the Health Care Financing Administration

Centigrade: *see* Celsius

central processing: also called specimen processing; where all specimens are received and prepared for testing

central processing unit (CPU): handles input/output (i.e., manipulation and calculation of data)

centrifugation: a process of separating substances of different densities, such as blood and urine, by using a centrifuge (a machine that spins substances at high speeds)

cephalic vein: the second-choice vein for venipuncture, located in the lateral aspect of the arm in the antecubital fossa

cerebrospinal fluid (CSF): a clear, colorless liquid that circulates in the cavities surrounding the brain and spinal cord, which has many of the same constituents as blood plasma

certification: a process that indicates the completion of defined academic and training requirements, and the attainment of a satisfactory score on a national examination

CEUs: continuing education units

chain-of-custody: special protocol for forensic specimens that must be strictly followed; requires documentation that the specimen is accounted for at all times

chain of infection: a series of related events that leads to infection

chordae tendineae: thin threads of tissue that attach the AV valves to the walls of the ventricles

circulatory system: also called the cardiovascular system; consists of the heart, blood, and blood vessels, along with the lymph, lymph vessels, and nodes (lymphatic system)

citrate-phosphate-dextrose (CPD): an additive used in collecting units of blood for transfusion purposes. The citrate serving as an anticoagulant, the phosphate stabilizes the pH, and the dextrose provides energy to the cells to keep them alive

civil law: the law of private rights between persons or parties

clean-catch: method of obtaining a urine sample so that it is free of contaminating matter from the external genital areas

CLIA '88: Clinical Laboratory Improvement Amendments

Clinical Laboratory Improvement Amendments (CLIA '88): a federal law signed in 1988, mandating that all laboratories be regulated using the same standards—regardless of their location, type, or size

clot activator: clot-enhancing substance, such as siliceous earth, silica, or celite

CMS: Center for Medicare and Medicaid Services

coagulation: blood-clotting process

coinsurance: a predetermined percentage of the bill in an indemnity plan that is the patient's portion. In HMOs, this portion is called a copayment.

cold agglutinin: an antibody that attaches to red blood cells and causes them to clump together or agglutinate at temperatures below body temperature

collapsed vein: an abnormal retraction of the vessel walls

collateral circulation: a process that allows tissue to be supplied with blood from an accessory vessel

College of American Pathologists (CAP): a medical society composed exclusively of pathologists and considered a leader in providing laboratory quality improvement programs

combining form: a word root, along with a combining vowel, that can be attached to a suffix or another word root

combining vowel: a vowel (usually an "o") that joins a word root to a suffix, or to another word root, to ease pronunciation

compatibility: able to be mixed together with favorable results, such as in blood transfusions

competencies: educational standards that were designed to improve student outcomes and maintain quality education; developed by NAACLS for the phlebotomy programs approval process

concentric circles: beginning from the center and moving outward in ever-widening even circles

confidentiality: the ethical cornerstone of professional behavior; the practice of regarding information concerning a patient as privileged and not to be disclosed to anyone without the patient's authorization

contact precautions: precautions used in addition to standard precautions when a patient is known or suspected to be infected or colonized with epidemiologically important microorganisms that can be transmitted by direct contact with the patient, or indirect contact with surfaces or patient-care items

continuing education units (CEUs): credits given for workshops and seminars, offered to continually upgrade skills and knowledge

Continuous Quality Improvement (CQI): an ongoing commitment by all levels of the administrative structure of an organization to improve all aspects of that organization. The objective of CQI in a healthcare facility is to enhance patient care and improve patient outcomes

coring: removal of a portion of the skin or vein

coronary arteries: the first branches off of the aorta, just beyond the aortic semilunar valve, which supply blood to the heart muscle

cost shifting: term used to describe how providers attempt to make up for reduced reimbursements from government-paid programs by charging more to other payers

CPD: citrate-phosphate-dextrose

CPR: cardiopulmonary resuscitation

CPT: Current Procedural Terminology

CPU: central processing unit

CQI: continuous quality improvement

criminal law: law that is designed to protect all members of society from injurious acts by others

crossmatch: a compatibility test performed before a unit of blood is determined to be suitable for transfusion

CRT: cathode ray tube

C&S: culture & sensitivity

CSF: cerebrospinal fluid

culture & sensitivity (C&S): the process by which organisms are grown on media and identified, and an antibiotic susceptibility (sensitivity) test is performed to determine which antibiotics will be effective against the organism

Current Procedural Terminology (CPT): a coding system developed by the AMA to provide a terminology and coding system for physician billing

cursor: a flashing marker on the CRT that indicates where the next key stroke will appear

cyanotic: pertaining to cyanosis or blue-gray discoloration of the skin due to lack of oxygen

data: information collected for analysis or computation

decimal system: system based on the number 10. In a decimal system, units larger or smaller than the basic units are arrived at by multiplying or dividing by 10 or powers of 10

defendant: in a lawsuit, person or people against whom the complaint is filed

delta check: a quality assurance procedure that compares current results of a lab test with previous results for the same test on the same patient

deposition: a process in which one party questions another under oath, while a court reporter records every word

dermis: corium or true skin; a layer composed of elastic and fibrous connective tissue

diabetes insipidus: a condition characterized by increased thirst and increased urine production, caused by inadequate secretion of ADH

diabetes mellitus: a condition in which there is impaired carbohydrate, fat, and protein metabolism because of a deficiency of insulin

diagnostic-related groups (DRGs): a system of disease classification used to determine PPS rates for reimbursement purposes

diaphragm: musculomembranous wall separating the abdomen from the thoracic cavity

diastole: the relaxation phase of the cardiac cycle

diastolic pressure: the pressure on the arteries during relaxation of the ventricles; averages 80 mm Hg and is an estimate of systemic vascular resistance

differential: determination of the number and characteristics of cells on a smear by staining and examining the cells under a microscope

discard tube: also called "clear tube." A tube used to collect and discard approximately 5 mL of blood, to prevent IV or tissue fluid contamination of a specimen

discovery: a process that involves taking depositions and interrogating parties involving litigation

disinfectants: solutions containing an agent intended to kill or irreversibly inactivate microorganisms (but not necessarily their spores). Disinfectants are used on surfaces and instruments, and generally are not safe for use on human skin

distal: farthest from the center of the body, origin, or point of attachment

diurnal (daily) variations: normal fluctuations throughout the day

dorsal: posterior or pertaining to the back

dorsal cavities: internal spaces located toward the back of the body

DRGs: diagnostic-related groups

droplet precautions: precautions used in addition to Standard Precautions for patients known or suspected to be infected with microorganisms transmitted by droplets (particles larger than 5 g in size), generated when a patient talks, coughs, or sneezes, and during certain procedures

ECG or EKG: electrocardiogram

edema: an accumulation of fluid in the tissues

electrocardiogram (EKG or ECG): an actual record of the electrical currents that correspond to each event in the heart muscle contraction

electrolytes: substances, such as potassium or sodium, that conduct electricity when dissolved in water

electrical safety: rules related to the safe use of electrical equipment

embolism: obstruction of a blood vessel by an embolus

embolus: a blood clot, part of a blood clot, or other mass of undissolved matter circulating in the blood stream

empathy: objective insight into the emotions and feelings of another person

endocardium: a thin membrane lining the heart that is continuous with the lining of the blood vessels

engineering controls: controls (such as sharps disposal containers, sharps with safety features, and needleless systems) that isolate or remove bloodborne pathogen hazards from the workplace

entitlement: a right earned by individuals through employment, such as Social Security or Worker's Compensation

Environmental Protection Agency (EPA): a federal agency that regulates the disposal of hazardous substances

EPA: Environmental Protection Agency

epicardium: the thin outer layer of the heart, continuous with the lining of the pericardium

epidermis: the outermost and thinnest layer of the skin

eosinophils (eos): granular leukocytes whose granules are beadlike and stain bright orange-red with the eosin acid stain

erythema: redness

erythrocyte: a mature, anuclear, biconcave, disk-shaped blood cell that is responsible for transporting oxygen to the cells of the body, and transporting carbon dioxide away from the cells; also called red blood cell (RBC)

erythropoietin: hormone secreted by the kidneys which stimulates red blood cell production

essentials: educational standards set forth by accrediting agencies

ethanol: ethyl or grain alcohol when referred to as part of a blood alcohol test

evacuated tubes: premeasured vacuum tubes that receive the patient's blood during the venipuncture procedure

expressed consent: consent expressed verbally or in writing and used for proposed treatment involving surgery, experimental drugs, or high-risk procedures. The written form must be signed by the person providing the treatment and the patient, and be witnessed by a third party. If consent is given verbally, the treatment provider should make an entry in the patient's chart of what was discussed with the patient

exsanguinate: loss of blood to the point at which life can no longer be sustained

external respiration: the process by which O_2 from the air enters the bloodstream in the lungs, and CO_2 leaves the bloodstream and is breathed into the air from the lungs

extrinsic pathway: a coagulation pathway initiated by the release of thromboplastin (factor III) from injured tissue and the activation of factor VII (proconvertin)

extravascular: outside the blood stream

ex vivo: outside the body

Fahrenheit: a scale used to measure body temperatures, based on the freezing point (32 degrees) and the boiling point (212 degrees) of water

fasting: abstinence from eating or drinking, except water, for approximately 12 hours before collection of the specimen

FDP: fibrin degradation products

feather: the thinnest area of a blood smear where the differential is performed

femoral artery: major systemic artery located superficially in the groin, lateral to the pubis bone

fibrin: a filamentous protein formed by the action of thrombin on fibrinogen

fibrin degradation products (FDP): small fragments of partially digested fibrin found in the blood stream

fibrinogen: also called factor I; a protein found in plasma that is essential for clotting of blood

fibrinolysis: process initiated by the activation of the clotting mechanism that releases substances that lead to the dissolution of the fibrin clot

fire tetrahedron: a new way of looking at the chemistry of fire in which the chemical reaction that actually produces fire is added as a fourth component to the traditional fire triangle components, fuel, heat, and oxygen

fistula: a tube passing from a cavity or vessel to a free surface or another cavity; also the term used to describe an artificial joining of an artery and a vein

flanges: extensions on the sides of an evacuated tube holder that aid in tube placement and removal

flea: small metal bar that is inserted into the tube after collection of a capillary blood gas specimen to aid in mixing the anticoagulant by means of a magnet

floor book: also called user manual; a manual of instruction provided to the unit by the laboratory that describes preparation of the patient and special instructions for specimen collection

fomite: any substance that adheres to and transmits infectious material

forensic specimen: specimen collected for legal reasons

fraud: a type of deceitful practice or willful plan resorted to with the intent to deprive another person of rights, or in some manner to cause that person injury

frontal plane: also called coronal plane; divides the body vertically into front and back portions

FUO: fever of unknown origin

gastric analysis: a laboratory test that examines gastric acid secretions to determine gastric function in terms of stomach acid production

gatekeeper: the primary care physician in a managed care plan, such as an HMO or PPO, who acts as the patient advocate in advising and coordinating the patient's health care needs

gauge: a standard for measuring the diameter of the lumen of a needle

germicide: an agent that kills pathogenic microorganisms

glucose: blood sugar

glucose monitoring: a means of observing and recording blood sugar for the purpose of maintaining a normal level

glucose tolerance test (GTT): a test used to diagnose carbohydrate metabolism problems

glycolysis: normal body process in which glucose is hydrolyzed or broken down by an enzyme

gram: the basic unit of weight in the metric system; approximately equal to a cubic centimeter or milliliter of water

granulocytes: WBCs with easily visible granules

great saphenous vein: the longest vein in the body, located in the leg

GTT: glucose tolerance test

guaiac test: also called occult blood; tests for blood in stool

hardware: CPU, monitor, and all peripherals, such as barcode readers, modems, and joysticks

HazCom: the abbreviation for the Hazardous Communication Standard, enacted in 1986 by OSHA, that requires employers to maintain documentation on all hazardous materials

HBV: hepatitis B virus

HCFA: Health Care Financing Administration, name has recently been changed to the Center for Medicare and Medicaid Services (CMS)

HCG: human chorionic gonadotropin

HCPCS: HCFA Common Procedure Coding System, widely used coding system of diagnoses in the United States

HCV: hepatitis C virus

health maintenance organization (HMO): group practice that is reimbursed on a prepaid, rather than a fee-for-service, basis

hematocrit (Hct): percentage by volume of red blood cells in whole blood

hematoma: a swelling or mass of blood (usually clotted) caused by blood leaking from a blood vessel during or following venipuncture or arterial puncture

hemochromatosis: a disease characterized by excess iron deposits in the tissues

hemoconcentration: a condition in which the plasma portion of the blood filters into the tissues, causing an increase in nonfilterable blood components such as RBCs, enzymes, iron, and calcium

hemoglobin (Hb or Hgb): an iron protein pigment found in red blood cells that carries O_2 and CO_2 in the blood stream

hemolysis: the destruction of RBCs and the liberation of hemoglobin into the fluid portion of the specimen, causing the serum or plasma to be pink (slight hemolysis) to red (gross hemolysis) in color

hemostasis: process by which the body stops the leakage of blood from the vascular system

hemostatic plug: fibrin clot

heparin: an anticoagulant that prevents clotting by inactivating the blood clotting agents thrombin and thromboplastin

heparin lock: a special winged needle set that can be left in a patient's vein for up to 48 hours, used to administer medication and draw blood

hepatitis: inflammation of the liver, from toxic or viral origin

hepatitis B virus (HBV): the virus that causes hepatitis B

hepatitis C virus (HCV): the virus that causes hepatitis C

HICPAC: Hospital Infection Control Practices Advisory Committee

HIV: human immunodeficiency virus

HMO: health maintenance organization

homeostasis: a "steady state" condition in which the body maintains its internal environment in a state of equilibrium or balance

Hospital Infection Control Practices Advisory Committee (HICPAC): federal organization, established in 1991, that advises the CDC on updating guidelines regarding prevention of nosocomial infection

hub: the end of the needle that attaches to the blood collection device

human chorionic gonadotropin (HCG): a hormone produced by the placenta that appears in both urine and serum, beginning approximately 10 days after conception

human immunodeficiency virus (HIV): the virus that causes acquired immunodeficiency syndrome (AIDS)

hyperglycemia: condition in which the blood sugar (glucose) is increased, as in diabetes mellitus

hypodermic needle: type of a needle that can be used to collect blood with a syringe or for a hypodermic injection

hypoglycemia: a condition in which the blood sugar (glucose) is abnormally low, as in hyperinsulinism

ICD-9-CM: International Classification of Diseases, Ninth Revision, Clinical Modification

icon: a small representative image used to access documents and software programs

ID band/bracelet: identification bracelet

ID code: a code given to a user along with a password. The ID code identifies each person entering data into the system; may not remain confidential because others may need to use the code to verify their collections

identification (ID) cards: clinic-issued cards containing a patient's name and other information identifying him or her as a clinic patient

immunoglobulins: antibodies that are released into the blood stream, where they circulate and attack foreign cells

impermeable: impenetrable, not allowing passage of fluids, as required in some lab coats

implied consent: consent implied by actions of the patient. For example, if a phlebotomist explains that he or she is there to collect a blood specimen, and the patient holds out his arm, consent is assumed

indemnity insurance: when the insurance company agrees to pay the health care provider a set amount of money

induration: hardness

indwelling line: tubing inserted into a main vein or artery, used primarily for administering fluids and medications

infection: invasion of a body by a pathogenic microorganism, resulting in injurious effects or disease

inferior: also referred to as caudal; beneath, lower, or toward the feet

inflammation: tissue reaction to injury, such as redness or swelling

informed consent: agreement by the patient to medical treatment after having received adequate information about the procedure, risks, and consequences

inpatient care: care performed in a health care setting where patients stay overnight

input: data that are entered into a CPU

interface: a device that enables two normally noncompatible circuits or parts to function together as in computers or computerized instrumentation

International Classification of Diseases, Ninth Revision, Clinical Modification (ICD-9-CM): the diagnosis coding system used by all major payers

intravascular: within the vascular system

intrinsic pathway: a coagulation pathway involving coagulation factors circulating within the blood stream, initiated with activation of factor XII

integumentary system: the skin and its appendages, including the hair and nails; also referred to as the largest organ of the body

internal respiration: the process by which O_2 leaves the blood stream and enters the cells, and CO_2 from the cells enters the blood stream

interstitial fluid: fluid found between cells, or in spaces within an organ or tissue

intracellular fluid: fluid found within cell membranes

iontophoresis: introduction of various ions into the skin by electrical stimulation from electrodes placed on the skin

ischemia: temporary lack of blood flow to the heart due to obstruction

isolation procedure: an infection control procedure that separates patients with certain transmissible infections or diseases from other patients

invasion of privacy: the violation of one's right to be left alone and to live without being subject to unwarranted or undesired publicity; includes the publishing or releasing of private information without the subject's permission

Ivy bleeding time: a bleeding time test modified by Ivy in 1941; performed on the volar (inner) surface of the forearm using a blood pressure cuff to maintain constant pressure

JCAHO: Joint Commission on Accreditation of Healthcare Organizations

Joint Commission on Accreditation of Healthcare Organizations (JCAHO): a voluntary, nongovernmental agency charged with, among other things, establishing standards for the operation of hospitals and other health-related facilities and services

K: potassium

keloid: fibrous tissue growth at scar area of the skin

kinesics: the study of body motion or language, such as facial expressions, gestures, and eye contact

kinesic slip: when nonverbal messages don't match verbal messages

Laboratory Information System (LIS): a complete software program for clinical laboratory specimen collection, reporting, and quality assurance

lancet: a sterile, disposable, sharp-pointed instrument used to pierce the skin to obtain droplets of blood used for testing

lateral: toward the side

leukemia: an increase in WBCs characterized by the presence of a large number of abnormal forms

leukocytosis: an abnormal increase in WBCs in the circulating blood

leukopenia: an abnormal decrease of WBCs in the circulating blood

leukocyte: also called white blood cell (WBC); round cell containing a nucleus whose main function is to combat infection and remove disintegrating tissue

licensure: a process similar to certification, but offered by a governmental agency, granted through examination to a person who can meet the requirements for education and experience in that field

lipemic: a term used to describe cloudy serum or plasma caused by increased lipid content in the blood

LIS: Laboratory Information System

liter: the basic unit of volume in the metric system, which is equivalent to 1,000 mL

local: restricted to one place or part

logging on: entering as a user on a computer system via a password

Luer adapter: in the Luer-Lok system, a device for connecting the syringe to the needle; when locked into place it gives a secure fit

lumen: the internal space of a vessel or tube

lymphocyte: a nongranular leukocyte; the second most numerous of the WBCs, composing approximately 15% to 30% of the WBC population

lymphostasis: a stoppage of lymph flow caused by lymph node removal

lysis: rupturing of red blood cells

malpractice: a claim of improper treatment or negligence brought against a professional person by means of a civil lawsuit

managed care: a variety of financial and organizational methods used to control the delivery of health care (i.e., a predetermined monthly payment for providing services to patients is set up with physicians, hospitals, and other health care agencies). Consequently, the financial risk lies with the provider and not the insurer

managed care organizations (MCO): local health care providers that offer a complete networks of services

material safety data sheets (MSDS): required written information on all products with a hazardous warning on the label

MCO: managed care organization

medial: toward the midline or middle

median cubital vein: the vein located in the middle of the antecubital fossa area of the arm; the first-choice vein for venipuncture

median cutaneous nerve: a major motor and sensory nerve in the arm that lies along the path of the brachial artery and in the vicinity of the basilic vein

Medicaid: a program funded by the state and federal governments for providing medical care to the poor

medical emergency (med emerg): designation replacing "stat" for requesting tests that are needed in critical or "life or death" situations

medical record number: the unique number given to a patient for purposes of identification

Medicare: a federally funded program, enacted in 1965, that provides health care to people older than age 65 years and to the disabled, regardless of financial status

megakaryocyte: a large cell that is formed in the bone marrow and is the precursor to platelet cells

meninges: membranes consisting of three layers of connective tissue that enclose and protect the brain and spinal cord

menu: a listing on the computer screen of options from which the user selects the program or process he or she needs

meter: the basic unit of linear measurement in the metric system; equal to 39.37 inches

metric system: a decimal system of weights and measures based on the basic meter, gram, and liter units

metabolism: the sum of all the chemical reactions necessary to sustain life

MI: myocardial infarction

microbes: microscopic organisms, or organisms not visible to the naked eye

microcollection containers or tubes: small plastic containers or tubes, often referred to as "bullets" because of their size and shape, that are primarily used to collect skin puncture blood specimens

microhematocrit tubes: disposable, narrow-bore glass or plastic tubes that fill by capillary action and are primarily used for hematocrit (packed cell volume) determinations on micro samples

midstream collection: specimen obtained during the middle of the urination rather than the beginning or end

military time: also called European time; based on a clock with 24 numbers instead of 12, eliminating the need for designating AM or PM

milliliter (mL): a unit of volume measurement which is approximately equal to a cubic centimeter (cc); the two terms are often used interchangeably

mitosis: a type of cell duplication that involves cell division and doubling of the DNA

mnemonic: memory-aiding code, such as the abbreviations used to request the appropriate computer program or function necessary to process data

mode of transmission: the route by which an organism is transferred from one host to another

monitor: a cathode-ray tube used for display of television or computer information

monocytes (monos): the largest of the leukocytes, comprising from 1% to 7% of the WBC population

MR number: medical record number used for patient identification

MSDS: material safety data sheets

multisample needle: a special blood drawing needle used with an evacuated tube system that allows the user to collect more than one tube of blood without contaminating the tubes or holder

myocardial infarction (MI): heart attack or death of heart muscle due to obstruction of the coronary artery

myocardium: the thick, muscle layer of the heart

Na: sodium

NAACLS: National Accrediting Agency for Clinical Laboratory Sciences

nasopharyngeal culture (NP): a sample collected using a special NP swab, inserted gently through the nose into the nasopharynx area, to detect the presence of microorganisms such as those which cause diphtheria, meningitis, whooping cough, and pneumonia

Natelson tubes: microcollection tubes that are approximately 47 mm in length, and that fill by capillary action to a capacity of approximately 250 g

National Accrediting Agency for Clinical Laboratory Sciences (NAACLS): an international agency for accreditation and approval of educational programs in the clinical laboratory sciences and related health professions

National Credentialing Agency (NCA): certifies all levels of clinical laboratory personnel

National Committee for Clinical Laboratory Standards (NCCLS): a national nonprofit organization, formed by representatives from the profession, industry, and government, that develops guidelines and sets standards for all areas of the laboratory

National Institute for Occupational Safety and Health (NIOSH): an agency that approves respirators to be used when entering rooms of patients with pulmonary tuberculosis and other diseases with airborne transmission

NCA: National Credentialing Agency

NCCLS: National Committee for Clinical Laboratory Standards

needle sheath: covering or cap of a needle

Needlestick Safety and Prevention Act: a law passed by Congress and signed into law November 6, 2000, that directed OSHA to revise the BBP standard in four key areas, including: revision and updating of the exposure control plan, selecting engineering and work practice controls with employee input, modification of engineering control definitions, and new record keeping requirements

negligence: the violation of a duty to exercise reasonable skill and care in performing a task

nephron: functional unit of the kidney. Each kidney contains nearly a million

networking: simple interoffice connections or connection of complex systems between several organizations in different cities or across continents

neutropenic: pertaining to an abnormally small number of neutrophil cells in the blood

neutrophils: normally the most numerous of the WBCs; averaging 65% of the total WBC count, with granules that are fine in texture and that stain lavender

newborn screening: tests performed on neonates (newborns) to check for the presence of genetic or inherited diseases, such as phenylketonuria (PKU), hypothyroidism, galactosemia, homocystinuria, maple syrup urine disease, and sickle cell

NIOSH: National Institute for Occupational Safety and Health

noninvasive: not penetrating the skin

nosocomial: pertaining to a hospital or place of care for the sick

nosocomial infection: an infection acquired in a health care institution

NP: nasopharyngeal culture

NPO: nothing by mouth (Latin: *nulla per os*)

O & P: ova & parasite

occlusion: obstruction

occult blood: *see* guaiac test

occupational exposure: an anticipated skin, eye, mucous membrane, or parenteral contact with blood or other potentially infectious materials that may result from the performance of the employee's duties

Occupational Safety and Health Administration (OSHA): a U.S. government agency that regulates the safety and health of workers

on-line: when a computer system is operational

order of draw: the special sequence in which multiple specimen tubes are collected during a draw or filled from a syringe; designed to reduce interference in specimen testing caused by carryover of additives between tubes, and to minimize the effects of tissue thromboplastin on coagulation specimens

OSHA: Occupational Safety and Health Administration

osteochondritis: inflammation of the bone and cartilage

osteomyelitis: inflammation of the bone (especially the bone marrow) caused by bacterial infection

outpatient care: *see* ambulatory care

output: any data that flow from a CPU to its peripherals

ova & parasite (O & P): a stool sample for diagnosis of intestinal parasites

oxyhemoglobin (HbO$_2$): hemoglobin combined with O$_2$

palmar surface: palm side of the hand

palpate: to examine by feel or touch

parenteral: any route other than the alimentary (digestive tract), i.e., intramuscular, intravenous, subcutaneous, or mucosal

password: a unique identification of a person that allows him or her to become a system user

patency: state of being freely open, as in a patient's veins

paternity test: a test to determine the probability that a specific individual fathered a particular child

pathogen: an organism or substance capable of causing disease

pathogenic: capable of causing disease

patient identification (ID): the process by which a health care worker verifies the fact that a patient is the same as the one described on a requisition or work order

Patient's Bill of Rights: the rights or privileges a patient has while in a hospital or other health care facility that are clearly defined in a document originally published in 1975 by the American Hospital Association

peak level: drug level collected when the highest serum concentration of the drug is anticipated, 15 to 30 minutes after administration of the drug

pediatric tubes: small evacuated tubes designed to be used on small veins

percutaneous: delivered through the skin

pericardial fluid: fluid aspirated from the cavity surrounding the heart

pericardium: a thin, fluid-filled sac surrounding the heart

peripherals: all additional equipment attached to a CPU

peritoneal fluid: fluid aspirated from the abdominal cavity

permucosal: through mucous membranes, a route through which infectious microorganisms and other biohazards can enter the body

personal protective equipment (PPE): disposable gloves, lab coats or aprons, and/or protective face gear, such as masks and goggles with side shields, required by OSHA to be worn when handling body fluids

petechiae: small, nonraised red spots which appear on a patient's skin under certain conditions, such as when a tourniquet is applied

phagocytosis: a process by which bacteria and antigens are surrounded and engulfed by WBCs

phalanges: bones of the fingers or toes

phlebitis: inflammation of a vein

phenylketonuria (PKU): a hereditary disease caused by the inability of the body to metabolize phenylalanine because of a defective enzyme; mental retardation results if not treated early

phlebotomy: the procedure for withdrawing blood from the body

physiology: the science of the functions of the living organism and its components

PHS: Public Health Service

PKU: phenylketonuria

plasma: a clear, pale yellow fluid that is nearly 90% water (H_2O)

plantar surface: bottom or sole of the foot

plaintiff: in a lawsuit, the party filing the complaint

plasma separator tube (PST): tube that contains the anticoagulant heparin

platelet adhesion: the process by which platelets stick to injured surfaces

platelet aggregation: the process by which platelets degranulate and stick to one another

platelet plug formation: platelet aggregation and adhesion to a blood vessel after an injury

pleural fluid: fluid aspirated from the pleural cavity, which surrounds the lungs

PMN: polymorphonuclear

point-of-care testing: testing done at the patient's bedside or virtually anywhere the patient happens to be, using portable or hand-carried instruments

polycythemia: a disease characterized by an overproduction of red blood cells

polymorphonuclear (PMN): a term used to describe a type of WBC whose nucleus has several lobes or segments

posterior: also called dorsal, refers to the back

post-op: after surgery

postprandial (PP): after a meal

potassium (K): a mineral that is essential for normal muscle activity and the conduction of nerve impulses

potassium/ammonium oxalate: an additive

povidone-iodine: a complex of iodine with povidone (a dispersing and suspending agent) used as a surgical scrub, aerosol spray, and in ointments and rubs

pneumatic tube: a unidirectional, continuously operating vacuum system that transfers specimens in plexiglas carriers from the patient units to the laboratory

PPD: purified protein derivative; *see* tuberculin test

PPE: personal protective equipment

PPS: Prospective Payment System

preanalytical: before analysis

preferred provider organization (PPO): an independent group of doctors and hospitals that offer their services to employers at discounted rates

prefix: a word part that precedes a word root and modifies its meaning

pre-op: before an operation or surgery

primary care: a type of service that originates with the family physician who offers the initial consult and related treatment

primary hemostasis: first part of the coagulation process, which involves formation of a platelet plug

procedural manual: a document required by JCAHO that states in detail the step-by-step procedure for each test or practice performed in the laboratory

professionalism: the conduct and qualities that characterize a professional person

proficiency testing: a form of quality assurance required by CLIA '88 in which the accuracy of a laboratory's performance is verified by testing samples submitted by an outside agency that compares the results obtained with those of other participating laboratories

prone: lying horizontal, with the face down; the opposite of supine. Also denotes the hand with the palm down

pronation: the act of lying prone or face downward

Prospective Payment System (PPS): a program begun in 1983 to standardize the Medicare/Medicaid payments made to hospitals by reimbursing hospitals a set amount for each patient procedure

prothrombin: protein in circulating blood, called factor II, that is involved in coagulation

proxemics: the study of an individual's concept and use of space

proximal: nearest to the center of the body, origin, or point of attachment

PST: plasma separator tube

psychoneuroimmunology (PNI): a new field of medicine that deals with the study of interactions among the brain, the endocrine system, and the immune system

Public Health Service: one of the principle units under the United States Department of Health and Human Services with agencies at the state and local level that monitor, screen, and educate the public about health issues

pulmonary circulation: the system that carries blood from the heart to the lungs to remove carbon dioxide, and returns oxygenated blood to the heart

pulse: a measurement of pressure created as the ventricles contract and blood is forced out of the heart and through the arteries

pumping: vigorous opening and closing of the fist

QA: quality assurance

QA indicator: a monitor for all aspects of patient care; indicators must be measurable and cover high-volume procedures and high-risk situations

QC: quality control

QNS: quantity not sufficient

quality assurance (QA): a complete program that guarantees quality client care by tracking outcomes through scheduled audits in which the hospital looks at the appropriateness, applicability, and timeliness of patient care

quality control (QC): a form of procedural control that is a component of a quality assurance program

QI (quality improvement): continuous review and tracking of outcomes so as to initiate process improvement

quantity not sufficient (QNS): insufficient amount of substance required for testing

radial artery: an artery located on the thumb side of the wrist, which is usually the first-choice, and therefore most common, site for arterial puncture

RAM: random access memory

random access memory (RAM): temporary storage of data in the CPU that will be lost when power is discontinued, unless transferred to permanent storage

read-only memory (ROM): firmware installed by the manufacturer; its purpose is to instruct the CPU on how to begin the necessary operations requested by the user

reciprocity: granting of corresponding privileges, such as a state recognizing another state's license

reference laboratory: an off-site laboratory to which specimens are referred for testing procedures not routinely done in-house

reference laboratory log book: a manual for recording information including patient ID, date sent out, and date results were received for specimens sent to a reference laboratory

reference laboratory manual: information on ordering, handling, packaging, and transporting specimens sent to a reference laboratory

reference values: normal values for lab tests, usually established using basal state specimens

reflux: a backward flow of blood into the patient's veins from the collection tube during the venipuncture procedure

requisition: forms on which test orders are entered and sent to the laboratory

resheathing: to recap or replace the sheath on a needle

respondeat superior: a Latin phrase that means "let the master respond." It is another way of saying that employers must answer for damages their employees cause within the scope of employment

reticulocytes: immature RBCs in the blood stream that contain nuclear remnants

Rh antigen: a substance that, when present on the surface of RBCs, causes the formation of antibodies that interact specifically with it

Rh immunoglobulins: a substance that, if given before and shortly after an Rh-negative mother delivers an Rh-positive baby, will prevent sensitization by destroying any Rh factor in the mother's blood stream

risk management: a department in organizations that identifies risk and oversees the protection of employees, employers, and patients from the chance of injury or loss associated with the risk

ROM: read-only memory

roman numeral: a letter used to represent a number

sagittal plane: divides the body vertically into right and left portions

sclerosed: hard, cordlike, and lacking resilience

secondary care: health care beyond primary care which until recently was considered inpatient service

secondary hemostasis: second stage of coagulation that involves formation of a tougher "fibrin" clot formed of RBCs, platelets, and fibrin

semen analysis: laboratory test used to assess fertility and to determine the effectiveness of sterilization after vasectomy

semilunar valves: the crescent-shaped valves that control blood exiting the ventricles of the heart

septicemia: blood poisoning or pathogenic bacteria in the blood

serum: a clear, pale yellow fluid that remains after blood clots and is separated; it has the same composition as plasma, except it does not contain fibrinogen

serum separator tube (SST): contains an inert synthetic substance that forms a physical barrier between the cells of a specimen and the serum or plasma when the specimen is centrifuged

service insurance: when the insurance company agrees to provide health care services in place of money to the patient

sexually transmitted diseases (STDs): diseases such as syphilis, gonorrhea, and genital herpes, which are usually transmitted by sexual contact

shaft: the cylindrical portion of a needle

sharps container: special puncture-resistant, leak-proof, disposable containers used to dispose of used needles, lancets and other sharp objects

silica: silicon dioxide, a substance found in some evacuated tubes that provides increased surface for platelet activity

sinoatrial (SA) node: a node, also called the pacemaker, located in the upper wall of the right atrium, which generates an electrical impulse that initiates contraction of the heart

skin antisepsis: destruction or inhibition of multiplication of microorganisms on the skin through use of antiseptics or germicides

skin puncture: collecting blood after puncturing the skin with a lancet or similar skin puncture device

skin test: intradermal injection of an allergenic substance to determine whether a patient has come in contact with a specific allergen (antigen) and developed antibodies against it

sodium (Na): an extracellular ion in the blood plasma that helps maintain fluid balance

sodium citrate: contained in light blue stopper tubes, used for coagulation specimens because it does the best job of preserving the coagulation factors

sodium fluoride: most common antiglycolytic agent may be used in combination with ammonium or potassium oxalate or lithium heparin; also used to inhibit the growth of bacteria

sodium polyanethol sulfonate (SPS): an additive in the yellow top tube that prevents coagulation by binding with calcium. It is used for blood culture collection because it inhibits complement and phagocytosis and reduces the activity of certain antibiotics

software: computer programs (i.e., word processing, graphics, and games)

solutes: dissolved substances

sphygmomanometer: blood pressure cuff

SPS: sodium polyanethol sulfonate

SST: serum separator tube

standard of care: a prevailing set of standards set by licensing and regulatory agencies

standard precautions: guidelines recommended by the CDC and HICPAC to minimize the risk and spread of infection in hospitals. Standard precautions apply to blood, *all* body fluids (including all secretions and excretions except sweat, whether or not they contain visible blood), nonintact skin, and mucous membranes. The guidelines replace universal precautions and are to be used for the care of all patients

STAT (stat): a term derived from the Latin word "statim," meaning immediately

statute of limitations: a time limit for filing a lawsuit after an alleged injury has occurred

STDs: sexually transmitted diseases

steady state: a stable condition; no exercise, suctioning, or respirator changes, for at least 30 minutes before obtaining blood gases

storage: in computer terminology, a place for keeping data. Outside the computer it is called secondary storage.

subcutaneous layer: a layer of connective and adipose tissue that connects the skin to the surface of muscles

suffix: the end of a word (word ending) that follows a word root and either changes the meaning of the word root or adds to it

superior: also referred to as cranial: higher, above, or toward the head

supine: lying on the back, face upward

supination: turning the arm or hand so the palm faces upward

suprapubic: collection of a urine specimen by inserting a needle into the urinary bladder and aspirating the urine directly from the bladder

surfactant: a coating fluid that lowers the surface tension on the walls of the alveoli and helps to stabilize them and keep them from collapsing due to the thinness of their walls

susceptible host: a person who has little resistance to an infectious disease

sweat chloride: a test that uses iontophoresis to stimulate sweat production to evaluate chloride content in sweat; the test is used to diagnose cystic fibrosis, primarily in children and adolescents younger than age 20 years

sweeps: hospital rounds that occur at regular intervals throughout the day

synovial fluid: fluid aspirated from joint cavities

syncope: fainting

systemic: affecting the entire body

systemic circulation: the system that carries oxygenated blood from the heart, along with nutrients, to all the cells of the body, and then returns to the heart carrying waste products from cellular metabolism

systole: the contraction phase of the cardiac cycle

systolic pressure: the pressure in the arteries during contraction of the ventricles, usually around 120 mm Hg

TAT: turnaround time

TDM: therapeutic drug monitoring

tech code: code given to computer users that uniquely identifies each user within the laboratory and is recorded with all entries on the system

tertiary care: highly complex services and therapy that are performed on an inpatient basis, requiring the patient to stay overnight or longer

test requisition: the form on which a test is ordered and sent to the lab

therapeutic drug monitoring (TDM): process used by the physician to determine an effective drug dosage and to manage individual patient drug treatment

therapeutic phlebotomy: the withdrawal of a large volume of blood as a treatment for certain medical conditions, such as polycythemia and hemochromatosis. It is performed in a manner similar to collecting blood from donors

third party payer: a fiscal intermediary; most often an insurance company that pools individual contributions for a common group objective (e.g., protection from financial disaster)

thixotropic gel: an inert (nonreacting) synthetic substance that prevents blood cells from continuing to metabolize substances in the serum or plasma by forming a physical barrier between the cellular portion of a specimen and the serum or plasma portion after the specimen is centrifuged

threshold values: acceptable level for a quality assurance indicator

thrombin: an enzyme formed from prothrombin that reacts with fibrinogen to form fibrin during the clotting process

thrombosed: denotes a vessel that contains a thrombus or clot

thrombocytes: also known as platelets; the smallest of the formed elements in the blood stream

thrombocytopenia: decreased platelets

thrombocytosis: increased platelets

thrombophlebitis: inflammation of a vein, particularly in the lower extremities, along with thrombus formation

thrombus formation: blood clot in a blood vessel

T-lymphocytes: specialized WBCs that play an important role in immunity by directly attacking infected cells

tolerance test: a test of the body's ability to absorb and use a particular substance

tort: a civil wrong or other breach of contract (i.e., negligence or battery)

total quality management (TQM): an institution-wide plan to assure quality care, mandated by JCAHO to be instituted by 1994, requiring all departments in the hospital to have ongoing evaluations that focus on quality of process rather than outcome

TQM: total quality management

trace elements: metals or minerals, including aluminum, arsenic, copper, lead, iron, and zinc, normally found in minute amounts

transfusion reaction: a response to an incompatible blood transfusion resulting in antigen/antibody reactions that cause agglutination or lysis of the RBCs

transmission-based precautions: precautions in addition to Standard Precautions to be followed for patients known or suspected to be infected or colonized with highly transmissible or epidemiologically significant pathogens. There are three transmission-based precautions: airborne, droplet, and contact

transport media: the medium or agent used to carry infective material to a laboratory for culturing

transverse plane: divides the body horizontally into upper and lower portions, often called a cross section

trough level: drug level collected when the lowest serum concentration of the drug is expected, usually immediately prior to administration of the next scheduled dose

tube additive: any substance placed within a tube other than the coating of the tube or tube stopper (closure)

tuberculin (TB) test: tuberculosis test also called PPD test; *see* PPD

tuberculosis (TB): infectious airborne disease affecting the respiratory system, caused by the bacteria *Mycobacterium tuberculosis*

tunica adventitia: the outer layer of blood vessels, made up of connective tissue, that is thicker in arteries than in veins

tunica intima: the inner layer or lining of blood vessels, made up of a single layer of endothelial cells

tunica media: the middle layer of blood vessels, made up of smooth muscle tissue, that is much thicker in arteries than in veins

turnaround time (TAT): specified amount of time for sample to be drawn and processed, and for test results to be sent to the floor or unit

Typenex ID band: a special three-part identification bracelet for a blood recipient that contains the same information and unique ID number for client confirmation on all three parts

UA: urinalysis

universal precautions: a set of rules established by the CDC, and adopted by OSHA, to control infection from body fluids in the healthcare setting

urinalysis (UA): a laboratory test that includes physical examination, and chemical and microscopic analysis of urine.

user manual: a manual containing specimen collection information, including the type of specimen required, minimum amount needed, special handling, reference values for the test, when testing is available, and the normal turnaround time (TAT)

UTI: urinary tract infection

VAD: vascular access device

vascular access device (VAD): tubing inserted into a main vein or artery, used primarily for administering fluids and medications, monitoring pressures, and drawing blood. It is also called an indwelling line

vasoconstriction: constriction of a blood vessel to decrease the flow of blood to an area

vector transmission: the transfer of the causative organisms of disease to a susceptible individual by an insect, arthropod, or animal

vehicle: contaminated food, water, or drugs that facilitates the transmission of an infective microbe to a susceptible individual; includes the transmission of hepatitis and HIV through blood transfusion

veins: vessels that return blood to the heart

vena cava: the largest vein in the body

venesection: slicing a vein in the forearm and collecting the specimen in a cup or bowl

venipuncture: collection of blood by penetrating a vein with a needle, syringe, or other collection apparatus

venous stasis: stagnation or stoppage of the normal blood flow

ventral: anterior or pertaining to the front

ventral cavities: internal space located in the front of the body

ventricles: lower chambers of the heart; also known as the delivering chambers of the heart, because they pump blood into the arteries

venules: the smallest veins at the junction of the capillaries

vicarious liability: institutions are liable for injury occurring as a result of negligent acts committed by independent contractors they have hired

virulence: the degree to which an organism is capable of causing disease

virulent: infectious or capable of overcoming the defensive mechanism of the host

whorls: circular pattern of a fingerprint formed by the ridges and grooves of the papillary dermis

winged infusion set (butterfly): a $1/2$- to $3/4$-inch stainless steel needle connected to a 5- to 12-inch length of tubing; it is called a butterfly because of its wing-shaped plastic extensions, which are used for gripping the needle

word root: foundation of all medical terms

work practice control: practices that alter the manner in which a task is performed to reduce the likelihood of exposure. Example of work practice controls are prohibiting needle bending, breaking, or recapping; requiring hand washing after glove removal; and prohibiting eating, drinking, smoking, or applying cosmetics in work areas of the laboratory

zones of comfort: in communication, the different distances around a person that are comfortable for intimate, personal, social, and public discourse

APPENDIX A

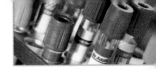

ANSWERS TO STUDY & REVIEW QUESTIONS

Chapter 1:

1. a
2. d
3. a
4. b
5. a
6. d
7. b
8. c
9. c
10. d
11. b
12. a
13. d
14. c
15. d

Chapter 2:

1. d
2. b
3. a
4. d
5. b
6. b
7. d
8. c
9. c
10. d

Chapter 3:

1. c
2. d
3. a
4. d
5. a
6. a
7. b
8. c
9. c

10. b
11. c
12. d

Chapter 4:

1. c
2. c
3. c
4. d
5. b
6. d
7. a
8. b
9. c
10. d
11. d
12. d

Chapter 5:

1. b
2. d
3. c
4. c
5. c
6. d
7. d
8. b
9. c
10. a
11. d
12. b

Chapter 6:

1. a
2. c
3. b
4. a
5. c

6. a
7. c
8. b
9. a
10. b
11. b
12. d
13. a
14. a
15. a
16. b
17. d
18. c

Chapter 7:

1. d
2. d
3. c
4. c
5. d
6. d
7. c
8. d
9. c
10. b
11. b
12. d

Chapter 8:

1. d
2. b
3. b
4. b
5. c
6. b
7. a
8. a
9. a
10. b

11. a
12. d
13. a
14. a
15. a
16. b
17. d

Chapter 9:

1. a
2. b
3. c
4. c
5. c
6. d
7. b
8. d
9. c
10. b

Chapter 10:

1. d
2. d
3. c
4. b
5. d
6. d
7. d
8. c
9. b
10. a
11. a
12. b

Chapter 11:	Chapter 12:	Chapter 13:	Chapter 14:
1. c	1. b	1. d	1. d
2. b	2. b	2. c	2. d
3. a	3. d	3. d	3. b
4. b	4. c	4. d	4. c
5. c	5. b	5. c	5. a
6. d	6. c	6. d	6. c
7. c	7. d	7. d	7. b
8. c	8. b	8. d	8. c
9. a	9. d	9. b	9. c
10. c	10. c	10. d	10. a
11. b			11. d
12. b			12. c

ANSWERS TO CASE STUDIES:

Chapter 1

No case study

Chapter 2

CASE STUDY 2-1: SCOPE OF DUTY

1. Although on the surface it seems like the proper thing to do, helping an inpatient walk to the bathroom is not in the phlebotomist's scope of duties and opens the phlebotomist up to liability issues as illustrated by this case. It would have been better to have nursing personnel, who are properly trained in this area, assist the patient.
2. The hospital may have liability for the injury because of the liquid spilled on the floor that caused the patient to slip.
3. Vicarious liability and respondeat superior could come into play if a lawsuit is filed on behalf of the patient. However, it is also possible for the phlebotomist to be seen as individually liable because helping the patient is not a normal duty of a phlebotomist.

Chapter 3

CASE STUDY 3-1: AN ACCIDENT WAITING TO HAPPEN

1. The first thing the phlebotomist needs to do is to wash the blood off of her arm, flushing the scratch site with water for 10 to 15 minutes.
2. The phlebotomist's actions that contributed to the accident included wearing heels and being in a hurry. It would have been better to wear appropriate shoes and change into heels just before going to lunch.
3. The phlebotomist should have covered the scratch with a waterproof bandage.
4. The type of exposure she received can be classified as a parenteral, nonintact skin contact exposure.

Chapters 4, 5, and 6

No case studies

Chapter 7

CASE STUDY 7-1: PROPER HANDLING OF ANTICOAGULANT TUBES

1. The clot in the CBC was most likely caused by the delay in mixing the specimen.
2. Yes. The problem with the second lavender top led to an even greater delay in mixing the specimen, which most likely contributed to the clotting problem.
3. If Chi had mixed the first lavender top as soon as he removed it from the holder and before laying it down, the problem with the second tube would not have had any effect on it.
4. Chi can prevent this from happening in the future by mixing all additive tubes as soon as they are removed from the tube holder.

CASE STUDY 7-2: ORDER OF DRAW

1. The green top for the stat electrolytes is compromised.

2. The specimen is compromised because it was drawn after the EDTA tube and may be contaminated by carryover of EDTA. Sodium or potassium levels (depending upon the type of EDTA) may be increased by EDTA contamination.

3. If the situation were to arise in the future, Chi could draw a few milliliters of blood into a plain discard tube to flush possible contamination from the needle before collecting the green stopper. Placing and removing the discard tube should help remove any EDTA residue on the outside of the needle. However, Chi should indicate how the specimen was collected in case interference is suspected by the laboratory.

CASE STUDY 7-3: BUTTERFLY USE AND ORDER OF DRAW

1. The protime was most likely rejected because the tube was not completely filled.

2. Mary collected the protime with a butterfly without using a clear tube. The air in the butterfly tubing displaces blood volume, preventing the tube from filling with blood to the proper level.

3. There is a critical 9:1 ratio of blood to anticoagulant needed for coagulation tests. Most laboratories will reject coagulation tubes that are not filled to within 90% of capacity.

4. To prevent this from happening again if a butterfly is used, Mary should draw a few milliliters of blood into a discard or "clear" tube before collecting the protime tube. This will remove air from the tubing and allow the tube to fill with blood to the proper level.

Chapter 8

CASE STUDY 8-1: PATIENT IDENTIFICATION

1. She didn't ask the patient to verbally state her name and date of birth.

2. She assumed that because the woman was the only one left in the waiting room, the woman was the right patient.

3. The patient may have been someone with a standing order who forgot to check in with the receptionist.

4. The real Jane Rogers can be drawn after a new requisition and labels have been created. The identity of the other patient may be discovered when a physician's office calls for results and there are none. The blood work on the unknown patient will have to be discarded; this is especially unfortunate because the patient was a difficult draw.

Chapter 9

CASE STUDY 9-1: PHYSIOLOGIC VARIABLES AND SITE SELECTION

1. Physiologic variables associated with this collection include: the patient is ill and may be dehydrated from vomiting, she is also overweight, has had a mastectomy on the left side, and is a difficult draw normally. Charles will be limited to drawing from the right arm. He will most likely need to draw the specimen using a butterfly and the smallest tubes available. He should check the cephalic vein if he does not find a suitable antecubital vein. He may need to draw from the right hand vein and he may need to warm the site to enhance blood

flow. Because it is a physician's office laboratory he should check with the patient's physician to see if it is advisable to offer the patient water because she is probably dehydrated, which makes it even more difficult to find a vein and collect a blood specimen.

2. Because the patient appears ill she should be asked to lie down to prevent her from fainting during specimen collection. An emesis basin should be close at hand in case she vomits.

3. Charles should check the antecubital area of the left arm first, paying particular attention to the area of the cephalic vein if the median cubital is not palpable. If no suitable vein is found he should check for a hand vein followed by veins in the dorsal wrist (never the ventral or palmar area of the wrist) and the forearm.

4. If Charles is unable to find a proper venipuncture site he should consider using skin puncture. Both the CBC and glucose can easily be collected by skin puncture. The site will need to be warmed to enhance blood flow because the patient may be dehydrated.

CASE STUDY 9-2: PROCEDURAL ERRORS

1. Blood most likely spurted into the tube because the needle was partly in the vein but also partly out; therefore, the tube quickly lost vacuum.

2. The hissing sound and the fact that the tube no longer fills with blood even after repositioning the needle are clues that the tube has lost vacuum.

3. Sara must position the needle in the vein, making certain that no part of the needle bevel is out of the skin, and then replace the tube with a new one.

CASE STUDY 9-3: COMPLICATIONS AND PROCEDURAL ERRORS

1. Site selection variables associated with this case include the presence of the IV in the left hand, the depth of the median cubital vein, and the prominence of the basilic vein. She properly chose the right arm over the arm with the IV. However, choosing the basilic vein was improper considering her inexperience at phlebotomy. She should have chosen a different vein, collected the specimen by skin puncture, or asked a more experienced phlebotomist to collect the specimen.

2. Drawing the basilic vein and not anchoring it properly to keep it from rolling were both procedural errors. (She was also unable to anchor it well on the redirect.) The fact that the vein rolled is a complication.

   The pain experienced by the patient was a complication. Failure to remove the needle when the patient exhibited classic symptoms of nerve involvement was a procedural error. The needle should have been removed regardless of the patient wanting to continue. A patient may not be aware of how serious nerve involvement can be. Another complication involved was possible inadvertent arterial puncture. In directing the needle Erica most likely hit an artery, evidenced by blood spurting into the tube. She failed to recognize blood spurting into the tube as a sign of possible inadvertent arterial puncture. She mistakenly rationalized that it was not arterial because the blood was dark in color. However, the patient was having difficulty breathing and was about to receive oxygen therapy. This should have been a clue to Erica that his arterial blood might not be of normal color.

Because she failed to recognize possible arterial puncture, she also failed to hold pressure herself and treat the site as an arterial puncture site. In addition the specimen should have been labeled as possible arterial blood since normal values for arterial specimens may differ from venous specimens.

Chapter 10

CASE STUDY 10-1: SKIN PUNCTURE COLLECTION

1. The phlebotomist tried to collect the specimen as it was running down the finger. A scooping or scraping motion during collection may have activated the platelets and caused them to clump. In addition, because the child was uncooperative, the specimen was not collected and mixed quickly, which may also have contributed to platelet clumping.
2. It appears that the phlebotomist started to collect the specimen without wiping away the first drop of blood. Alcohol residue may have caused the hemolysis. Trying to collect the specimen as it ran down

the finger may have resulted in scraping the blood from the skin, which could also have caused hemolysis.
3. Improper direction of puncture and presence of alcohol residue may have contributed to the blood running down the finger, making it more difficult to collect the specimen. The phlebotomist's inexperience with children may have contributed to the child being uncooperative. In addition, if the phlebotomist had been more experienced with skin puncture in children, he may have held the hand differently and prevented the child from pulling away.

Chapter 11

CASE STUDY 11-1: PERFORMANCE OF A GLUCOSE TOLERANCE TEST

1. Mr. Smith should finish drinking the glucose beverage within 5 minutes.
2. The timing for all specimens begins when the patient finishes the glucose beverage. The patient was given the beverage at 5:25 AM. If he finished it on time at 5:30, the 1-hour specimen would be collected at 6:30.
3. No. A level of 300 mg/dL at 30 minutes is abnormal according to the graph in Figure 11-10.
4. If the patient vomits within the first 30 minutes of the procedure, the test should be rescheduled. The patient's physician should be consulted to determine if the test should be continued.

Chapter 12

CASE STUDY 12-1: ABG PUNCTURE COMPLICATIONS

1. The patient's nurse should be alerted to the problem.
2. A thrombus may be affecting blood flow and affecting the pulse.
3. The patient moving his arm very likely resulted in the phlebotomist missing the artery. In addition, the restless and agitated state of the patient may have contributed to arteriospasm and made it harder to hit the artery.
4. The phlebotomist should have made an attempt to calm the patient. In addition, he or she should have been prepared for movement by the patient or have asked the nurse to help steady the arm because the patient was restless and agitated.
5. Although the specimen appears dark in color the phlebotomist can be fairly certain the specimen is arterial because it pulsed into the tube. It is probably dark in color because the patient has breathing difficulties.

Chapter 13

CASE STUDY 13-1: 24-HOUR URINE SPECIMEN COLLECTION

1. No. The specimen is missing a critical portion of urine.
2. The phlebotomist should not accept the specimen without first consulting a supervisor. Whether or not the specimen will be accepted depends upon the type of test and individual lab policy, and may require consultation with the patient's physician. If it is determined that the specimen will be accepted, the phlebotomist should note the discrepancy in collection time and identify the person who authorized acceptance on the requisition or computer entry.
3. Patients should be given verbal and written instructions on 24-hour collection procedures and verbal feedback should be obtained to ensure that they have complete understanding of the procedure. Patients should be made aware of the importance of timing and reminded to set an alarm if necessary.

Chapter 14

CASE STUDY 14-1: USE OF BARCODED PATIENT ID SPECIMEN LABELS

1. Nurse Susan may have used the label for Betty Smith on the specimens she collected on Mr. Jones.
2. The lab reports results according to the identification on the specimen, with the assumption that it is correctly labeled.
3. Nurse Susan will have to follow hospital protocol, which typically involves reprinting a lab slip and recollecting the specimen.
4. The results on Mrs. Smith will have to be removed from all records and the reason why documented according to laboratory protocol.

APPENDIX B

CONVERSATIONAL PHRASES IN ENGLISH AND SPANISH

The following remarks or sentences are designed to assist the phlebotomist when conversing with a patient who speaks only Spanish. Before approaching the patient, these basic phrases should be said aloud several times to a person who could correct the pronunciation, if necessary. If these phrases are said incorrectly, the meanings could be changed enough to insult or bewilder the patient.

Hello	¡Hola!	(Ō-lah)
Good morning	Buenos días	(BWĀ-nos DĒ-ahs)
Good afternoon	Buenas tardes	(BWĀ-nahs TAHR-dās)
Good evening	Buenas noches	(BWĀ-nahs NO-chās)
I am from the laboratory	Soy del laboratorio	(soy dāl lah-bō-rah-tō-RĒ-ō)
My name is	Me llamo	(mā YAH-mō)
I am here to take a blood sample	Estoy aquí para tomarle una prueba de sangre	(ās-TOY ah-KĒ PAHR-ah tō-MAHR-lā UN-ah prū-bah dā SAHN-grā)
What is your name?	¿Cual es su nombre? OR ¿Como se llama?	(kwahl ās sū NŌM-brā?) (CŌ-mō sā YAH-mah?)
May I see your wristband?	¿Me permite ver su identificación?	(mā pār-MĒ-tā vār sū ē-dān-tē-fē-cah-sē-ŌN?)
Mr. or Sir	Señor	(sā-NYOR)
Mrs. or Madame	Señora	(sā-NYŌ-rah)
Ms. or Miss	Señorita	(sā-nyō-RĒ-tah)
Okay	Muy bien	(MŪ-ē- byān)
You are the person I need	Usted es la persona que necesito	(ūs-TĒD ās lah pār-SŌN-ah kā na-sā-SĒ-tō)
I am going to put a tourniquet on your arm	le voy a poner un torniquete en el brazo	(lā voy ah pō-NĀR ūn tor-nē-KĀ-tā ān el BRAH-sō)
Please	Por favor	(por fah-VOR)
close your hand	cierra la mano	(SYĀ-rah lah MAH-nō)

A-8

open your hand	abra la mano	(AH-brah lah MAH-nō)
straighten your arm	enderezca el brazo	(en-dār-ĀZ-kah el BRAH-sō)
	OR estire el brazo	(ās-TĒ-rā sū BRAH-sō)
bend your arm	doble el brazo	(DŌ-blā el BRAH-sō)
relax	relájese	(rā-lah HĀ-sā)
sit there	siéntese aquí	(syān-TĀ-sā ah-KĒ)
Your doctor ordered this	Su doctor ordeno esto	(sū dōc-TOR or DĀ-nō ĀS-tō)
You need to ask your doctor	Necesita preguntarle a su doctor	(nā-sā-SĒ-tah prā-gūn-TAHR-lā ah sū dōc-TOR)
Have you eaten?	¿Ha comido?	(ah cō-MĒ-dō)
It will hurt a little	Le dolerá un poco	(lā dō-lā-RAH ūn PŌ-kō)
I will get the nurse	Buscaré a la enfermera	(būs-cah-RĀ ah lah ām-fār-MĀ-rah)
Thank you	¡Gracias!	(GRAH-syahs)
Have a good day	Que le vaya bien	(kā lā VĪ-yah byān)
Someone will be back in a few minutes	Alguien regresará en un momento	(ahl-GWĒ-ān rā-grā-sah-RAH ān ūn mō-MĀN-tō)
Make a fist	haga un puño	(HAH-ga ūn pun yo)

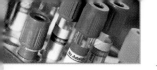

APPENDIX C

AHA MANAGEMENT ADVISORY

A Patient's Bill of Rights

A Patient's Bill of Rights was first adopted by the American Hospital Association in 1973. This revision was approved by the AHA Board of Trustees on October 21, 1992.

Introduction

Effective health care requires collaboration between patients and physicians and other health care professionals. Open and honest communication, respect for personal and professional values, and sensitivity to differences are integral to optimal patient care. As the setting for the provision of health services, hospitals must provide a foundation for understanding and respecting the rights and responsibilities of patients, their families, physicians, and other caregivers. Hospitals must ensure a health care ethic that respects the role of patients in decision making about treatment choices and other aspects of their care. Hospitals must be sensitive to cultural, racial, linguistic, religious, age, gender, and other differences as well as the needs of persons with disabilities.

The American Hospital Association presents A Patient's Bill of Rights with the expectation that it will contribute to more effective patient care and be supported by the hospital on behalf of the institution, its medical staff, employees, and patients. The American Hospital Association encourages health care institutions to tailor this bill of rights to their patient community by translating and/or simplifying the language of this bill of rights as may be necessary to ensure that patients and their families understand their rights and responsibilities.

Bill of Rights

These rights can be exercised on the patient's behalf by a designated surrogate or proxy decision maker if the patient lacks decision-making capacity, is legally incompetent, or is a minor.

1. The patient has the right to considerate and respectful care.
2. The patient has the right to and is encouraged to obtain from physicians and other direct caregivers relevant, current, and understandable information concerning diagnosis, treatment, and prognosis.

    Except in emergencies when the patient lacks decision-making capacity and the need for treatment is urgent, the patient is entitled to the opportunity to discuss and request information related to the specific procedures and/or treatments, the risks involved, the possible length of recuperation, and the medically reasonable alternatives and their accompanying risks and benefits.

    Patients have the right to know the identity of physicians, nurses, and others involved in their care, as well as when those involved are students, residents, or other trainees. The patient also has the right to know the immediate and long-term financial implications of treatment choices, insofar as they are known.

3. The patient has the right to make decisions about the plan of care prior to and during the course of treatment and to refuse a recommended treatment or plan of care to the extent permitted by law and hospital policy and to be informed of the medical consequences of this action. In case of such refusal, the patient is entitled to other appropriate care and services that the hospital provides or transfer to another hospital. The hospital should notify patients of any policy that might affect patient choice within the institution.

4. The patient has the right to have an advance directive (such as a living will, health care proxy, or durable power of attorney for health care) concerning treatment or designating a surrogate decision maker with the expectation that the hospital will honor the intent of that directive to the extent permitted by law and hospital policy.

   Health care institutions must advise patients of their rights under state law and hospital policy to make informed medical choices, ask if the patient has an advance directive, and include that information in patient records. The patient has the right to timely information about hospital policy that may limit its ability to implement fully a legally valid advance directive.

5. The patient has the right to every consideration of privacy. Case discussion, consultation, examination, and treatment should be conducted so as to protect each patient's privacy.

6. The patient has the right to expect that all communications and records pertaining to his/her care will be treated as confidential by the hospital, except in cases such as suspected abuse and public health hazards when reporting is permitted or required by law. The patient has the right to expect that the hospital will emphasize the confidentiality of this information when it releases it to any other parties entitled to review information in these records.

7. The patient has the right to review the records pertaining to his/her medical care and to have the information explained or interpreted as necessary, except when restricted by law.

8. The patient has the right to expect that, within its capacity and policies, a hospital will make reasonable response to the request of a patient for appropriate and medically indicated care and services. The hospital must provide evaluation, service, and/or referral as indicated by the urgency of the case. When medically appropriate and legally permissible, or when a patient has so requested, a patient may be transferred to another facility. The institution to which the patient is to be transferred must first have accepted the patient for transfer. The patient must also have the benefit of complete information and explanation concerning the need for, risks, benefits, and alternatives to such a transfer.

9. The patient has the right to ask and be informed of the existence of business relationships among the hospital, educational institutions, other health care providers, or payers that may influence the patient's treatment and care.

10. The patient has the right to consent to or decline to participate in proposed research studies or human experimentation affecting care and treatment or requiring direct patient involvement, and to have those studies fully explained

prior to consent. A patient who declines to participate in research or experimentation is entitled to the most effective care that the hospital can otherwise provide.

11. The patient has the right to expect reasonable continuity of care when appropriate and to be informed by physicians and other caregivers of available and realistic patient care options when hospital care is no longer appropriate.

12. The patient has the right to be informed of hospital policies and practices that relate to patient care, treatment, and responsibilities. The patient has the right to be informed of available resources for resolving disputes, grievances, and conflicts, such as ethics committees, patient representatives, or other mechanisms available in the institution. The patient has the right to be informed of the hospital's charges for services and available payment methods.

The collaborative nature of health care requires that patients, or their families/surrogates, participate in their care. The effectiveness of care and patient satisfaction with the course of treatment depend, in part, on the patient fulfilling certain responsibilities. Patients are responsible for providing information about past illnesses, hospitalizations, medications, and other matters related to health status. To participate effectively in decision making, patients must be encouraged to take responsibility for requesting additional information or clarification about their health status or treatment when they do not fully understand information and instructions. Patients are also responsible for ensuring that the health care institution has a copy of their written advance directive if they have one. Patients are responsible for informing their physicians and other caregivers if they anticipate problems in following prescribed treatment.

Patients should also be aware of the hospital's obligation to be reasonably efficient and equitable in providing care to other patients and the community. The hospital's rules and regulations are designed to help the hospital meet this obligation. Patients and their families are responsible for making reasonable accommodations to the needs of the hospital, other patients, medical staff, and hospital employees. Patients are responsible for providing necessary information for insurance claims and for working with the hospital to make payment arrangements, when necessary.

A person's health depends on much more than health care services. Patients are responsible for recognizing the impact of their life-style on their personal health.

Conclusion

Hospitals have many functions to perform, including the enhancement of health status, health promotion, and the prevention and treatment of injury and disease; the immediate and ongoing care and rehabilitation of patients; the education of health professionals, patients, and the community; and research. All these activities must be conducted with an overriding concern for the values and dignity of patients.

Source: AHA Management Advisory. "A Patient's Bill of Rights." "A Patient's Bill of Rights" was first adopted by the American Hospital Association in 1973. This revision was approved by the AHA Board of Trustees on October 21, 1992.
http://www.aha.org/z_webmaster/resource/pbillofrights.asp. Accessed April 4, 2002 9:47:09 PM GMT.

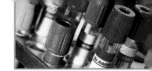

LISTING OF DEPARTMENTS AND TESTS

Chemistry

Tube Types Used	Additives
SST	Inert gel and silica
Green	Sodium heparin
	Lithium heparin
	Ammonia heparin
Gray	Sodium fluoride and potassium oxalate
Royal blue (red label)	Free of trace elements and no additive
Royal blue (green label)	Free of trace elements with heparin
Royal blue (lavender label)	Free of trace elements with EDTA
Red (glass	Nonadditive
Red (plastic)	Clot activator

Listing of Tests Performed in Chemistry Department

Test	Abbreviation	Sample considerations	Clinical correlation
Acid phosphatase	Acid p'tase	SST, centrifuge, separate and freeze serum. Transport frozen.	Cancer of the prostate
Alanine transferase	ALT (SGPT)	SST, centrifuge for complete separation and refrigerate.	Evaluate hepatic disease
Alcohol	ETOH	Gray, use nonalcohol germicidal solution to cleanse skin; chain-of-custody required if for legal purposes.	Intoxication
Aldosterone		Plain red top, centrifuge, separate and refrigerate serum. Draw "upright" sample at least ½ hour after patient sits up.	Overproduction of this hormone

continued

Listing of Tests Performed in Chemistry Department (continued)

Test	Abbreviation	Sample considerations	Clinical correlation
Alkaline phosphatase	Alk phos or ALP	SST, centrifuge for complete separation. Fasting 8-12 hours is required.	Liver function
Alpha-fetoprotein	AFP	SST, avoid hemolysis; do not freeze; can be performed on amniotic fluid.	Fetal abnormalities, adult hepatic carcinomas
Aluminum	Al	Royal blue tube; EDTA. Submit original unopened tube. Avoid all sources of external contamination. If no additive royal blue is used, serum must be transferred to a plastic tube within 45 minutes of collection.	Trace metal contamination, dialysis complication
Ammonia	NH4	Green-top tube placed immediately on ice slurry; centrifuge within 15 minutes without removing stopper; separate plasma and freeze in plastic vial using dry ice.	Evaluates liver function. High levels in the blood lead to a problem known as hepatic encephalopathy.
Amylase		SST, centrifuge, and refrigerate serum. Avoid hemolysis and lipemia.	Acute pancreatitis
Aspirate transferase	AST	SST, centrifuge for complete separation and refrigerate.	Acute and chronic liver disease

Listing of Tests Performed in Chemistry Department (continued)

Test	Abbreviation	Sample considerations	Clinical correlation
B_{12} and folate		SST, centrifuge, separate, and refrigerate. Avoid hemolysis. If testing is delayed, freeze specimen in plastic vial.	Macrocytic anemia
Basic metabolic panel	BMP	SST, refrigerate unopened spun barrier tube. Separate within 45 minutes of venipuncture. Fasting 8-12 hours is required.	A designated number of tests covering a certain body system
Bilirubin, total and direct	Bili	Wrap in foil to protect from light; refrigerate.	Increased with types of jaundice (i.e., obstructive, hepatic, or hemolytic; hepatitis or cirrhosis)
Blood urea nitrogen	BUN	SST, centrifuge for complete separation, and refrigerate.	Kidney function
Calcitonin		Plain red, centrifuge, separate, and freeze immediately in plastic vial. Overnight fasting preferred.	Evaluate suspected medullary carcinoma of the thyroid and is characterized by hypersecretion of calcitonin
Carbon monoxide (carboxyhemoglobin)	CO level	Fill lavender tube completely. Submit at room temperature.	Carboxyhemoglobin intoxication
Carcinogenic antigen	Ca 125	Refrigerate; freeze if testing is delayed.	Tumor marker primarily for ovarian carcinoma

continued

Listing of Tests Performed in Chemistry Department (continued)

Test	Abbreviation	Sample considerations	Clinical correlation
Calcium, ionized		Allow blood to clot for 20 minutes; centrifuge with cap on; do not pour over; refrigerate.	Bone cancer, nephritis, multiple myeloma
Carcinoembryonic antigen	CEA	Refrigerated serum.	Monitoring of patients with diagnosed malignancies; malignant or benign liver disease; indicator of tumors
Carotene		Refrigerated serum. Wrap in aluminum foil to protect from light. Overnight fasting is preferred.	Carotenemia
Cholesterol	Chol	Refrigerated serum.	Evaluates risk of coronary heart disease (CHD)
Chromium	Cr level	Royal blue—no additive; metal-free, separate and refrigerate immediately.	Associated with diabetes and aspartame toxicity
Cold agglutinins		Collect serum, must be kept warm, deliver to lab STAT, and alert the lab personnel. Store and ship at room temperature.	To diagnose primary atypical pneumonia caused by *Mycoplasma pneumoniae*
Copper	Cu level	Royal blue—no additive; separate and refrigerate immediately.	Wilson's disease or nephritic syndrome
Cortisol, timed		Refrigerated serum; clearly note time drawn.	Cushing's syndrome

Listing of Tests Performed in Chemistry Department *(continued)*

Test	Abbreviation	Sample considerations	Clinical correlation
Creatine kinase	CK	Refrigerated serum.	Muscular dystrophy and trauma to skeletal muscle
Creatine kinase MB	CK-MB	Refrigerated serum.	Organ differentiation and to rule out myocardial infarction
Creatinine		Refrigerated serum.	Kidney function
Cyclosporin		Whole blood or serum refrigerated. NOTE: use same type of specimen each time analyte is measured.	Immunosuppressive drug for organ transplants
Cryoglobulin		Draw and process at room temperature; should be fasting.	Associated with immunological diseases (i.e., multiple myeloma or rheumatoid arthritis)
Drug Monitoring Amikacin		Gel barrier not suggested. Centrifuge and separate within 1 hour and transfer to plastic transfer tube.	Broad-spectrum antibiotic
Carbamazepine (Tegretol)		Gel barrier not suggested. Centrifuge and separate within 1 hour and transfer to plastic transfer tube.	Mood-stabilizing drug in bipolar affective disorder

continued

Listing of Tests Performed in Chemistry Department (continued)

Test	Abbreviation	Sample considerations	Clinical correlation
Digoxin (Lanoxin)		Red top or SST. If red-stoppered tube is used, transfer separated serum to a plastic transport tube.	Heart stimulant
Dilantin (Phenytoin)		Gel barrier not suggested. Centrifuge and separate within 1 hour and transfer to plastic transfer tube.	Treatment of epilepsy
Gentamicin		Gel barrier not suggested. Centrifuge and separate within 1 hour and transfer to plastic transfer tube.	Broad-spectrum antibiotic
Lithium	Li	Red top or SST. If red-stoppered tube is used, transfer separated serum to a plastic transport tube.	Manic-depression medication
Phenobarbital (barbiturates)		Gel barrier not suggested. Centrifuge and separate within 1 hour and transfer to plastic transfer tube.	Anticonvulsant for seizures
Salicylates (aspirin)		Gel barrier not suggested. Centrifuge and separate within 1 hour and transfer to plastic transfer tube.	Evaluation of therapy
Theophylline		Gel barrier not suggested. Centrifuge and separate within 1 hour and transfer to plastic transfer tube.	Asthma medication

Listing of Tests Performed in Chemistry Department (continued)

Test	Abbreviation	Sample considerations	Clinical correlation
Tobramycin		Gel barrier not suggested. Centrifuge and separate within 1 hour and transfer to plastic transfer tube.	Broad-spectrum antibiotic
Vancomycin		Gel barrier not suggested. Centrifuge and separate within 1 hour and transfer to plastic transfer tube.	Broad-spectrum antibiotic
Electrolytes	Na+, K+, Cl−, CO_2, lytes	Spun barrier tube. Centrifuge within 30 minutes after drawing. Avoid hemolysis and lipemia.	Fluid balance, cardiotoxicity, heart failure, edema
Ferritin		Refrigerated serum.	Hemachromatosis, iron deficiency
Gamma-glutamyl transpeptidase	GGTP	Refrigerated serum.	Assists in the diagnosis of liver problems; specific for hepatobiliary problems
Gastrin		Overnight fasting is required; separate serum from cells within 1 hour after collection; freeze serum.	Stomach disorders
Glucose	FBS (fasting blood sugar), RBS (random blood sugar)	Separate from cells within one hour or use gray-top tube.	Diabetes, hypoglycemia
Glycosylated hemoglobin	Hgb A1c	Lavender tube.	Monitoring diabetes mellitus
Glucose-6-phosphate dehydrogenase	G-6-PD	Lavender tube; do not freeze.	Drug-induced anemias

continued

Listing of Tests Performed in Chemistry Department (continued)

Test	Abbreviation	Sample considerations	Clinical correlation
Hemoglobin electrophoresis		Refrigerate; whole blood; do not spin.	Hemoglobino-pathies and thalassemia
Human leukocyte antigen typing A & B	HLA A & B	Yellow-top (ACD) tubes; do not freeze or refriger-ate; ethnic origin must be included.	Tested for disease association, matching prior to organ trans-plantation, and platelet transfu-sion, and pater-nity and forensic evaluation
Human chorionic gonadotropin	HCG	Refrigerated serum.	Pregnancy, testicular cancer
Immunoglobulins	IgA IgG IgM	Refrigerated serum.	Measurement of proteins capable of becoming an-tibodies, chronic liver disease, myeloma
Iron + iron binding capacity	TIBC & Fe	Refrigerated serum. Separate from cells within 1 hour of collection. Fasting morning specimen is preferred.	Assist in diagnosis of anemia
Lactic acid (blood lactate)		Draw whole blood from a stasis-free vein into a gray-top tube. Centrifuge and separate plasma within 15 minutes of collection.	Measurement of anaerobic gly-colysis due to strenuous exer-cise; increased lactic acid can occur in liver disease
Lactic dehydrogenase	LD	Serum, avoid hemolysis—do not freeze or refrigerate.	Cardiac injury and other mus-cle damage

Listing of Tests Performed in Chemistry Department (continued)

Test	Abbreviation	Sample considerations	Clinical correlation
Lead	Pb	Royal blue EDTA or tan-top lead-free tube; use of other evacuated tubes or transfer tubes may produce falsely elevated results due to contamination.	Lead toxicity, which can lead to neurologic dysfunction and possible permanent brain damage
Lipase		Refrigerated serum.	Used to distinguish between abdominal pain and that owing to acute pancreatitis
Lipoproteins High-density lipoprotein	HDL	Refrigerated serum. Must be fasting a minimum of 12 hours.	Evaluates lipid disorders and coronary artery disease risk
Low-density lipoprotein	LDL	Must be fasting a minimum of 12 hours.	Evaluates lipid disorders and coronary artery disease risk
Magnesium	Mg	Separate from cells within 45 minutes. Maintain specimen at room temperature.	Mineral metabolism, kidney function
Phosphorus	P	Separate from cells within 45 minutes. Maintain specimen at room temperature.	Thyroid function, bone disorders, and kidney disease
Prostatic specific antigen, total & free	PSA	Separate and freeze immediately in a plastic vial. Transport frozen.	Screen for the presence of prostate cancer, to monitor the progression of the disease and monitor the response to treatment for prostate cancer.

continued

Listing of Tests Performed in Chemistry Department (continued)

Test	Abbreviation	Sample considerations	Clinical correlation
Serum protein electrophoresis	SPEP or PEP	Refrigerated serum.	Abnormal protein detection
Sweat electrolytes (iontophoresis)		Fluid collected is sweat.	Cystic fibrosis
Thyroid profile (comprehensive)	FTI, T_3, T_4, TSH	SST or red-stoppered tube that must be separated to plastic transfer tube.	Hyper- or hypothyroid conditions
Triglycerides		Refrigerated serum. Strict fasting 12-14 hours (water only) is required.	Used to evaluate risk of coronary heart disease
Uric acid	UA	SST or red-stoppered tube that must be separated within 45 minutes; maintain specimen at room temperature.	Gout
Zinc	Zn	Royal blue, no additive or EDTA. If serum, should be separated within 45 minutes and transferred to plastic transport tube.	Liver dysfunction

Hematology

Tube Type	Additive
Lavender	Ethylenediaminetetraacetate (EDTA)

Listing of Tests Performed in Hematology Department

Test	Abbreviation	Sample considerations	Clinical correlation
Complete blood count	CBC	Lavender top. Invert gently 6-8 times immediately after drawing; includes WBC, RBC, Hgb, Hct, indices, platelets, and diff.	Blood dyscrasias
Differential	Diff	Blood smear stained with Wright's stain.	Classifying types of leukocytes, describing erythrocytes, and estimation of platelets
Eosinophil count	Eos. Ct.	Lavender top, invert gently 6-8 times immediately after drawing.	Allergy studies
Erythrocyte sedimentation rate	ESR, sed rate	Lavender top, invert gently 6-8 times immediately after drawing.	Abnormal protein linkage
Hematocrit	Hct	Lavender top, invert gently 6-8 times immediately after drawing	Anemia
Hemoglobin	Hgb	Lavender top, invert gently 6-8 times immediately after drawing.	Anemia
Hemoglobin electrophoresis		Refrigerated lavender top. Invert gently 6-8 times immediately after drawing.	Abnormal hemoglobin
Indices	MCV, MCH, MCHC	Lavender top, invert gently 6-8 times immediately after drawing.	Indicates mean cell hemoglobin (MCH), hemoglobin concentration (MCHC), and volume
Platelet count	Plt Ct	Lavender top, invert gently 6-8 times immediately after drawing.	Bleeding disorders
Red cell count	RBC	Lavender top, invert gently 6-8 times immediately after drawing.	Anemia
Reticulocyte count	Retic	Lavender top, invert gently 6-8 times immediately after drawing.	Anemia
White cell count	WBC	Lavender top, invert gently 6-8 times immediately after drawing.	Infection (viral or bacterial)

Coagulation

Tube Type Used	Additive
Light blue	Sodium citrate Tube must be completely filled by vacuum for all tests

Listing of Tests Performed in Coagulation Department

Test	Abbreviation	Sample considerations	Clinical correlation
Antithrombin III	AT-III	Light blue top, centrifuge, separate, and freeze plasma immediately in plastic vials. Transport frozen.	Clotting factor deficiency
D-Dimer	D-D1	1 mL frozen citrated plasma from a light blue. Separate and freeze plasma immediately in plastic vials. Transport frozen.	DIC and thrombotic episodes such as pulmonary emboli
Disseminated intravascular coagulation panel	DIC panel	Light blue top, centrifuge, separate, and freeze plasma immediately in plastic vials. Transport frozen.	Distortion of the normal coagulation and fibrinolytic mechanisms
Factor assay		Light blue top, centrifuge, separate, and freeze plasma immediately in plastic vials. 1 mL aliquot for each factor.	To determine the actual percentage of a specific coagulation factor
Fibrinogen		Completely filled light blue top, centrifuge 15 minutes, separate, and freeze immediately. Place in plastic vial and transport frozen.	To investigate suspected bleeding disorders
Fibrin split products/ fibrin degradation product	FSP/FDP	1 light blue top completely filled and inverted 6 times. Immediately centrifuge for 15 minutes, separate and freeze. Transport frozen.	DIC and thrombotic episodes, valuable early diagnostic sign of increased rate of fibrin deposition

Listing of Tests Performed in Coagulation Department (continued)

Test	Abbreviation	Sample considerations	Clinical correlation
Platelet aggregation	Plt Agg	4-5 mL sodium citrate tubes. Do not centrifuge. Do not refrigerate. Notify the lab before collection. Specimen must be received within 1 hour of collection.	Hemostasis and thrombus formation
Plasminogen		Blue top centrifuge, separate, and freeze plasma immediately in plastic vials. Transport frozen.	Fibrin clot formation prevention
Prothrombin time	PT	Completely filled blue top, invert 6-8 times immediately after drawing. Do not centrifuge or freeze if the sample needs to be transported.	Clotting factor deficiency, monitoring warfarin therapy
Partial thromboplastin time (activated PTT)	PTT (APPT)	Completely filled blue top, invert 6-8 times immediately after drawing. Do not centrifuge or freeze if the sample needs to be transported.	Clotting factor deficiency, monitoring heparin therapy

Immunology/Serology

Tube Types Used	Additive
Red/gray	Clot activator and inert silicon gel
Gold	Clot activator and inert silicon gel
Red	No additive

Listing of Tests Performed in Serology/Immunology Department

Test	Abbreviation	Sample considerations	Clinical correlation
Antinuclear antibodies	ANA (screen or titer)	Refrigerated serum, avoid hemolysis and lipemia.	Systemic lupus erythematosus and other autoimmune connective tissue diseases
Antistreptolysin O test	ASO	Refrigerate or freeze serum if not performed immediately.	Group A streptococcal infection
Cold agglutinins		In a collection tube containing no additives that has been prewarmed to 37°C. Do NOT refrigerate.	Viral and atypical pneumonia caused by *Mycoplasma pneumoniae*
Chlamydia antibody panel	IgM, IgG, IgA	Refrigerate serum collected using aseptic technique. Centrifuge and separate serum from clot within 4 hours of collection.	For trachoma, psittacosis, LGV, and pneumoniae
C-reactive protein	CRP	Refrigerated serum.	Chronic inflammation
Cytomegalovirus screen	CMV	Refrigerate serum.	Screens donors and blood products for transplant programs
Epstein-Barr virus	EBV	Refrigerated serum.	Mononucleosis
Febrile agglutinins		Random serum specimen; avoid hemolysis.	Screens for *Salmonella, Tularemia, Rickettsia,* and *Brucella* organism antibodies

Listing of Tests Performed in Serology/Immunology Department (continued)

Test	Abbreviation	Sample considerations	Clinical correlation
Fluorescent treponemal antibody-absorption	FTA-ABS	Refrigerated serum.	Syphilis
Hepatitis B surface antibody	HBsAb	Refrigerated serum.	Determination of previous infection and immunity by hepatitis B
Hepatitis B surface antigen	HBsAg	Refrigerated serum.	Diagnosis of acute or some chronic stages of infection and carrier status of hepatitis B
Human immunodeficiency virus antigen	HIV-1	Refrigerated serum—do not ship in glass tubes. Protect patient's confidentiality by using a code number in place of patient's name.	Screen for donated blood and plasma as an aid in the diagnosis of HIV-1 infection
Mononucleosis screen	Mono-test	Refrigerated serum.	Infectious mononucleosis
Radioallergosorbent test	RAST	Refrigerated serum. No fasting required.	Allergies
Rheumatoid factor	RF	Refrigerated serum. Overnight fasting is preferred.	Arthritic conditions
Rapid plasmin reagin	RPR	Refrigerated serum. Hemolysis and lipemia may alter test results.	Syphilis

Immunohematology/Blood Bank

Tube Types Used	Additive
Pink	Ethylenediaminetetraacetate (EDTA)
Plain red	No additive
Lavender	Ethylenediaminetetraacetate (EDTA)

Listing of Tests Performed in Immunohematology/Blood Bank

Test	Abbreviation	Sample considerations	Clinical correlation
Antibody screen	Coombs' test, indirect	Special ID procedure.	Identify any atypical antibodies present
Blood group & Rh type	ABO & Rh	Dedicated lavender top. Special ID procedure.	Detection of ABO and Rh antigens on the red blood cells
Cord blood		Refrigerate serum.	Group and type baby's blood to detect the presence of incompatibilities, or mother for possible Rh immune globulin
Direct antiglobulin test	DAT, Coombs' test, direct	Dedicated lavender top. Special ID procedure.	Detects antibodies attached to the patient's red blood cells
Indirect antiglobulin test	IAT	Special ID procedure.	Detects antibody sensitization, either acquired or inherited, which is present in serum
Anti-Rh antibody preparation	RhoGAM workup	Special ID procedure.	Administered to Rh-negative mothers to prevent Rh immunization
Type & screen	T & S	Special ID procedure—hand label with Typenex band.	Group and type and detect atypical antibodies for prenatal screen or crossmatch
Type & crossmatch	T & C	Special ID procedure—hand label with Typenex band.	Group and type and crossmatch with donor unit

Microbiology

Tube Types Used	Additive
Yellow	Sodium polyanetholesulfonate (SPS)
Isolator	Lysing agent, anticoagulant, HIV inactivator

Listing of Tests Performed In Microbiology Department

The following tests are collected in various collection equipment as specified.

Test	Abbreviation	Sample considerations	Clinical correlation
Acid-fast bacillus culture	AFB	Isolator tube or refrigerated green-top tube.	To differentiate the type of mycobacteria and to determine appropriate treatment. Used to diagnosis tuberculosis.
Blood cultures	BC	Yellow tube or two blood culture bottles: one anaerobic and one aerobic from two different sites. Do not refrigerate.	To confirm the presence in the blood, bacteremia or septicemia
Culture and sensitivity	C & S	Collect the appropriate fluid or tissue using culture swab transport media. Indicate on the requisition location of culture.	Identification of infective agent and appropriate antibiotic treatment
Screening for: Gonorrhea	GC	Taken from the urethra of male or endocervical canal from female	Sexually transmitted disease
Streptococcus	Strep	Submit culturette	Strep throat
Sputum		True sputum—early morning sample	Tuberculosis

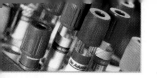

APPENDIX E

Laboratory Mathematics

The Metric System

The metric system is the system of measurement used in the health care industry. The metric system derives its name from its fundamental unit of distance, the meter (M or m). In the metric system, the meter is the basic unit of linear measure, the gram (G or g) is the basic unit of weight, and the liter (L or l) is the basic unit of volume. The metric system is a decimal system (a system based on the number 10). In a decimal system, units larger or smaller than the basic units are arrived at by multiplying or dividing by 10 or powers of 10.

In the metric system, prefixes added to the basic units indicate larger or smaller units. Prefixes are the same whether or not the units are meters, grams, or liters. Table E-1 shows prefixes commonly used in the medical laboratory. Basic metric units (grams, meters, liters) can be converted to larger units by moving the decimal point to the left according to the appropriate multiple. The multiple is the value of the exponent. The exponent is a number that indicates how many times a number is multiplied by itself. For example, a kilogram is 1,000 or 10 3 10 3 10 or 103 g. The multiple, determined by the exponent, is three.

Example: Convert 100 grams to kilograms.

From Table E-1 we determine that 1 kg is equal to 1,000 or 10^3 g. The multiple is three. Therefore, to convert 100 grams to kilograms, move the decimal point three places to the left:

$$100 \text{ g} = \underset{\smile}{100.0} = 0.1 \text{ kg}$$

To convert basic metric units to smaller units, move the decimal point to the right the appropriate multiple.

Example: Convert 100 g to mg.

From Table E-1, we see that 1 mg is equal to 10^{-3} g. The multiple is a minus three. We therefore move the decimal point three spaces to the right:

$$100 \text{ g} = \underset{\smile}{100.000} = 100,000 \text{ mg}$$

Metric units other than basic units can be converted to larger units by moving the decimal point to the left according to the appropriate multiple, determined by subtracting the value of the exponent of the desired unit from the value of the exponent of the existing unit.

Example: Convert 200 mg to kg.

From Table E-1, we determine that 1 mg is 10^{-3} and 1 kg is 10^3. The desired unit is kilograms; therefore, subtract -3 from 3 to determine the multiple:

$$3 - (-3) = 3 + 3 = 6$$

We are going from a smaller unit to a larger unit, so the decimal point moves to the left six spaces.

$$200 \text{ mg} = \underline{000200.} = 0.0002 \text{ kg}$$

Metric units other than basic units can be converted to smaller units by moving the decimal point to the right according to the appropriate multiple, determined by subtracting the value of the exponent of the desired unit from the value of the exponent of the existing unit.

Example: Convert 25 cm to μm.

From Table E-1, we determine that 1 cm is 10^{-2} and 1 μm is 10^{-6}. The desired unit is micrometers; therefore subtract -6 from -2 to determine the multiple:

$$-2 - (-6) = -2 + 6 = 4$$

We are going from a larger unit to a smaller unit, so the decimal point moves to the right four spaces.

$$25 \text{ cm} = 25.0000 = 250,000 \text{ μm}$$

It is often necessary to convert our English system of units to metric units. Table E-2 lists English units and their metric equivalents commonly encountered in the health-care setting.

To convert from English units to metric units, multiply by the factor listed. Metric units can be converted back to English units by dividing by the same factor or multiplying by the factor in the metric conversion chart.

Example: Convert 200 lb to kg.

1 pound is equal to 0.454 kg.

Therefore, multiply 200 × .454 to arrive at 90.8 kg.

Table E-3 shows the common equivalents for converting metric units to English units. To convert metric units to English units, multiply by the factor listed. To convert English units back to metric, divide by the same factor or multiply by the factor in the English unit conversion chart.

Example: Convert 15 mL to tsp.

1.0 mL is equal to $\frac{1}{5}$ tsp.

Therefore, multiply $15 \times \frac{1}{5}$ to arrive at $\frac{15}{5}$
or 3 tsp (or $15 \times 0.2 = 3.0$ tsp).

Military Time

Most hospitals use military (or European) time, which is based on a clock with 24 numbers instead of 12 (Fig. E-1). Twenty-four-hour time eliminates the need for designating AM or PM. Each time is expressed by four digits. The first two digits represent hours, and the second two digits represent minutes. 1200 hours is noon and 2400 hours is midnight. One AM is 0100, 2 AM is 0200, and so on.

Noon is 1200; 1 PM is 1300.

To convert regular (12-hour) time to 24-hour time, add 12 hours to the time from 1 PM on.

Example: 1:00 PM becomes 1:00 + 12 hours = 1300 hours.
5:30 PM becomes 5:30 + 12 hours = 1730 hours.

To convert 24-hour time to 12-hour time, subtract 12 hours after 1 PM.

Example: 1300 hours becomes 1300 − 12 hours = 1:00 PM.

Temperature Measurement

Two different temperature scales (Fig. E-2) are used in the health care setting. The Fahrenheit (F) scale is used to measure body temperature, whereas the Celsius (C), also known as the centigrade, scale is used to measure temperatures in the laboratory.

- Fahrenheit: The freezing point of water is 32°F, and the boiling point is 212°F. Normal body temperature expressed in Fahrenheit is 98.6°F.
- Celsius/centigrade: The freezing point of water is zero (0°C) and the boiling point is 100°C. Normal body temperature expressed in the Celsius scale is 37°C.

The following formulas can be used to convert from one temperature scale to the other:

$$\text{Celsius temperature} = \tfrac{5}{9}\,(°F - 32)$$

$$\text{Fahrenheit temperature} = \tfrac{9}{5}°C + 32$$

Roman Numerals

In the Roman numeral system, letters represent numbers. Roman numerals may be encountered in procedure outlines, in physician's orders or prescriptions, and in the identification of values or substances such as coagulation factors.

The basic Roman numeral system consists of the following seven capital (or lower-case) letters:

I (i)	= 1	C (c)	= 100
V (v)	= 5	D (d)	= 500
X (x)	= 10	M (m)	= 1,000
L (l)	= 50		

GUIDELINES FOR INTERPRETING ROMAN NUMERALS

1. When numerals of the same value follow in sequence, the values should be added. There should never be more than three of the same numeral in a sequence.

   Example: III = 1 + 1 + 1 = 3

   XX = 10 + 10 = 20

2. When a lower-value numeral precedes a numeral with a higher value, the lower value should be subtracted from the higher value. Numerals V, L, and D are never subtracted. No more than one lower value number should precede a higher value number.

   Example: IV = 5 − 1 = 4

   IX = 10 − 1 = 9

3. When a numeral is followed by one or more numerals of lower value, the values should be added.

Example: XI = 10 + 1 = 11

VII = 5 + 1 + 1 = 7

4. When a lower value numeral comes between two higher value numerals, it is subtracted from the numeral following it.

Example: XIX = 10 + 10 − 1 = 19

XXIV = 10 + 10 + 5 − 1 = 24

5. Roman numerals are written from left to right in order of decreasing value (except for numerals that are to be subtracted from subsequent numerals).

Example: XXVII = 10 + 10 + 5 + 1 + 1 = 27

MCMXCII = 1,000 + (1,000 − 100) + (100 − 10) + 1 + 1 = 1992

6. A line over a Roman numeral means multiply the numeral by 1,000.

Example: $\overline{V}$ = V × 1,000 = 5,000

Percent

Percent means per 100 and is represented by the symbol %. Two values are involved when a number is expressed as a percentage. They are the number itself, and 100.

Example: 10% means 10 per 100 or 10 parts in a total of 100 parts.
To change a fraction to a percentage, multiply by 100
and add a percent sign to the result.

Example: Change ¾ to a percentage.

$$\frac{3}{4} \times \frac{100}{1} = \frac{300}{4} = 4\overline{)300}^{\,75} = 75\%$$

Dilutions

The concentration of laboratory reagents is often expressed as a percentage. For example, a solution of 70% isopropyl alcohol is used in skin cleansing before blood collection.

A 10% dilution of bleach (5.25% sodium hypochlorite) is used to disinfect countertops and other surfaces. A 10% dilution of bleach means that there are 10 parts of bleach in a solution containing a total of 100 parts. The above dilution can also be expressed as a ratio, showing the relationship between the part of the solution and the total solution. A 10% solution is also a 1:10 (1 to 10) solution or one part bleach in a total of 10 parts solution. A dilution of 10 parts in a total of 100 parts is the same as 1 part in a total of 100 parts, or a 1:10 dilution. A 10% dilution of bleach can be prepared by adding 10 mL bleach to 90 mL water, resulting in a total of 100 mL of bleach solution. The same percentage dilution would result from adding 1 mL bleach to 9 mL water, 20 mL bleach to 180 mL water, and so on.

Blood Volume

Blood volume in adults is generally stated as 5.0 quarts or 4.75 liters (L). Because people are not the same size, common sense tells us that they should not all have 5 quarts of blood. Actual blood volume is based on weight. Blood volume can be calculated for any size person from infant to adult, as long as the weight of the person is known.

Adult Blood Volume

Adult blood volume is 70 mL per kg of weight.

Example: Calculate the amount of blood volume
for a man who weighs 250 lb.

1. Change the weight in pounds to kilograms.

Because 1 lb = .454 kg, you need to multiply 250 lb
by .454 to arrive at 113.5 kg.

2. Next, multiply the number of kilograms by 70 because there are 70 mL of blood for each kg of weight.

113.5 kg × 70 mL/kg = 7,945 mL

3. Because blood volume is reported in liters rather than milliliters, divide the total number of mL by 1,000 (1 liter = 1000 mL).

Blood volume = 7,945 mL/1,000 mL = 7.945 L or 7.9 L

Infant Blood Volume

It is very important to be able to estimate the blood volume of an infant, especially if that infant is in an intensive care unit where blood samples may be taken several times a day. A very small infant can become anemic if not monitored closely. Removal of more than 10% of an infant's blood volume in a short amount of time can lead to serious consequences, including cardiac arrest.

An infant's blood volume is 100 mL per kg.

Example: Calculate the blood volume of a baby
who weighs 5.5 lb.

1. Change the weight from pounds to kilograms using the same formula as for adults.

5.5 lb × .454 = 2.5 kg

2. Multiply 2.5 kg by 100 for total blood volume in milliliters.

2.5 kg × 100 = 250 mL

3. Change blood volume in mL/kg to liters.

250 mL/1,000 mL = 0.25 L

Military Time
or
European Time

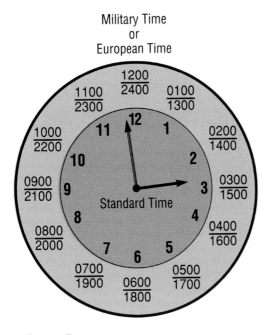

■ FIGURE E-1 ■

Clock showing 24-hour (military) time.

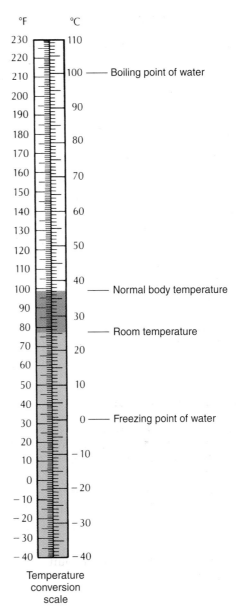

Temperature
conversion
scale

■ FIGURE E-2 ■

Thermometer showing both Fahrenheit
and Celsius degrees.   (Memmler RL, Cohen
BJ, Wood DL.)

Table E-1

Commonly Used Measurement Prefixes

Prefix	Multiple	Meter (m)	Unit of Measure Gram (g)	Liter (l)
Kilo- (k)	1,000 (10^3)	km	kg	kL
Deci- (d)	1/10 (10^{-1})	dm	dg	dL
Centi- (c)	1/100 (10^{-2})	cm	cg	cL
Milli- (m)	1/1,000 (10^{-3})	mm	mg	mL
Micro- (μ)	1/1,000,000 (10^{-6})	μm	μg	μL

Table E-2

Metric–English Equivalents

	English		Metric
Distance	Yard (yd)	=	0.9 meters (m)
	Inch (in)	=	2.54 centimeters (cm)
Weight	Pound (lb)	=	0.454 kilograms (kg) or 454 grams (g)
	Ounce (oz)	=	28 grams (g)
Volume	Quart (qt)	=	0.95 liters (L)
	Fluid ounce (fl oz)	=	30 milliliters (mL)
	Tablespoon (tbsp)	=	15 millimeters (mL)
	Teaspoon (tsp)	=	5 milliliters (mL)

Table E-3

English–Metric Equivalents

	Metric		English
Distance	Meter (m)	=	3.3 feet/39.37 inches
	Centimeter (cm)	=	0.4 inches
	Millimeter (mm)	=	0.04 inches
Weight	Gram (g)	=	.0022 pounds
	Kilogram (kg)	=	2.2 pounds
Volume	Liter (L)	=	1.06 quarts
	Milliliter (mL)	=	.03 fluid ounces
	Milliliter (mL)	=	.20 or 1/5 tsp

Note: A milliliter (mL) is approximately equal to a cubic centimeter (cc), and the two terms are often used interchangeably.

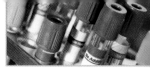

Conditions Requiring Work Restrictions for Health Care Employees

Condition	Work Restriction
Chicken pox (Varicella)	Off work until 7 days after appearance of first eruption and lesions are dry and crusted
Hepatitis A	Off work until cleared by a physician
Hepatitis B	Off work until cleared by a physician
Herpes zoster	May work if no patient contact
Influenza	Work status determined by Employee Health Department depending on work area
Impetigo	Off work or no patient contact until crusts are gone
Measles	Off work until rash is gone (minimum 4 days)
Mononucleosis	Off work until cleared by a physician
MRSA (methicillin-resistant *Staphylococcus aureus*)	May work, but no patient care until treatment is successful
Pink eye (acute conjunctivitis)	Off work until treatment is successful
Positive PPD test	May work depending upon evaluation and follow-up by Employee Health Department
Pregnancy	May work, but avoid contact with patients with rickettsial or viral infections, patients in isolation, and patients being treated with radioactive isotopes. Avoid areas with radioactive hazard symbol.
Tuberculosis (active)	Off work until treated and AFB smears are negative for 2 weeks
Rubella (German measles)	Off work until rash is gone (minimum 5 days)
Salmonella	Varies depending on symptoms, treatment results, and Employee Health Department evaluation
Scabies	Off work until treated
Shigella	Varies depending on symptoms, treatment results, and Employee Health Department evaluation
Strep throat (group A)	Off work until 24 hours after antibiotic therapy is started and symptoms are gone
URI (upper respiratory infection)	Work status determined by Employee Health Department

INDEX

Note: Page numbers followed by "f" indicate figures; page numbers followed by "t" indicate tables; page numbers followed by "b" indicated boxed material; and page numbers preceded by "A" indicate material in appendices at end of the book.

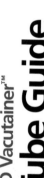

BD Vacutainer™
Tube Guide

A full line of BD Vacutainer Blood Collection Needles, Needle Holders and Blood Collection Sets is also available.

BD Indispensable to human health

BD Vacutainer™ Tubes With Hemogard™ Closure	BD Vacutainer™ Tubes With Conventional Stopper	Additive	Inversions at Blood Collection*	Laboratory Use	Your Lab's Draw Volume/Remarks
Gold	Red/Black	• Clot activator and gel for serum separation	5	BD Vacutainer™ SST™ Tube for serum determinations in chemistry. Tube inversions ensure mixing of clot activator with blood. Blood clotting time 30 minutes.	
Light Green	Green/Gray	• Lithium heparin and gel for plasma separation	8	BD Vacutainer™ PST™ Tube for plasma determinations in chemistry. Tube inversions prevent clotting.	
Red	Red	• None (glass) • Clot activator (plastic tube with Hemogard closure)	0 5	For serum determinations in chemistry and serology. Glass serum tubes are recommended for blood banking. Plastic tubes contain clot activator and are **not** recommended for blood banking. Tube inversions ensure mixing of clot activator with blood and clotting within 60 minutes.	
Orange	Gray/Yellow	• Thrombin	8	For stat serum determinations in chemistry. Tube inversions ensure complete clotting which usually occurs in less than 5 minutes.	
Royal Blue		• Sodium heparin • Na_2EDTA • None (serum tube)	8 8 0	For trace-element, toxicology and nutritional-chemistry determinations. Special stopper formulation provides low levels of trace elements (see package insert).	
Green		• Sodium heparin • Lithium heparin	8 8	For plasma determinations in chemistry. Tube inversions prevent clotting.	
Gray		• Potassium oxalate/sodium fluoride • Sodium fluoride/Na_2 EDTA • Sodium fluoride (serum tube)	8 8 8	For glucose determinations. Oxalate and EDTA anticoagulants will give plasma samples. Sodium fluoride is the antiglycolytic agent. Tube inversions ensure proper mixing of additive and blood.	
Tan		• Sodium heparin (glass) • K_2EDTA (plastic)	8 8	For lead determinations. This tube is certified to contain less than .01 µg/mL(ppm) lead. Tube inversions prevent clotting.	

Closure color	Additive	Inversions	Laboratory use
Yellow	• Sodium polyanethol sulfonate (SPS)	8	SPS for blood culture specimen collections in micro-biology. Tube inversions prevent clotting.
	• Acid citrate dextrose additives (ACD): **Solution A -** 22.0g/L trisodium citrate, 8.0g/L citric acid, 24.5g/L dextrose **Solution B -** 13.2g/L trisodium citrate, 4.8g/L citric acid, 14.7g/L dextrose	8 8	ACD for use in blood bank studies, HLA phenotyping, DNA and paternity testing.
Lavender	• Liquid K_3EDTA (glass) • Spray-dried K_2EDTA (plastic)	8 8	K_3EDTA for whole blood hematology determinations. K_2EDTA for whole blood hematology determinations and immunohematology testing (ABO grouping, Rh typing, antibody screening). Tube inversions prevent clotting.
Pink	• Spray-dried K_2EDTA	8	For whole blood hematology determinations and immunohematology testing (ABO grouping, Rh typing, antibody screening). Designed with special cross-match label for required patient information by the AABB. Tube inversions prevent clotting.
Light Blue	• .105M sodium citrate(≈3.2%) • .129M sodium citrate(3.8%) • Citrate, theophylline, adenosine, dipyridamole (CTAD)	3-4 3-4 3-4	For coagulation determinations. NOTE: Certain tests may require chilled specimens. Follow your institution's recommended procedures for collection and transport. CTAD for selected platelet function assays and routine coagulation determination. Tube inversions prevent clotting.

Partial-draw Tubes   Small-volume Pediatric Tubes
(2ml and 3 ml: 13 x 75 mm) (2ml: 10.25 x 47 mm, 3ml: 10.25 x 64 mm)

Closure color	Additive	Inversions	Laboratory use
Red	• None	0	For serum determinations in chemistry and serology. Glass serum tubes are recommended for blood banking. Plastic tubes contain clot activator and are not recommended for blood banking. Tube inversions ensure mixing of clot activator with blood and clotting within 60 minutes.
Green	• Sodium heparin • Lithium heparin	8 8	For plasma determinations in chemistry. Tube inversions prevent clotting.
Lavender	• Liquid K_3EDTA (glass) • Spray-dried K_2EDTA (plastic)	8 8	K_3EDTA for whole blood hematology determinations. K_2EDTA for whole blood hematology determinations and immunohematology testing (ABO grouping, Rh typing, antibody screening). Tube inversions prevent clotting.
Light Blue	• .105M sodium citrate (≈3.2%) • .129M sodium citrate (3.8%)	3-4	For coagulation determinations. Tube inversions prevent clotting. NOTE: Certain tests may require chilled specimens. Follow your institution's recommended procedures for collection and transport of specimen.

* Invert gently, do not shake

BD, BD Logo and all other trademarks are property of Becton, Dickinson and Company. ©2002 BD.
Printed in USA   01/02   VS5229-4

BD Vacutainer Systems
Preanalytical Solutions
1 Becton Drive
Franklin Lakes, NJ 07417 USA
www.bd.com

BD Technical Services: 800.631.0174

NEW

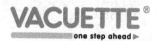 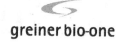

Tube Guide

Vacuette® tube type	colour-coding of cap	additive	intended purpose
Serum		Clot activator	Determinations in serum for clinical chemistry, microbiological serology, immunology, TDM
Serum Gel		Clot activator and Gel	Determinations in serum for clinical chemistry, microbiological serology, immunology, TDM
Serum Beads		Clot activator and Beads	Determinations in serum for clinical chemistry, microbiological serology, immunology
Serum Crossmatch		Clot activator	Determinations in serum for crossmatch testing
Plasma		Sodium Heparin Lithium Heparin Ammonium Heparin	Determinations in heparinised plasma for clinical chemistry
Plasma Gel		Lithium Heparin and Gel	Determinations in heparinised plasma for clinical chemistry
EDTA		K_2 EDTA K_3 EDTA	Determinations in EDTA whole blood for haematology
EDTA Crossmatch		K_3 EDTA	Determinations in EDTA whole blood for crossmatch testing
EDTA Gel		K_2 EDTA / Gel	Determinations in EDTA plasma for molecular biological identification of viruses, parasites und bacteria
Coagulation		Citrate Solution (3.2%) Citrate Solution (3.8%)	Determinations in citrated plasma for coagulation testing
CTAD		CTAD (3.2%)	Determinations in citrated plasma for coagulation testing where the artificial entry of platelet factors into the plasma is avoided
Glucose		Anticoagulant Glycolysis inhibitor	Determinations in stabilised anticoagulated whole blood or plasma for glucose and lactate testing
Trace Elements		Clot activator Sodium Heparin	Determinations in serum / heparinised plasma for trace elements testing
Blood Grouping		ACD-A ACD-B CPDA	Determinations in ACD / CPDA whole blood for blood grouping

greiner bio-one

Headquarter: Greiner Bio-One GmbH, 4550 Kremsmünster, Austria
Greiner Vacuette North America Inc., 4238 Capital Drive, Monroe, NC 28112, U.S.A.
For further information please visit
www.vacuette.com

Courtesy, Greiner Bio-One, Kremsmuenster, Austria